PRAISE FOR

Even Better Data , Better Decisions:
Advanced Business Intelligence for Medical Practices

Nate is once again on the cutting edge of the healthcare technology curve. The truth is, MS Excel can't handle the new stream of big data and Access lacks the power and processing speed. SQL is the perfect solution as it combines the ability to manage massive databases with built-in mathematical and statistical formulae to make it through any analysis. And when it comes to business intelligence and the creation of custom reports and dashboards, SQL is the only game in town. Kudos to Nate for bringing his knowledge and experience as a SQL programmer to the forefront. This book is not just for data analysts and scientists, but for anyone in leadership that needs to take their business intelligence up to the next level.

FRANK COHEN, MBB, MPA
Director, analytics
DOCTORS MANAGEMENT LLC, CLEARWATER, FLA.

•

Nate's experience as a practice administrator, expertise in Microsoft Excel and SQL Server technology and his passion to share his knowledge with the industry makes him an invaluable resource to MGMA's members. His newest book provides a road map to implement automated reporting to achieve next generation of business intelligence in medical practices.

TODD EVENSON, MBA
Chief operating officer
MGMA

•

Nate Moore's best-selling, *Better Data, Better Decisions*, just got turbocharged with new updated information to give medical practice executives more of the tools and resources they need to manage with data in this turbulent environment. Nate's new edition – *Even Better Data, Better Decisions: Advanced Business Intelligence for Medical Practices*, leverages his expertise and experience to present more real-world solutions to the problems, shortfalls and glitches that can plague attempts to manage vital information with systems that lack reporting or which necessitate trained data techs just to generate standard reports. Moore not only provides you with an array of tools to translate data into business intelligence, he gives you a road map for integrating this new approach into your practice. Data is no longer a 'nice-to-have' in medical practice management; it's how you manage. Pulling, manipulating and analyzing data about your medical practice becomes a reality using Nate Moore's principles. If you want to manage a medical practice today's climate, you need this book.

ELIZABETH W. WOODCOCK, MBA, FACMPE, CPC
Principal
WOODCOCK & ASSOCIATES, ATLANTA, GA.

EVEN BETTER DATA, BETTER DECISIONS:

Advanced Business Intelligence for Medical Practices

Medical Group Management Association
104 Inverness Terrace East
Englewood, CO 80112-5306
877.275.6462
mgma.com

MGMA
Medical Group Management Association®

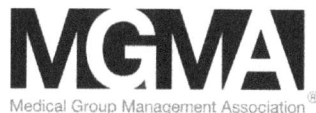

Library of Congress Cataloging-in-Publication Data

Names: Moore, Nate, author. | Medical Group Management Association, issuing
   body.
Title: Even better data, better decisions : advanced business intelligence
   for the medical practice / by Nate Moore.
Description: Englewood, CO : Medical Group Management Association, [2018] |
   Includes index.
Identifiers: LCCN 2017051734 (print) | LCCN 2017052074 (ebook) | ISBN
   9781568295404 (e-book) | ISBN 9781568295398 (pbk.)
Subjects: | MESH: Practice Management, Medical--organization & administration
   | Medical Informatics | Software | Office Management--organization &
   administration
Classification: LCC R855.3 (ebook) | LCC R855.3 (print) | NLM W 80 | DDC
   610.285--dc23
LC record available at https://lccn.loc.gov/2017051734

Moore, Nate
MGMA (Association); publisher.
EGZ Publications; production.

Dedication

To Larraine, my best friend and wife for 26 years. To our amazing children, Charity, Joy, and Henry Moore.

Contents

CHAPTER 7

CHAPTER 8

CHAPTER 9

Foreword

I met Nate Moore, in 2009 at an MGMA annual meeting. He was trying desperately to present some Excel tips that would help medical practice managers save time and better utilize Excel. We were all so eager to learn and asking so many questions that there is no way he covered his intended material. He showed all of us a way to save hours of time every month – and now there was no end to where our imaginations would go next. This was the day that Nate's fan club was born, and all of those present for his session are now charter members.

After running in to him another time or two, I asked Nate to visit my office (Ortho NorthEast) and teach a few of us how to better use Excel. As the Director of Administrative Operations for a large orthopedic practice, I often struggled to find time to gather data and the competing priorities of the entire organization often overwhelmed the IT resources. I wanted to get the data I needed. But perhaps more importantly, I needed to be liberated from the data often included in my canned software reports that caused unnecessary repetitive work for me and my staff. During that visit Nate overwhelmed us with the hidden possibilities within Excel, and what a little extra SQL coding & programing could do to reduce our overhead, reduce frustration and improve stakeholder satisfaction. It is safe to say our practice would not be the same if we had never hired Nate. Our entire leadership team now trusts that every problem we have should be evaluated to determine if an Excel, SQL program (or some other IT solution) can permanently solve a problem – especially before adding to staff headcount.

A few years ago, I suggested to Nate that he and I should write a book together. I began a relentless campaign to get a book out there for our colleagues. Practices need to learn to use data to solve problems. I was very anxious to share much of what we had learned and accomplished together. Finally, Nate agreed. And together we wrote the first *Better Data, Better Decisions: Using*

Business Intelligence in the Medical Practice. The point of the first book was to liberate practices from expensive re-working of Excel, manual upgrades to spreadsheets, and to assure practice leaders that they should expect their data to be at their fingertips or automatically delivered to their in-box. The practice manager should not have to choose between two off the shelf solutions that are either much more software (and cost) than they need or a less expensive option that falls short of what they need

Since the publishing of our first book, the most frequent question that I heard from people when they read our book or when I showed them our new business intelligence tools, was "How did you do that?" This second book, *Even Better Data, Better Decisions: Advanced Business Intelligence for Medical Practices*, answers the question of "how" for the do-it-yourself crowd. This second book can be used help bridge the communication gap between leaders and programmers, IT or vendors.

Much like the first book, *Even Better Data* is filled with examples of homegrown BI solutions that were made in a relatively short period of time to solve a problem. Many examples illustrate how to use data to solve problems at the root-cause, allowing customization to help practices prevent or mitigate issues before the claim is denied, monitor staff productivity, and much more. The solutions in both books are simple and were produced in weeks, without spending a fortune. They can be used to meet unique practice problems as well as to measure the key performance indicators that are standard in our industry. I encourage the readers think creatively and design their own BI tools to free up time, meet the challenges of the new payment systems, reduce staffing costs, eliminate claim denials, scheduling mistakes or any other problem that presents.

Within this book, there is a contract payment manager BI tool that identifies underpaid claims. Nate worked with our practice and helped to bring this to fruition. This tool has been awarded a productivity award by our practice management software vendor. More importantly, this tool has helped us recoup significant underpayments from our contracted payers. Quite honestly, we started out with a small idea – look at a few things, and the idea grew beyond our wildest expectations.

Without hesitation, my own career would be far less meaningful without having met Nate, and having benefited from the advice he has provided to me. I speak for many of my colleagues at Ortho NorthEast when I say that we would still be dealing with many of the same issues we struggled with back in 2009, without Nate's assistance and solutions. But, more importantly, Nate has provided me with a listening ear and friendship that I value as much if not more. Enjoy *Even Better Data*.

Mona Reimers

Preface

This book is designed to be a continuation of the concepts introduced in the first book in the Better Data, Better Decisions series. The first book, *Better Data, Better Decisions: Using Business Intelligence in the Medical Practice* focused on how PivotTables can change the way practices see their data. This content is all-new and builds on the foundation of *Better Data, Better Decisions*.

Shortly after publishing *Better Data, Better Decisions*, I spoke at a meeting in Savannah, Georgia. After the presentation, Kevin Burris introduced himself and said, "You have a lot of smart clients." He was absolutely right. Kevin is now a good friend and one of those smart clients. The main reason to write a second book is that my smart clients have only gotten smarter and there are more smart clients generating game-changing ideas for Business Intelligence. I write the code to pull the data out of the Practice Management (PM) and Electronic Health Record (EHR) systems, but most of the examples in this book started with a need identified by a smart client.

This book will focus on a tool called SQL Server Reporting Services (SSRS). While PivotTables and Excel work very well for analyzing data, you and your users must remember (and have the time) to open Excel and analyze the data. SSRS works differently. Instead of pulling the information from a spreadsheet, SSRS can push the data to you and your team with scheduled emails. SSRS also builds dashboards available inside the practice's network. The ability to push information to users using SSRS is a huge advantage. If you want to interact with the data, Excel is generally a better choice. If your end users are not as familiar with Excel, SSRS is an effective way to get those users the data they need.

Now, if you use Excel but do not use PivotTables, get *Better Data, Better Decisions* and start using PivotTables today. There is no better way to quickly analyze hundreds of thousands of rows of medical practice data. You will get more insights from one well designed PivotTable than you will get from dozens of canned reports.

Better Data, Better Decisions offered many examples how PivotTables would look using sample medical practice data. This book takes a different approach. There are many more screen captures of actual reports used by practices across America. Names are masked, patient information, numbers and dates have been altered, but the format and structure of the examples is what smart medical practice executives use daily to succeed. It's hard to publicly express gratitude for their willingness to share without identifying their data, but practice after practice has allowed me to do just that. Thank you.

That said, my friend Mona Reimers read drafts of this book and provided invaluable ideas, corrections, and insight that made the book so much better. Mona and I wrote the first book in the *Better Data, Better Decisions* series together. We have worked together, presented at MGMA conferences together, and changed medical practices for the better. Pay attention to what Mona has to say. She is innovative, insightful, and intelligent. Thank you, Mona.

If you have heard me speak at a conference, you will not be surprised to hear that after a recent MGMA Annual Conference, a physician in attendance suggested a little Adderall to settle me down a bit. I am passionate about Business Intelligence in medical practices. I have seen better data drive better decisions and better results for practices across America. It's hard not to get excited when practices see game-changing results or when practices can finally access critical data that has been buried in their software for years. I hope this book fuels your passion with opportunities and ideas to apply to your unique situation.

Acknowledgements

Craig Wiberg coordinates those speaking engagements. Craig has been my MGMA contact for years and has consistently advocated my work as he advocates for the best educational opportunities for medical practice managers in America. Craig and his team, especially Isabel Penraeth and Jody McDonald, are consummate professionals who get the job done. All three made this book better with their recommendations, editing, and support. Michelle Mattingly, MGMA's Data Solutions Manager, graciously gave me access to data from the 2016 Practice Operations Report in Chapters 6 and 7. Erica Betz and Mariann Lowery added MGMA Stat data to enhance Chapter 4. Thank you.

Most importantly, I'm very grateful for the love of my dear wife, Larraine, and our three children, Charity, Joy, and Henry. They have consistently and unfailingly supported me as I have pursued my dream of taking Business Intelligence to medical practices. Sometimes that dream means long hours and frequent travel, but other days that dream leads us to Hawaii to get more Aloha shirts. None of this happens without their support and encouragement. I cannot tell you how many times Larraine has mowed the lawn, managed the house, and helped the kids while I have worked to meet a deadline. We are in this together. My parents, Wayne and Eileen Moore, taught me to work hard and to have faith. They have been behind me all the way. Each has been a tremendous blessing in my life.

Overview

Getting Better Data to Make Better Decisions

If you could have a daily one-page email highlighting critical metrics in your practice, what would be on that email? What do you need to see to drive growth and improve your practice's bottom line? What would that email reveal about practice finances, patient care, upcoming appointments, or quality metrics?

What if you could send a separate email to your providers, your managers, your front desk staff, or your nurses? What game-changing data would be on each email? What would change physician behavior the most? What would increase front desk collections, reduce days in accounts receivable, or deliver better patient care? How would each email align with your overall practice strategy?

What if you could customize daily, weekly, and monthly versions of these emails? What trends would become apparent? What new initiatives would finally take hold and change performance the most? What would you finally be able to see clearly? If emails were sent out each day that would identify potential discrepancies in data entry, how many claim or care errors could you quickly mitigate? How would that vision dramatically impact practice operations?

These questions should have you thinking about seeing your data differently; referring not just to seeing different data, but also in using tools to manipulate how the data is analyzed and presented, via customizable emails and dashboards. Medical practices across America are implementing ideas described in this book to see their data in new and exciting ways. This has resulted in more efficient, more profitable, more flexible, and more responsive medical practices that deliver higher-quality patient care.

A Vision for Business Intelligence in a Medical Practice.

PivotTables, spreadsheets, dashboards, emails, maps, visualizations, and other tools that drive practice performance, automatically refresh and can be customized by end users without IT support.

Chapter 2 offers a description of the tools listed in that vision statement. You certainly do not need to master every tool to get started, but you do need data to work with and a tool or two to consume that data. Understanding these tools, their advantages and disadvantages and how each fits into your practice's technical environment is essential. If your practice is just starting with Business Intelligence, spreadsheet-based tools are a low-cost but powerful way to get started.

Business Intelligence is not just a fancy name for the same old kind of canned reporting. Business Intelligence needs to drive practice performance. The tools must deliver mission-critical data exactly when the data is needed, without sorting through pages and pages and columns and columns of unneeded data. A major difference between Business Intelligence and generating canned reports is that many of the Business Intelligence examples in this book combine data from two discrete datasets. The data might combine upcoming appointments with historical clinical data or front desk collections with staffing data. Part 2 of this book is full of ways that practices around the country are combining data to deliver actionable insights and drive performance in their unique practice situations.

Dumping canned reports to Excel, cleaning up the data, and then creating an analysis is inefficient. The tools introduced in this chapter are designed to connect directly to the underlying sources of data, most often a PM or EHR system. The data refreshes automatically every time you open the tool. All the time you used to spend dumping, cleaning and creating is now available to spend acting on the data instead. The ability to customize reports without IT support is also a huge benefit.

After refining your Business Intelligence vision, Chapter 3 will prepare you to communicate your vision to IT, other administrators, managers and staff. IT teams are rightly concerned about anything affecting their data, fearing data will be corrupted, precious resources will be consumed, or their workload will be increased. Chapter 3 reveals a three-step process to succeed with IT. First, how to communicate a vision and anticipate possible concerns in terms IT will understand. Second, how to comfort IT's concerns that Business Intelligence will add to their workload or slow down the system. Finally, how to convince IT that Business Intelligence will actually reduce their workload by offloading most of the report requests and customizations that IT is currently buried under.

But IT isn't the only group that needs convincing. Administrators and physicians may be justifiably reluctant to spend money on reporting. The best strategy may be to meet their needs first. Show administrators data they have never been able to see before, or data that once took hours to compile being emailed to them automatically. Show physicians data that directly impacts their compensation. Even if other reports seem to be more pressing or have more potential upside, strategically it may be best to meet administrators' and physicians' needs first to get the widespread buy-in your Business Intelligence project needs.

Managers and staff also need to buy in to a Business Intelligence project. The goal isn't to eliminate jobs, but to eliminate unnecessary busy work. Replace the time spent tediously running canned reports containing half the information the team really needs. Instead, provide managers and staff the information they need to do their jobs well at the time they need to see that information. Rather than having staff search for the next accounts receivable balance, pre-authorization, or upcoming appointment they need to work on, provide the information automatically with exactly the information they need to see. You will also need to manage the organization's expectations about Business Intelligence to ensure success.

This book is a continuation and expansion of the ideas presented in Better Data, Better Decisions. That first book of the series introduced datasets and PivotTables, two fundamental tools to speed report development and increase flexibility. Chapter 3 introduces SQL Server Reporting Services

(SSRS), a tool most practices already own, that can email data to users as often as needed. SSRS uses the same datasets the PivotTables do. SSRS reports can also be delivered as an internal web page dashboard. Build one dataset, and now you have an analysis tool (PivotTables) and a distribution tool (SSRS) to develop better reports faster.

Chapter 3 also discusses new developments in analyzing and delivering data, including Power BI and PowerPivot. Power BI allows users to interact with data on mobile devices and browsers. PowerPivot removes the million-row limit for Excel data in Pivot Tables. Now you can analyze millions of rows of data in a PowerPivot Pivot Table, thanks to the new Excel Data Model. The latest versions of Excel now allow practices to map data in Excel. The ability to see geographic information like new patients and referral patterns is dramatically improved when viewed on a map. This chapter also introduces two other tools that, like SSRS, come bundled with almost all versions of SQL Server. SQL Server Integration Services (SSIS) imports and exports data from SQL Server. If you have data you need to get into SQL Server to take advantage of the reporting and analysis tools, SSIS can make that happen. SQL Server Analysis Services (SSAS) creates cubes, a very efficient way to store millions of rows of practice data. SSAS also has analysis tools for data mining. What's presented in this chapter is an overview, more technical details about SSRS and the other Business Intelligence tools can be found in the appendices.

Chapter 4 concentrates on payer contracting. You will find ideas on how to set contracted rates with payers and how to ensure that claims are being paid according to contract. There are examples from practices that track denied claims, adjustment reason codes, and successful appeals. Chapter 4 also has ideas on how to set billed charges as practices' fees become more transparent and comparable among providers. This chapter concludes with a section on the future of payer contracting, including a primary care practice's efforts to manage payer incentive programs. The section gives readers a sense for where payer contracting is heading and how to succeed in the new environment.

Attracting patients to your practice is the focus in Chapter 5, featuring examples of tracking and trending referral sources over time. Tracking new patients is important, but tracking procedures is also critically important for many practices. Through maps, patterns and opportunities in patient data will be revealed. In this chapter, you'll see how to use publicly available data to analyze whether referring physicians are sending patients to your physicians or your competition. You can also use publicly available Centers for Medicare and Medicaid Services (CMS) data to see how many procedures are being performed in your market for Medicare patients.

Chapter 6, longest chapters in the book, focuses on using appointment data to see and manage the practice's future. Practice managers need determine:

- How many patient appointments go unsold, and what can be done to use providers' time more efficiently?

- How many patients do not show for their appointments?

- How can appointment information reduce the number of no shows?

- How can patient access to providers be measured and improved?

- What obstacles can we identify in future appointments, and how can those problems be solved before the patient arrives?

- How can appointment data be used to improve practice efficiency?

Chapter 7 turns to measuring productivity, both for providers and other staff members. You will find a discussion of productivity metrics and learn about ways practices are communicating productivity throughout their organization. Ideas for helping a practice be more efficient range from measuring lag days to submit claims to tracking the number of claims coded. There is an example of how a practice measures their appointment duration, the total amount of time a patient spends from arriving at the clinic through check out. The example allows for options to visualize the data while taking some common variations of patient treatments and pathways through the clinic into consideration. Reducing patient appointment duration can increase the number of patients seen in a practice, see patterns of scheduling that cause clinic delays, and decrease the staff and space needed to care for those patients. Of course, shorter patient visits are a big patient satisfier as well. Working in a practice where patients are happier makes the clinic staff happier. When clinic staff know how to schedule to avoid delays and are not fighting against the clock to go home on time, staff retention can improve dramatically.

Chapter 8 describes automating and simplifying reports. Some of the examples shown are designed to make existing reporting run faster. Other reports are designed to pull together data from different sources to quickly give managers a sense for how their departments are doing. Many of the reports discussed in this chapter began either as a manual process or a time-consuming series of steps to combine data from different canned reports. You will find ideas on streamlining the entire pre-authorization process and giving more visibility to potential difficulties in pre-authorization. You will also find examples of simple reports designed to help staff consistently do the right thing.

Chapter 9 covers the use of Business Intelligence tools to leverage clinical data. Many of these reports integrate clinical data with practice management data to better serve patients. For example, a report that tracks patients who have a serious medical condition but have missed or cancelled their last appointment. There is an example of practice that combined clinical data about patients who need an x-ray with appointment data to dramatically reduce costs and save time in an x-ray department. Another example combines clinical data with appointment data to track upcoming appointments missing clinical data like labs or pathology.

Compliance with government and payer mandates is only getting more time-consuming. Chapter 10 has examples of reports tracking Medicare credit balances and quality codes for Medicare programs. This is one of several chapters in the book featuring lots of exception reports. An exception report only shows readers what they need to act on immediately. For example, instead of showing all accounts receivable balances or all credit balances, the Medicare credit balance report only shows credit balances for Medicare claims. Instead of showing all quality codes, only show claims without quality codes or claims with quality codes that indicate that compliance objectives were not met. Make compliance easier by only showing staff claims, charges, or balances that do not meet stated criteria.

Chapter 11 has a wide variety of dashboards from practices across the country that are seeing their data like they never have before. Some of the dashboards respond to a CPA's desire to manage by the numbers. Other dashboards are focused on patient access, visits, and trends in accounts receivable. Each dashboard is tailored to the specific needs of the practice. Many of the dashboards automate a process that once took days to compile the information. Some dashboards are designed for senior management. Other dashboards are designed at a middle management or even a staff level. Those dashboards can then roll up information to support practice-wide dashboards and objectives. You will see plenty of ideas to implement dashboards in your practice throughout Chapter 11.

Chapter 12 concludes with ideas to begin Business Intelligence in your practice, including suggestions for overcoming hurdles to getting started. There are also suggestions on how to successfully implement your first Business Intelligence project that will lead to future successes. Start small, but get started is the message.

As you begin, please remember that this book is intended to be an idea book, not a recipe book. There will be plenty of ideas of how practices are using their data to solve business and clinical challenges, but there will not be specific code to pull certain data out of a given PM or EHR system. The examples in this book come from a variety of different PM and EHR software packages. Those systems have hundreds if not thousands, of tables of data. Some are reasonably well organized. Others need a lot of help. One system which will remain anonymous requires searching through 90 separate tables to figure out which providers have open appointments next week. Explaining the hurdles in any PM and EHR systems is beyond the scope of this book.

Your practice is unique. You know the strengths, weaknesses, opportunities, and threats your physicians face. This book is designed to give you ideas about how other smart practices have addressed similar challenges that can be adapted to your needs. Rather than tell you how to run your practice, the intent is to give you the tools to implement your own ideas, and thus run your practice as efficiently and effectively as possible.

PART 1

THE VISION AND THE TOOLS TO ACHIEVE IT

This book is divided into two parts. This first section outlines a vision for Business Intelligence in a medical practice. The second, larger section, offers real world examples from practices across America that embrace that vision. Technical details of the tools used and examples are available in the appendices.

Many practice managers may not have the time, the background, or the interest in examining the technical aspects related to this topic. CHAPTER 3 briefly describes the Business Intelligence tools than can give practice managers a sufficient fundamental understanding to communicate more effectively with their IT department (many small to mid-size medical practices outsource their IT). Whether your IT team are employees or contractors, Part 1 will provide you ample enough information to take to, manage, and leverage your IT team.

Many medical practice managers are frustrated with the data in their Practice Management (PM) and Electronic Health Records (EHR). You might relate with a chief operations officer who recently said, "Not sure why (major PM/EHR software system) has to be so user unfriendly at times." She wanted to know how many unsold appointments the practice had, and sort them by resource, location, date, day of the week, appointment type, and more. (For example, how many appointments were unsold because of a no show?) She also wanted to know how many of those unsold appointments were a result of an appointment cancellation with so little notice that it may as well have been a no show. Requests like these are specific enough that it is very difficult for a PM or EHR system to build reports that answer these questions.

Your PM system may come with hundreds of pre-built or canned reports, but having so many can actually make it difficult to find the report you need. Often the information desired is scattered among several reports with no easy way to combine and pull only the data you need. The bigger challenge is that your practice is unique. The way a practice is owned, the way the business office is managed, and the way the physicians are compensated vary widely from practice to practice. That says nothing about a physicians' specialty, the size of a practice, and the nature of the business. Even if you use specialty-specific software, the fast-changing medical practice environment makes it difficult to decide what to report on next. Software vendors are bombarded with an ever-changing list of acronyms that takes development time and energy to comply with. The demanding requirements of the previous ICD-10, MU and PQRS initiatives, now compounded with MIPS and APM, push reporting down on the priority list until practices are stuck with nothing but a common set of generic canned reports.

Add-on reporting systems are available, but those systems often come with a learning curve of their own. The systems are typically technical and require time and training to master. Many people have ground though days of training, only to struggle to create their first report effectively. And despite the quality of their information, they are getting, at best, one report.

One report is never enough. A slightly different report might be required for this provider or that location. A similar report might be required using almost the same columns or filters, but that still means producing a new report. The number of reports multiplies like rabbits, making the task of finding the right report even harder.

Some practices have turned to cloud-based reporting tools that function independently of the PM or EHR system. The premise is that the reports are available from anywhere, and some of these systems have done a lot of good for medical practices. Because these stand-alone reporting tools are typically highly focused on reporting instead of all the compliance distractions the PM and EHR vendors face, the reports are better. Some of these stand-alone reporting systems also slow down considerably as the number of physicians increases. The ability to access reports from anywhere too often means that you can wait anywhere as the report loads and loads each time you change a filter. Though these reports are generally much better than the canned reports, they are not easily customizable beyond the ability to filter. Practice managers still end up exporting to Excel and massaging the data to get the insights they need.

Burned by this whole process, administrators and physicians are often reluctant to throw more money at reporting. The PM and EHR software is usually expensive to start with. Physicians, administrators, and staff can find it very difficult to make time to analyze the practice, let alone taking the time to run a report, clean up the data, and organize the information in a meaningful way. And even the "good" reports that were influential in the past tend to grow stale over time as obstacles facing the practice evolve. If you do not have time to act on the data, why take the time to get a report in the first place? This is even more potent if the report requires significant time to clean, massage, and organize the data to act on the information.

Fortunately, there is a better way.

CHAPTER 1

GETTING STARTED

W**hat** is Business Intelligence? You can look in any direction at a medical conference exhibit hall and see a vendor selling a product they describe as a Business Intelligence tool, but what does a Business Intelligence tool do? Business Intelligence is more than just fancy jargon applied to the same old canned reports. Business Intelligence for major corporations generally means expensive systems pulling data from across the organization to support decision making in real time. These systems are often very sophisticated, proprietary, and supported by a large group of IT professionals. That approach can work very well in large businesses, but medical practice environments are often quite different. The unique requirements of PM and EHR software are more specialized than many businesses, but the distinguishing factor is that most medical practices cannot justify a system that is very sophisticated, proprietary, or supported by a large group of IT professionals. Many medical practice groups outsource IT and most of those IT vendors support a variety of different industries besides healthcare. Many practice leaders think that they have already spent more than they would have liked to have spent on IT already.

What do you need to get started with Business Intelligence in a medical practice? The first step is a clear picture of the destination. The vision from the Overview is:

PivotTables, spreadsheets, dashboards, emails, maps, visualizations, and other tools that drive practice performance, automatically refresh and can be customized by end users without IT support.

TOOLS

The vision starts with tools to gather, analyze and distribute your data. *Better Data, Better Decisions* focused on spreadsheets, especially PivotTables.

PivotTables are a terrific way to analyze large quantities of data. If you have not used PivotTables, please pick up a copy of *Better Data, Better Decisions: Using Business Intelligence in the Medical Practice*, also published by MGMA. If you are looking for trends or want to drill down and understand data, PivotTables are very hard to beat.

The good news is that most practices own Microsoft Excel and many people are reasonably familiar with it. Excel makes it easy to chart, compare, and summarize data. Business Intelligence tools typically utilize multiple datasets, and Excel makes it easy to integrate data from multiple sources (like PM and EHR data) into one spreadsheet for analysis. As an example, the payer contracting tools in Chapter 4 use an Excel function called VLOOKUP to get all the contracts on one page. Lining up each procedure code and the allowed amount from each payer allows better comparison of payers for contracting. If you or your team are not familiar with Excel, there are over 500 free, short videos at mooresolutionsinc.com to get you up to speed in Excel quickly. Excel is often the first step in visualizing the health of your practice, so being efficient in the program will make it easier to quickly understand your practice data.

Chapter 11 includes a variety of dashboards, from complex, CPA-designed festivals of numbers to simpler dashboards focused on one concern. The tools listed in the vision are not necessarily in order, but a basic place to start is with spreadsheets, especially PivotTables. Dashboards are important and valuable, but without tools to direct staff and improve numbers, dashboards simply report that practice metrics are the same, month after month. Begin by giving the staff PivotTables to see their performance and to help them know what to focus on next. Also provide administrators with PivotTables that focus on overall trends and issues in the practice. Once you know what the staff or the administrators need to see, that data can be summarized in a dashboard. Dashboards are more of a reporting tool. PivotTables and spreadsheets are more of an analysis tool.

The ability to automate mission-critical data via email is a critically important. Rather than rely on physicians, administrators, or staff to remember to open a spreadsheet or a dashboard, SSRS lets you push the data to whomever needs to the see the data via email (many practices allow business email to be accessed on personal devices, so be careful not to include Protected Health Information [PHI] in the email). Email can be a powerful way to motivate staff and communicate priorities. Examples throughout this book are sent as daily email. Copy the email to supervisors and managers so that everyone is clear on priorities and those priorities can be managed appropriately. Transparently measuring and reporting objectives across the organization is key to motivating behavior. The beauty of SSRS is that a dashboard and an email are the same underlying report. For example, an SSRS report can be scheduled to be delivered weekly but can also be available on an internal web page during the week with updates. SSRS is a major part of this book. SSRS is introduced in Chapter 3 and covered in much more detail in Appendix 1.

Particularly for something like zip codes, there is no substitute for seeing data displayed geographically. The ability to map data has come a very long way with the introduction of Excel 2013. Excel 2013's Power Map feature allowed users to map data effectively, though the feature only existed in Excel's professional versions. Excel 2016 and Office 365's data mapping feature is now called 3D Map and is available in Excel Standard and Professional. Chapter 5 has examples of using maps to attract patients to a practice. Adding maps to an analysis is well within the skills of an average Excel user.

Visualizations includes new ways to see your data beyond the traditional spreadsheet rows and columns. Microsoft built a Power View tool into the professional version of Excel 2013 that introduced visualizations. Power View has been replaced by Microsoft's Power BI tool. Power BI offers visualization tools that are not available in Excel or SSRS. New versions and updates of Power BI are released frequently and Power BI is showing great potential. Power BI is also discussed in Chapter 3, with more detail in Appendix 2.

Reports, as part of the vision, might be a catch-all for data communicated in a way other than with the tools already mentioned. For some practices, this still means a printed page. Other practices design tools that work well in a dual-monitor environment. Staff can have the report on one monitor and the PM or EHR open on the other monitor, making it easy to follow along and work the report.

This book will not attempt to prescribe which tool is best for each application. The objective is to describe the different tools that are available and then encourage readers to customize the approach to meet your practice needs. There are numerous examples in Part 2 showing different tools in action.

DRIVE PRACTICE PERFORMANCE

The "Business" part of Business Intelligence means that the tools must help practices run their businesses like a business, regardless of the ownership structure. Even a not-for-profit organization needs to run efficiently to keep serving patients within a limited budget. Running a practice like a business means that the tools help physicians and administrators identify opportunities to increase revenues and decrease costs. Running a practice like a business also means the tools address important issues to all the stakeholders in the practice, including patients, physicians, and staff.

Reporting tools need to drive practice performance, not simply report on practice performance. It's nice to *know* the score at the end of the day (or the week, the month, or the year), but it is much more helpful to *influence* the score. A report that simply says this month was as bad as last month does not tell a practice what they need to change. Driving practice performance also means measuring the success of changes made. If a practice has decided to reduce lag days and bill more quickly, how is that objective being measured? How often is it being measured, and who sees the measurements? What are the obstacles to reducing lag days, and how can progress be measured to reduce those obstacles? Is the issue a factor of physicians documenting procedures or the billing office generating claims?

Driving practice performance means giving critical, game-changing information to the people who can actually change the game. Rather than build reports exclusively for management, give staff tools that will move the needle on management's reports. Many of the reports throughout this book are designed for front-line, patient-facing employees. A good example is the front-desk balances-to-collect reports, highlighted in Chapter 7. These are designed to be delivered as an email or a dashboard to the front desk staff and managers. There are two separate reports. The first shows who is coming in today with a copay or a patient balance. The second shows how the front desk performed collecting the previous day's amounts, subtotaled by who collected the balance. Daily feedback by staff member is the key to driving front desk collections.

Driving practice performance means showing people who can influence results only the data they need to see, when they need to see it. Including too much information from multiple objectives on the same report can lead to misunderstandings and misplaced priorities. The front-desk collections reports only show the relevant information on the relevant day. For example, the report does not show all patients with an appointment; it is filtered to only show patients that the front desk needs to collect from. Patients who are not projected to owe a copay and do not owe a patient balance should not be on the report. Too many canned reports go on for pages and pages with superfluous information that a busy staff does not need. Look instead for exception reports. An exception report only shows what the reader needs to see. Filter out information, and reduce the number of columns in the report as well. Make the reports easy for the staff to act on. As Mona Reimers says, "Make it easy for staff do the right thing." Design tools to make it easy for staff to drive practice performance. Examples of making it easy for staff to do the right thing appear throughout Part 2 of this book.

AUTOMATICALLY REFRESH

Building tools that automatically refresh means that once you build an analysis in a PivotTable, spreadsheet, dashboard, or other tool, that tool is connected to your data warehouse. Every time users open the tool, they see the same analysis they created last time, updated with current numbers. Exhibit 1.1 is from the Data tab on the Excel Ribbon, under Connections. Excel is set to refresh data in the background every time the spreadsheet is opened. The spreadsheet may take a little longer to open depending on the size of the data to be refreshed, but think of the time savings compared to saving a report as a Comma Separated Value (csv) file, importing the csv file into Excel, cleaning up the data, and creating the report.

EXHIBIT 1.1 EXCEL RIBBON: DATA TAB

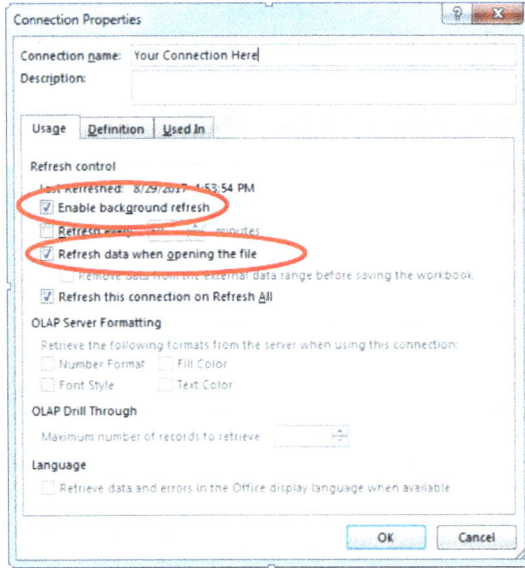

EXHIBIT 1.2 CANNED REPORTS

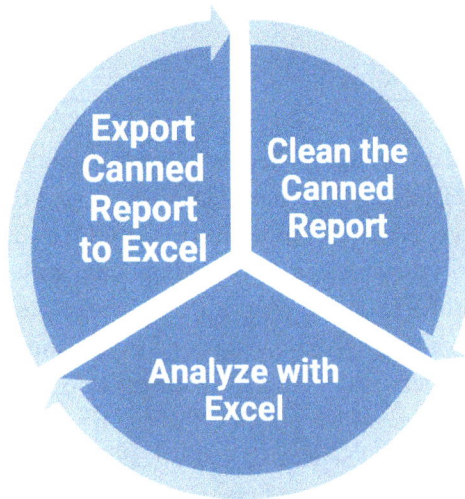

Every time you want to analyze data from a canned report, you must export the report to Excel—and this is before you even see the data. Cleaning the canned report refers to getting rid of the all the artifacts that come with it that you do not need in your analysis. For example, a PivotTable can summarize data, but if the canned report already totals the data, you will double-count your numbers if you include the canned report totals in your PivotTable. Besides unwanted totals, other columns of data may also not be needed. Some canned reports export the data to Excel in a way that tries to preserve the printed report format, resulting in a bunch of blank, space-holding columns. Often header and footer data (sometimes on each printed page!) appears that needs to be deleted before the data can be analyzed. The process of cleaning the canned report can be time-consuming and tedious without adding any value.

Once the data is cleaned, analysis can then proceed in Excel via PivotTables, charts, or analyses. The complication is that each time you want to do the analysis, you must re-export the data, re-clean the data, and re-create the PivotTable, chart, or any other components in your analysis. The process is so time intensive that reports that should be ideally run daily are run weekly. Reports that should be run weekly are run monthly, and the process snowballs.

The key is to have the tool connected to the data warehouse so that exporting, cleaning or rebuilding any analysis is unnecessary. Build the analysis once, connect the analysis to the data source, and all you ever need to do is open the tool to get the results you want. The time originally spent preparing the data for analysis to can now be used to analyze the data. The potential time savings is tremendous. Automatically refreshing the data also dramatically reduces the chance for errors to creep into your spreadsheet due to manually preparing the data. Other Business Intelligence tools can automatically refresh data by connecting to SQL Server. Faster, more accurate analysis is hard to beat!

Another advantage of automatically refreshing from the data warehouse is that time consuming calculations can be scheduled to run overnight. If a spreadsheet or other tool takes several minutes to open due to a data refresh, schedule all the calculations to occur overnight, refreshing dramatically faster the next day when you need that data. Part 2 contains examples of overnight calculations that speed up daily operations.

CUSTOMIZED BY END USERS WITHOUT IT SUPPORT

"Customized without IT support" means that that once these tools and the underlying datasets are created, end users can modify at least some of the report without needing an IT expert or a budget increase every time the next data request surfaces. IT is a scarce resource at medical practices, pulled multiple ways by competing demands, all of which are set aside if a critical server goes down. Good IT people are in high demand, let alone IT people who understand healthcare. It can be especially hard to find someone who understands your business and your clinical needs. And for too many practices technology to solve those challenges is prohibitively expensive. For too many practices, the timeframe to get the data you need is months and months, with no guarantee that your timeframe will be met or that the finally delivered report will still be relevant. The key is to use your IT resources wisely.

One way to use IT resources—whether internal or external—wisely, is to have IT build datasets and then have end users use tools to customize the way they consume the data. A dataset is simply a collection of data organized into rows and columns. For example, a billed charges dataset would have a row for every procedure code and each column tells you something about that procedure. Columns could be things like:

- Patient
- Rendering provider
- Referring provider
- Procedure code
- Modifiers
- Date of service
- Date of entry
- Location

- Primary insurance
- Secondary insurance
- Diagnosis codes
- Encounter number
- And more

Users can take that one billed charges dataset and build dozens of reports around productivity, charge utilization, the number and characteristics of new patients, days to enter charges, and much more.

It takes IT support to create the dataset in a data warehouse. Building the dataset typically involves a deep understanding of the structure of the PM or EHR data, as well as knowledge to extract the data using SQL queries. Generally, that specialized knowledge is beyond the scope of other staff in a medical practice. Internal IT departments supporting one PM or EHR software package are much more likely to have detailed information about the structure of the data necessary to write queries. External IT departments supporting multiple software packages or multiple industries have less incentive to take the time to dig into the structure of the underlying data to know enough to query the data.

Software vendors may be an option. They understand the structure of the PM and EHR information and know how to retrieve data. The difficulty with software vendors is that typically they do not support a separate data warehouse. Vendor solutions are too often one-off reports, not a dataset that connects to a tool to automatically refresh data. Vendors can be costly and a slow way to get to the data. One practice in the Southwest recently got a quote from a vendor that was 7-10 weeks to produce a single report. One viable solution is to send your IT department to vendor-sponsored training to understand the PM or EHR database structure. That solution works best when the IT department understands SQL Server. Sending non-technical staff to learn how to run reports using the vendor's software has not met this book's vision for Business Intelligence.

Once the practice has datasets, then "customized by end users without IT support" can become more and more of a reality. Spreadsheets are a perfect example of this. Once practice managers, billing staff, or clinical leaders understand the data, Excel training is relatively fast and inexpensive. The IT department could provide training to get started connecting the data warehouse to tools. After being trained, the end users' responsibility is to learn those tools so that most requests for data can be solved by the requestor, not by IT. End users may not necessarily know what they want the final product to look like until they see the initial draft of the report. Rather than go back to IT time and again for small report changes, empower staff to make those changes themselves. Save the IT resources to add more data to the data warehouse.

If you do not have internal IT, or you do have internal IT but they are booked a year in advance, Business Intelligence is still well within reach. Many medical practices, even mid-size groups, do not have internal IT. Depending on how you outsource your Business Intelligence, you may move a little slower than groups with internal IT, but remember that you and your team can only consume so much data at once. Throughout this book, the advice is to start small. Get one or two datasets you understand and can work with. Learn one tool. Start customizing your own data without IT support. As soon as you are comfortable with the tool and the data, add more data or a new tool. If you understand Excel, learn PivotTables, SSRS, maps, or another tool. Business Intelligence does not require internal, dedicated IT staff. Find a way to get a dataset and get started.

THE CLOUD

What if your data is in the cloud? For the purposes of this book, simply define the cloud as meaning the practice does not own or control the server or network that stores the practice's data. The word control is critical. If your data is stored offsite but you own your data, meaning you can control who has access to the raw data, for purposes of this discussion your data isn't in the cloud. Some hosting companies create separate servers and separate networks offsite such that it's easy to give practices access to their raw data. Other hosting solutions combine the data in such a way that it's almost impossible to give the practice access to their data.

If you do not control access to your own data, for the purposes of this book, your data is in the cloud. To paraphrase Dante, "abandon most hope, ye who enter here." If you can get to your data, and that is a big if, then you're in a good place—leveraging practice data is a competitive advantage, though Business Intelligence projects will take longer and cost more. Knowing how to use your data is a powerful way to differentiate yourself from other practices and to compete in today's marketplace. Do not give up that competitive advantage by losing control over your data.

The phrase was "abandon *most* hope," not *all* hope. Physician groups have successfully changed their workflow or built creative ways to get to their data. A good example is anesthesia. Those providers are almost always working on another entity's system, either a hospital or a surgical center. One anesthesia group in the Midwest controls their PM system in-house, but does not control the hospital data they need to submit quality data. They built a system to capture that quality data with the anesthesia billing data, which is then stored in a separate data warehouse and integrated with the PM data to successfully submit data to the Anesthesia Quality Institute (AQI).

Another Midwest anesthesia practice had an inexpensive cloud-based system. One of the things the AQI requires is the start and end time of each anesthesia case. The cloud vendor quote was thousands of dollars and several months to access the practice's own data about start and end times. The practice ended up downloading what data they could get from the cloud to three separate spreadsheets, combining those spreadsheets into one spreadsheet, entering data like start and end times into the combined spreadsheet, and uploading the revised data to SQL Server to submit the quality data. If that sounds painful, it was. The practice was frustrated, the process was very labor intensive, but they successfully submitted the quality data.

Yet another practice was frustrated with the inability of their cloud-based system to give them access to data they had entered into the EHR. The EHR stored the data, but none of the available canned reports gave them sufficient access to their own data. The EHR also did not have the flexibility to store the all quality data they needed to see to care for their patients. They ended up building a separate, stand-alone system to capture and report on the data. The downside for this practice is that all the data must be entered twice, once into the patient record in the cloud-based EHR and once into the quality system. Having their data in the cloud made the process frustrating. The upside is that the practice successfully met the quality reporting requirements.

What if you own your data, but your data isn't based in SQL Server? A dermatology practice owned the PM system and data in an SQL Server-based system, but the cosmetic software was not SQL-based. Several examples of this situation appear in Appendix 2, which discusses SQL Server Integration Services (SSIS). SSIS can get data from a non-SQL Server environment into a data warehouse. One way to deal with cloud-based systems is to get the cloud vendor to give you a nightly or a weekly data dump and use SSIS to get that data into the data warehouse.

Once you have a vision for Business Intelligence and a plan to access the data you need, the next step is to sell that vision to stakeholders throughout your practice. There is a financial aspect, but IT needs to cooperate in getting to the data, managers need to use the new reports, and staff may need to adjust to new tools and workflows. Communicating that vision to those stakeholders is the subject of Chapter 2.

CHAPTER 2

COMMUNICATING YOUR BUSINESS INTELLIGENCE VISION

For some practices, capturing a vision and a direction is the easy part. The harder part is communicating that vision so that physicians and administrators support it. Part of the buy in requires a financial commitment, but just as important as being willing to pay for Business Intelligence is being willing to leverage the data to improve practice operations. Management approval isn't enough. The staff need to understand and appreciate that Business Intelligence will make their jobs easier and less frustrating. The IT department also needs convincing. Many IT departments, especially internal IT departments, are often nervous about protecting the practice data. Since IT is the gatekeeper to the data you need, this chapter starts with ideas on how to work with an IT department to access the data. If you have ever taken a box of doughnuts to an IT department to get a report done, keep reading.

COMMUNICATING THE VISION TO IT

The practice's IT department can be either an internal team (practice employees) or outsourced to an external IT vendor. Your practice can implement Business Intelligence without having internal IT. If the internal IT department is too busy, adapt to the issue via an external vendor for Business Intelligence projects. Most internal IT departments are busy enough trying to maintain the status quo. Keeping the current network and software packages running is often a more than full-time job between software updates, hardware changes, staff turnover, security, compliance, and more. The last thing IT needs is one more project, especially a project that accesses and potentially impacts PM and EHR data.

The first step is to share the vision of tools that end users can customize without IT support. The result of a Business Intelligence project should be to reduce IT's workload—that's not necessarily a primary objective of the vision, but many IT departments are just swamped with requests for data and reports. Also, many of the tools IT currently uses to deliver reports only deliver one report at a time. Exhibits 2.1 and 2.2 are from MGMA presentations about communicating with IT departments.

The old model is each time anyone requests a report, IT or the PM vendor builds a report to meet that specific request only. It might be possible to share underlying code or logic between reports, but building one report typically results in one report.

EXHIBIT 2.1 REPORTS: OLD MODEL

Old Model

Build One Report **=** Get One Report

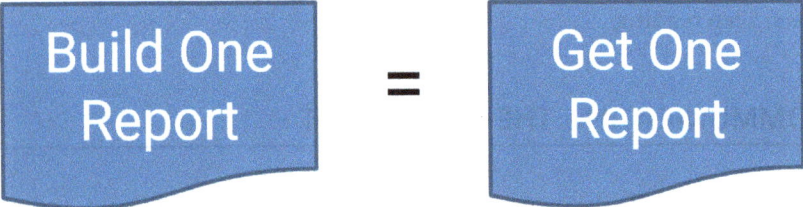

The new model is to build datasets, as discussed in Chapter 1. Datasets are the secret sauce of Business Intelligence for medical practices. One dataset can drive dozens and dozens of reports. Part of the value of datasets is that IT only needs to pull data from the PM or EHR system once instead of each time a report is requested, but there is more to it. The key is to use different tools to consume the data in the dataset. Some tools, especially those that come with PM and EHR systems, are designed to build a single report. The tools also take significant training time and often require a technical background and a knowledge of the underlying data in the PM or EHR being reported on. The tools introduced in Chapter 3 are very different. End users either know how to use spreadsheets or can quickly come up to speed on spreadsheets. One well-designed dataset/spreadsheet combination can be used in many ways by different departments. Most of the other tools are well within the grasp of a medical practice.

EXHIBIT 2.2 REPORTS: NEW MODEL

New Model

Build One Dataset = Get Dozens of Report

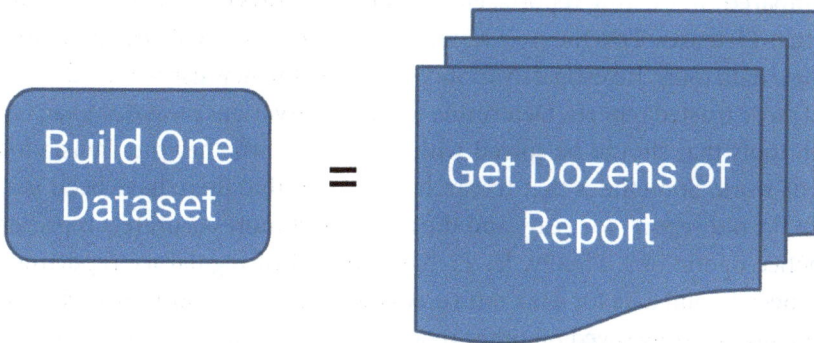

Having users create or modify their own reports saves IT time, but there is another big, time-saving advantage. Users know their needs better. Many times, IT will build a report they think meets a user's needs, only to find out that the report isn't quite what the user had in mind. This disconnect causes culture issues. The issue isn't that the user did a poor job explaining the report or that IT did a poor job implementing the request. The user feels that they did not get what they wanted after waiting what feels like forever and IT report creators feel like they worked hard on something that is now just trashed. To be fair, sometimes a user needs to see an example of a report before realizing how the report could be improved. Other times putting the report into practice for a couple of weeks reveals changes that would make the report far more useful. Take away the iterative and time-consuming process of going from users to IT and back again by training users to design and customize their own reports.

Savvy IT departments will appropriately raise data quality issues. If users run their own reports, they are more like to make mistakes in applying the data, creating formulas, and understanding business logic. Solve part of these concerns with training on the tools (how to use Excel, for example) as well as how to use the datasets. For example, users could understand that the Billed Charges Dataset has a row for every procedure code charged. Counting charges isn't the same as counting patient visits, since many patients will have more than one charge per visit. Train users to validate their reports (compared) to existing reports, either canned reports or reports designed by IT that IT trusts. Test the new reports repeatedly, especially early iterations of new data tools. Investigate variances between the new user-created reports and those trusted reports. Determine whether the variance was due to an issue with tools that should be solved with training or whether the dataset logic needs work. Sometimes that research will reveal that there have been issues with the old reports for years and the new report more accurately represents practice operations. Finally, let IT have control of regulatory reporting. If you need to pull data for a tax return, Medicare quality reporting, or a similar need, use the time saved on other reports to let IT manage these needs.

Another common IT concern is that accessing PM or EHR data directly from SQL Server will slow down the system. This is a very valid concern for many practices. Solve this issue by using a data warehouse. Let IT run any backup or maintenance routines overnight. When those routines finish, pull a copy of the data you need to populate the datasets into a separate SQL Server database. Depending on the size of the practice and hardware configurations, the data warehouse could reside on the same server or on a different server. Some practices are small enough that they only have one SQL Server installation and the same server can hold both the live, production data and the data warehouse. Larger practices will benefit from a separate SQL Server. Some vendors like NextGen® frequently sell a report server in addition to the production server. (The production server holds the live PM and EHR data used by the practice.) Initially, a second server can manage without the latest and greatest hardware and software. Many practices put their data warehouse on an older, underutilized server. The idea is to pull the data overnight and to store it in a way that you can run reports all day long without slowing down the PM and EHR.

Some practices want data more often than an overnight pull can provide. For 95-99% of reports, overnight data is better than anything that the practice has had before and is current enough. If you do want data to refresh throughout the day, medical practices have successfully use a SQL Server technology called log shipping to move data from the production server to a data warehouse periodically during the day. Log shipping is beyond the scope of this book. Plan on onsite, full-time IT employees to manage log shipping if you choose to consider that technology. SQL Server 2017 makes refreshing data even easier.

Wherever you store the data warehouse, your only access to production data should be read-only access. Always ask for read-only access. Tell your IT departments, "Don't call me if it breaks, because I cannot break it." Read-only access cannot change or delete data, so the integrity of the PM and EHR data is never compromised. If a data warehouse is inadvertently deleted or changed, it can be restored the following night. Restoring production data from a backup is a much more time-consuming hassle.

Data warehouses can often be faster than pulling data from production data since IT can write code to compile, analyze, and group data overnight. If you need a complex query that requires a lot of processing, run the query and store the results overnight in a separate table. Reports running off that separate table run significantly faster than reports that must compile data before running. Data warehouses are usually much faster at combining data from multiple sources (separate PM and EHR systems, eligibility and benefits data, outside systems like labs or pathology, etc.) as well.

Data warehouses also allow for custom logic. Read-only access to production data means you cannot save anything, so there is no place to save custom logic. Save custom logic in a data warehouse instead. For example, the Denied Claims spreadsheet in Chapter 4 includes a tickler column that counts down the number of days to appeal the claim with the insurance carrier. The logic for the tickler column isn't in the PM system. To make the tickler column work, there is a separate table in the data warehouse that stores appeal times by insurance group. Some of the logic could be implemented on a report-by-report basis, but then any time the logic changed each report that references the logic would also need to be updated. Using a data warehouse for custom logic is much more efficient and SQL Server generally crunches the numbers more quickly than trying to add custom logic to spreadsheets.

Speaking of crunching numbers, data warehouses are faster and more efficient at storing data than spreadsheets. Spreadsheets are a fantastic way to consume data, but are not as good at storing very large amounts of data. Certified Public Accountants do very complex things to store a tremendous amount of data in spreadsheets. One practice in the Southeast has spreadsheet which stores a massive amount of data about a practice, sliced and analyzed several different ways. It takes hours and hours every year to prepare the spreadsheet for the coming year's data. It takes more hours every month to enter the data into the spreadsheet. Those spreadsheets posing as a data warehouse are at a heightened risk for calculation and transposition errors due to their size and complexity. Use SQL Server to store data, it's what you pay SQL Server to do. Use spreadsheets to analyze the stored data. That approach is far more efficient.

The good news is that once the datasets are loaded in the data warehouse and end users are trained, IT can move on to the next pressing project on their list. More good news is that the practice likely owns most of the tools users need to build their own reports. There may be some training (and retraining) to get started, but users who can fill most of their reporting needs independently will save IT hours of time. Staff efficiency and effectiveness will increase at the same time. The Business Intelligence solution in medical practices isn't simply, "Call IT." Wisely leveraging IT resources can deliver Business Intelligence more quickly and more cost effectively than practices have done in the past.

Transforming a medical practice into a data-driven organization may well decrease IT's workload in the ways described, but good data is addicting. IT may save time building one-off reports, but the need for more data, especially value-added analysis of that data, will likely increase the IT department workload. The trade-off for IT isn't just job security as data needs increase, but the type and importance of IT's role in the organization changes dramatically—and for the better. Data becomes a competitive advantage for the practice, and IT holds the keys to that advantage. Instead of responding to the clinic's headaches with one-time reports, IT becomes much more proactively involved in business strategy.

Exhibit 2.3 is another picture from MGMA presentations. If all else fails with IT, fried carbohydrates work every time! For even better results, frost the fried carbohydrates!

EXHIBIT 2.3 FRIED CARBOHYDRATES

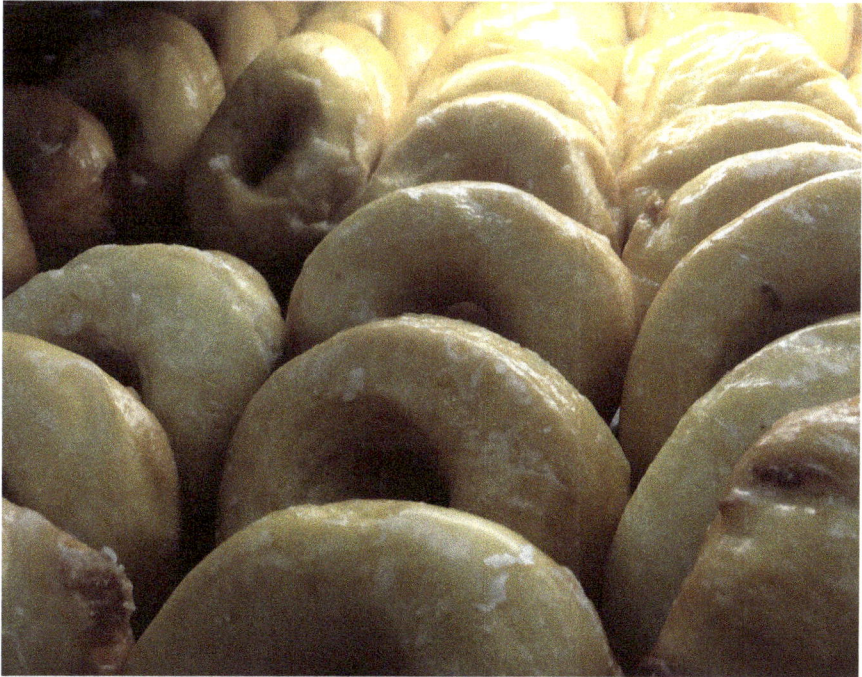

COMMUNICATING THE VISION TO ADMINISTRATORS AND PHYSICIANS

IT departments are concerned about protecting their data and about not creating additional work. Administrators and physicians have broader concerns, and it helps to listen carefully to discover their concerns. A place to start might be the question from Chapter 1. "If you could have a daily one-page email highlighting critical metrics in your practice, what would be on it?" You may focus on the physician compensation system. How are the physicians compensated and what data drives the physician compensation model? For example, in a Relative Value Unit (RVU) based system, the one-page email might have data comparing current RVUs to last week, last month, or the same period last year. You may even be able to project compensation levels and incentivize physician productivity in that email.

Medical practice administrators are constantly pressed for time. Thus administrators might appreciate automating a report that takes hours if not days to compile. Several of the dashboards in Chapter 11 are based on automating existing data and freeing up administrator's time to act on the numbers instead of simply compiling them. Some of these reports may involve combining data from different areas of the practice, like following up on appointment cancellations and no shows for certain clinical diagnoses in Chapter 9. These reports take a long time to compile because combining data from multiple practice areas means dumping multiple reports to a spreadsheet to clean before the data can be combined for analysis. The days to third next available reports in Chapter 6 are examples of data that used to have to be stored manually every day and is now easily available to analyze. Also look for data that is in the PM or EHR, but not currently available in existing reports.

Another approach to win over administrators and physicians is to resolve an issue in the practice. One practice's billing office was overwhelmed with old accounts receivable balances. Getting those old accounts receivable balances back under control and collected was a priority. Regulatory requirements often create crises that require an unreasonable number of hours of manual work that can be solved much more quickly with Business Intelligence. Quality reporting systems and Medicare credit balance requirements are examples of time-consuming regulatory necessities and are another good place to start. Once the crisis is averted, use data to solve other difficulties before they hit a crisis level.

Patient feedback may capture physicians' attention. A patient who reports that it took 60 days to get in to see the physician may prompt a discussion about patient access issues that can be addressed with reports in Chapter 6. A patient who was prescribed narcotics without an appointment (Chapter 9) or a patient who appears for an appointment without having the necessary labs or pathology (Chapter 9) may also prompt a Business Intelligence project.

Competitive advantage is another place to look for ideas to get started with Business Intelligence. A good topic at many practices is determining where patients are coming from and what can be done to increase new patient admission. Chapter 5 has several examples of how to get started with attracting patients to the practice. The size or unique specialties in the practice may give the practice a competitive advantage in payer contracting. Chapter 4 has a variety of examples of using Business Intelligence in payer contracting.

This book and *Better Data, Better Decisions* are also sources of ideas for physicians and administrators. Medical groups across America have found inspiration from reviewing examples in these books. The sample ideas are helpful, but they are much more impactful if the example is customized to the needs of the practice. Start with the examples, but do not end there. Your practice may make a few customizing tweaks that make the difference between a good report and a game-changing report.

If you are the administrator and the physicians or owners have different priorities, let the boss win. Start with what the boss wants in order to establish Business Intelligence and a culture of using data to make decisions in the practice. To build what the boss wants, the practice will likely end up with a data warehouse and tools that can be used for future projects as well. Make that first project successful, and future projects will follow.

As you are communicating your Business Intelligence vision to administrators, physicians, and owners, it might help to ask this question. "Do you want a fancy dashboard for management that shows the same results month after month or do you start with tools for the staff that will change the results month after month?" You will not be the first practice administrator who started out thinking they wanted a dashboard and started with staff tools first. It might seem unselfish to meet staff needs first, but the results of giving the staff better tools to do their jobs can impact the bottom line more than a fancy dashboard can.

COMMUNICATING THE VISION TO MANAGERS

The first step in communicating the vision to front-line managers is simply to schedule a time to communicate. A large practice in the Southeast scheduled a meeting in the conference room with managers and the IT team. Managers in medical practices are very busy and the IT team is also swamped with projects. This practice was no different. Just facilitating a meeting between the managers and the IT team resulted in several immediate benefits. End users identified existing reports that the IT team could easily modify to better meet needs. They discovered existing PM functionality that could be used to meet another manager's pressing need. The practice also found a very time-consuming process to automate and simplify. Now a data warehouse project is underway to build datasets and link those datasets to spreadsheets and SSRS. The starting point was to schedule a time for IT and managers to brainstorm together about the Business Intelligence vision for the practice.

Some managers will be excited about the tremendous time savings possible by customizing their own reports instead of having to get in IT's queue. Other managers might be intimidated by the new reporting tools and wondering where they will find the time to learn one more thing. Start with the first group of managers. Find an early adopting manager who senses the need for better reports and who is comfortable with technology and the tools they can use to customize the report. Following are several ideas to get that manager engaged with Business Intelligence.

Staff productivity is a common concern of managers. Look at some of the reports that measure productivity in Chapter 7. If you can show a manager which team members enter the most claims, check in the most patients, appeal the most claims or collect the most copays, you will convert that manager to Business Intelligence quickly. Giving managers better tools to measure productivity is a very effective way to share a vision. Managers will also be excited to trend improvement in productivity over time. Managers will appreciate spending less time creating reports and more time analyzing the practice, doing what the practice pays the manager to do. SSRS reports that are automatically delivered to managers instead of managers having to remember to run reports will also be big selling point. Even the most change-averse managers will start to see the value in the early-adopting managers' productivity reports.

A key idea in communicating the Business Intelligence vision to managers is to make sure everyone understands that some projects require workflow changes to store necessary data. For example, to track how many appeals are done each week, the practice may need staff to record appeals in the PM system with a specific transaction code. Staff may be used to storing notes in their own words about the appeal, but a specific appeal transaction code can be mined to know who did the appeal and when the appeal was done. The appeal transaction code may also define what kind of issue was appealed. Managers can help implement workflow changes so that staff enter data correctly.

Managers are uniquely qualified to support Business Intelligence projects because they understand the practice administrators' priorities and they also understand what the front-line employees do every day. Many managers used to do the jobs and tasks they now manage. This perspective helps them identify tools that make employees' jobs easier and that meet management objectives. Many of the best ideas for Business Intelligence come from managers.

COMMUNICATING THE VISION TO STAFF

As staff come to understand how Business Intelligence can make their lives easier, they will begin suggesting better tools to do their job. A staff member at a busy orthopedic practice suggested tracking pre-authorizations for procedure codes that were billed but not pre-authorized. Having the staff member suggest the report was helpful for several reasons. She recognized the need, but she also recognized that the pre-authorizations did not always have the pre-authorized procedure codes listed. She knew what needed to be changed and was motivated to list the pre-authorized procedure codes and make the change happen.

Having staff suggest ideas for reports and tools offers particular benefits. The reports and tools are more likely to be used by the staff because they are practical and were invented by the staff instead of being imposed by administration. Staff realize that the new tool will help the practice and also make their jobs easier. The practice culture benefits in at least two ways. The staff know that they are being listened to. The administrative team also sends a clear message about the value of using data to make better decisions throughout the practice, not just in board meetings.

As with managers, it may help to have a technologically savvy staff member as an early adopter and cheerleader to help the rest of the team understand how much faster and easier their jobs will be. Having early champions and their momentum are invaluable. That staff member can also help iron out any bugs before the entire staff adopts the new tools. As you will hear throughout this book, the objective is to make it easy for staff to do the right thing. Employees' jobs will get easier and less mundane in some respects, but they will also be able to be much more productive.

Business Intelligence allows clinics to do more with less. One practice has seen 10 percent more patients each year for several years without adding front desk staff. Business Intelligence does not require staff to be replaced with automation. It means that staff will be able to do more work more accurately because they have better tools.

Some employees who resist change will likely resist Business Intelligence. They may have an "always done it this way" mentality, or they may be concerned about not being up to speed on the new tools for reporting. Management can help by being clear with the Business Intelligence objectives, which is to run the practice more like a business, and not to reduce staff count. One practice in the Midwest turned off old canned reports to motivate the employees to start using new reports. Free training to help staff learn basic, intermediate, and progressively advanced Excel skills is available at mooresolutionsinc. com. Finally, a more experienced staff may also be concerned over a big mistake occurring (that they will be held accountable for) when the new tools are implemented. They need to be reassured while they try out the tool and be given an opportunity ask questions to gain trust. One big advantage of SSRS is that your staff don't have to know Excel since the reports are delivered via email and dashboards. The next chapter has more information about SSRS.

MANAGING EXPECTATIONS

As you sell your vision of Business Intelligence throughout the organization, manage expectations of what Business Intelligence will not do:

- It will not be perfect. Especially at first, the data in your PM and EHR will not be clean. You might see a date of service in 2081 instead of 2018. Every now and then you might see that 2081 charge paid! You might find claims for providers who do not offer that service or for providers at the wrong location. That is entirely normal. Part of the difficulty is that the practice has never been able to see data like this before and so has never seen the errors before. The Business Intelligence process helps practices discover and fix incorrect data. Make a reasonable effort to clean up mistakes and move forward.

- It will not compensate for inconsistent workflow. Garbage in means garbage out. The analysis is only as good as the data that feeds the analysis. If different staff members in the billing office use different codes to describe the same thing, trends will be very difficult to see. Consistent data is much easier to analyze. If data has not been consistent or workflows have not been clearly defined or followed in the past, then start today. Previous data may not be especially reliable, but that's no reason to wait for all practice workflows to be perfect before starting.

- It won't ever be "done." You may think you have all the reports your practice needs, but the healthcare environment is incredibly fluid. You are building an organizational culture and foundation to adapt, and thus survive over the long run. With the data stored in a data warehouse, it's just a matter of changing that data as practice needs change or adding new data to the data warehouse. You will know how to use the tools and you will have all layers of the organization thinking about new tools to meet any new threats and opportunities that arise.

- It will involve more rigorous emphasis on data governance. In simple terms, the practice agrees what each key field means in the PM and EHR system and everyone follows those guidelines. For example, what goes in the referring physician field? Is it the last provider to see the patient, the last provider outside the practice to see the patient, or the patient's primary care provider? Getting these details consistent will dramatically improve the quality of the analyzable data.

- It will not compensate for poor staff training. Poor staff training will make the Business Intelligence less reliable and trustworthy. Once workflows have been agreed upon and data governance rules have been set, staff need to be trained to consistently follow the guidelines. Some departments in the practice with high turnover may need frequent training to get the data entered correctly. Design a custom report to ensure that the data is consistently entered and identify training gaps.

- It will not be one size fits all. What works for another practice, even in the same market, the same specialty, and the same size, may not work for you. What matters is the data that will drive practice performance in your unique situation. Do not let the perfect be the enemy of progress. Start with something. Start collecting data. If the data does not tell you what you need to know to drive the practice, collect different data. Let the examples in part 2 of this book send you in the right direction.

- It will not take forever. Business Intelligence projects take weeks, not months. Do not bite off more than you can chew. That means not trying to build every dataset your practice will ever need at once. Start with a dataset or two. Those projects take weeks. Also, do not overwhelming your team with dozens of spreadsheets and emails initially. Start with one or two reports and build from there. Give the users time to learn a tool, test it out, and seek out feedback from the users and managers. Nothing is worse than developing a new tool only to find out it was never implemented, or that it was shelved after a few days due to one tiny flaw.

- It shouldn't cost a fortune. Typical projects start in the thousands of dollars, not tens or hundreds of thousands. Start small. Build a foundation of a data warehouse, a dataset or two, and a tool to use the data. Build on that foundation with additional datasets and tools over time. What are you waiting for?

TEST, TEST, TEST

Testing cannot be overemphasized. Validate the data before you ever show the reports to physicians and administrators. There are no second chances at first impressions. As you start, introduce the data as a rough draft or a first take. Compare the data to canned reports to make sure your data is reasonable. That said, the canned report may not necessarily be "right."

A physician group in the Southeast was concerned when the new dataset did not match their canned report. Since the canned report was part of the system, it must be "right." It turned out that the canned report included voided charges, while the new dataset specifically excluded voided charges. There may not be a right answer so much as a preference regarding how to handle voided charges. The canned report included both the voided transaction and the original transaction, as well as the date the void occurred. The new dataset filtered out the voided transaction and the transaction that was voided.

A practice in Texas accidentally entered a $1 million charge. Including a similar voided charge in this practice would inflate charges by $1 million in the month the charge was entered and reduce charges by $1 million in the month the error was discovered. A million-dollar mistake is a big variance to explain. On the other hand, if the charge was entered, financials were run, and then the charge was voided, there is a potential for numbers to change after the month is closed. Hopefully both sides of the argument are clear. The point isn't to exactly match canned reports. The key is to understand what the canned reports do, how that logic affects your practice, and choose accordingly.

CRAWL, WALK, RUN

As Mona Reimers, Director of Revenue Services at Ortho NorthEast in Fort Wayne, Indiana, says "Crawl, walk, run." She often says this to describe the process of getting started with Business Intelligence. She was in a meeting with the practice's finance director several years ago to discuss a complex project. He suggested that sometimes even before you crawl, you might need to slither. Her point is that you need to start small and grow over time, but most importantly that you need to start.

Start crawling by catching the vision of what Business Intelligence can mean in your practice. Keep crawling by identifying the datasets and tools you will use to produce that Business Intelligence. Communicate that vision to enough people in your organization to build enough momentum to get that first project underway. Once the first project is underway, decide whether to add information to the dataset you have or think about building another dataset. Spreadsheets are so common that they are often the easiest tool to start crawling (though there are other tools as well that can really leverage the value of your data). Email and dashboards are a natural next step, and will be discussed more in the next chapter. But the key thing is to keep crawling, and soon you will walk, and who knows, even run!

CHAPTER 3

BUSINESS INTELLIGENCE TOOLS

This chapter is designed to a be high-level summary of the Business Intelligence tools described throughout this book. Practice administrators who want more than a general understanding of each tool should review the appendices. SSRS is the focus of Appendix 1 and the other tools are described in Appendix 2. The right balance of where a practice administrator stops and the IT department takes over will vary with the environment in each practice, but this chapter will provide enough information to get a conversation with IT started.

PIVOT TABLES

PivotTables were the focus of *Better Data, Better Decisions*. There is no faster, simpler, more accessible way to analyze a large amount of data for the average practice than a PivotTable. They are the tool of choice to quickly understand and act on a large of amount of charges, collections, receivables, appointments, or other medical practice data. The secret sauce of a dataset connected to a PivotTable that refreshes every time the spreadsheet is opened is very hard to beat. One well-designed PivotTable can replace dozens of canned reports.

Provide PivotTable training to as many levels of your practice as is feasible. Push that limit to include teams from the front desk through executives and physicians. Do this for two reasons. First, PivotTables are not difficult to work with. Even if you must design PivotTables for users who are not very familiar with Excel, the learning curve to understand PivotTables isn't hard and free resources are available online. Many state MGMA associations also provide PivotTable training as part of their conferences.

Second, PivotTables ultimately enable end users to run their own reports and answer their own questions. The front desk can see how many people are scheduled tomorrow by location, how many copayments were collected yesterday by cashier, or how long front desk wait times were last month.

The executive team can drill down to understand why charges increased last month, why collections were down in the South location, or what the trend in referring physicians or payers looks like this month. PivotTables combined with datasets can make end users more self-sufficient report producers, a big part of the Business Intelligence vision of this book. Once PivotTables have identified trends to monitor and have tracked progress on key performance indicators, the next step will likely be SSRS.

SQL SERVER REPORTING SERVICES

SSRS is the major Business Intelligence tool discussed in this book. If the objective is to analyze and interact with data, PivotTables are the tool of choice. Once the objective moves from analyzing data to communicating results, SSRS is an effective way to deliver information to everyone from the front desk to the physicians. Best of all, SSRS is included with almost every version of SQL Server, so practices that own their data in SQL Server already own SSRS at no additional cost.

SSRS reports are more challenging to create than Excel spreadsheets. The fundamental building blocks of an SSRS report are tables and matrices. A matrix looks much like a PivotTable. SSRS also offers a wide variety of charts, sparklines, indicators (such as arrows and other colored symbols), maps, and gauges to focus users' attention and add color to your reports. These features are described in Appendix 1. It will likely take IT help to get started, though interested practice administrators or data analysts can learn to create their own reports with a tool called Report Builder, also described in Appendix 1.

A time-saving feature of SSRS is that the same report can be shared on an internal web page dashboard and emailed throughout the organization. In other words, build a dashboard in SSRS and you can subscribe to have the report delivered via email as often as you prefer. SSRS can deliver the report in the body of the email or can attach the report as a PDF. The advantage of including the information in the body of the email is that users only need to open the email to see the data. A sample SSRS report embedded in the body of the email is shown in Chapter 9. Saving the report as a PDF works better for complex reports that need to be viewed consistently on-screen sizes ranging from phones and tablets to desktops.

SSRS reports include a feature called parameters, a way to filter the data. Many of the dashboards in Chapter 11 are designed with parameters so that the same practice-wide dashboard can be filtered by provider, location, payer or any other variable for more in-depth analysis. When you subscribe to an SSRS report with parameters, SSRS will allow you to use the parameters to filter the report so that Dr. Smith's email only contains Dr. Smith's data, for example.

Many of the SSRS reports in this book are designed as exception reports, limiting the data to only show charges, claims, appointments, or other data that fall outside a normal, expected range. If the exception does not happen frequently but the exception report is delivered via email, users would end up opening SSRS emails that show no data so often that they may stop opening the email altogether. To solve the problem of emails reporting that there are no exceptions to report, SSRS email subscriptions can also be data-driven, so that emails are only sent when the report contains data. Make exception reports data-driven emails so that users learn that when they see that email, there is an important exception to be reviewed and addressed.

Appendix 1 is a demonstration and discussion of SSRS. The remaining tools below are described in Appendix 2.

POWER BI

Power BI is Microsoft's new tool to interact with data on mobile devices or via a desktop browser. The objective is to provide users an environment for self-service Business Intelligence. Users can drag fields (similar to a PivotTable field list) onto a graphical interface and choose from an expanding array of visualizations, different ways to see data. A list of visualizations and some examples are included in Appendix 2. Visualizations range from charts that will be very familiar to Excel users to treemaps and waterfall charts. Appendix 2 has a detailed example of a treemap.

Where SSRS is limited to some filtering options, users have a much more interactive environment in Power BI. For example, Excel PivotTable users may be familiar with slicers, a visual way to filter data. In Excel, a slicer is simply a list of fields that users can select from. Power BI takes the slicer concept further by allowing a chart to function as a slicer. Rather than simply displaying fields to choose from, Power BI charts those fields. In other words, an Excel slicer for charges could list the years available to filter data, such 2017, 2018, and 2019. A Power BI slicer would chart the charge data for each of those years so that one could see charges by year. Users who tap on 2018 would see related charts in the same visualization change to reflect 2018 data. A sample Power BI dashboard in the web-based design interface is shown in Exhibit 3.1. Each of the four charts functions like a slicer that filters the other three charts.

EXHIBIT 3.1 SAMPLE POWER BI DASHBOARD

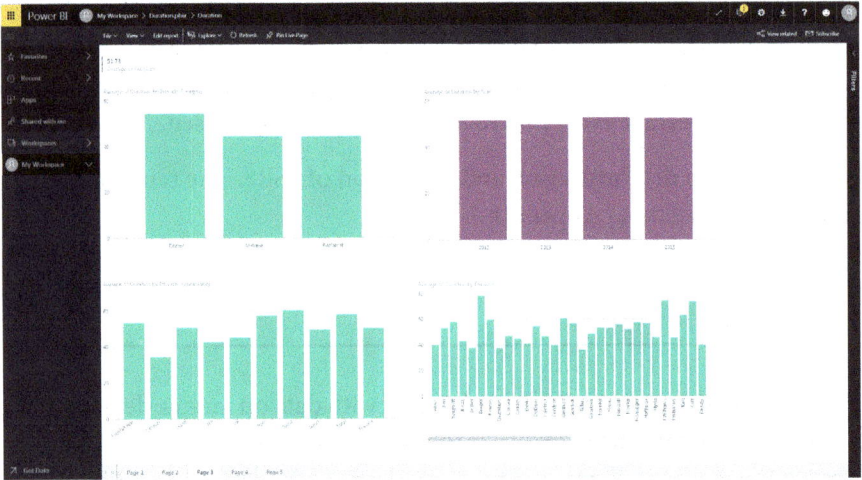

Power BI also allows a more graphical drill-down experience compared to an Excel PivotTable. One of the most powerful features in a PivotTable is the ability to double-click a value and have Excel show the detail that comprises the value selected. Power BI takes this functionality further by allowing users to drill down and up from charts and display the resulting data as a chart, rather than just displaying a raw table of detail as Excel does.

Power BI also includes a natural-language Q&A tool that allows users to type questions in English. Power BI responds with an answer to the question. For example, a user could type "2018 charges by provider" and Power BI would chart 2018 charges by provider. Typing "2018 charges by provider column" would prompt Power BI to respond with a column chart displaying 2018 charges by provider. The natural language syntax takes some getting used to and users need to know the names of the underlying fields (billed charges data might be called "charges," instead of "billed charges" or "fees"), but the potential for users to create their own reports and for self-service BI is there. Microsoft is making a concerted effort to update the Power BI apps and tools monthly. Even so, there are plenty of calculations, formulas, and formatting that can only be done in traditional Excel.

Power BI can deliver practice data on mobile devices. As with all the Business Intelligence tools in this book, ensure that Protected Health Information (PHI) is safeguarded in accordance with the practice's policies and procedures. As employees can consume data on more and more personal devices, PHI needs to be monitored vigilantly.

POWER PIVOT AND THE EXCEL DATA MODEL

PivotTables are powerful when analyzing lots of data, but if you have too much data, PivotTables run up against the million-row limit in Excel. If your data is getting to be that large, Power Pivot may be just the solution. The Power Pivot example in Appendix 2 has 60 million rows of data. Power Pivot can handle that much data without any trouble. Power Pivot is an advanced data analysis tool that is included Professional versions of Excel (not in the traditional, standard version).

Power Pivot is designed to use Microsoft's new Excel Data Model. The Excel Data Model allows for the handling of much more data than traditional Excel can handle. The Excel Data Model also allows users to combine data sources in Excel without resorting to formulas like VLOOKUP that Excel users have needed in the past. A traditional Excel PivotTable can only pivot data from one table at a time. The Excel Data Model uses a feature called relationships to join multiple tables into one source that feeds a Power Pivot Table. A sample screenshot from CMS provider utilization data is shown in Exhibit 3.2.

Exhibit 3.2 Excel Data Model Sample

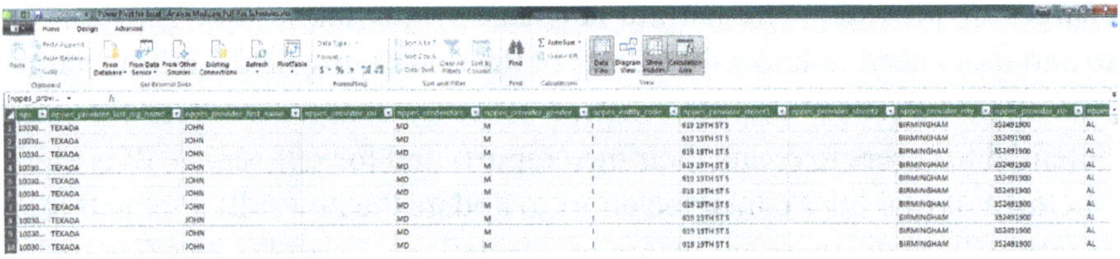

The Excel Data Model introduces a new programming language known as DAX. Expressions in DAX are more complicated and more powerful than traditional Excel formulas. Despite the learning curve, DAX can be helpful, especially for date-related functions. For example, comparing year-to-date data to prior year-to-date data is difficult in a traditional PivotTable, but simple to do in PowerPivot once the underlying DAX formulas have been built.

MAPS

The ability is see spatial data on a map can be a very helpful way to spot trends and opportunities. The Office 365 and 2016 versions of Excel include a feature called 3D Map that will display data geographically. The mapping tool requires internet access so that Microsoft can use Bing's mapping data. The 3D Map interface can recognize zip codes as well as city, county, and state information. The ability to see new patients or referred patients on a map, such as examples in Chapter 5, changes the way practices see their data.

Like Power BI, 3D Map also has a field list shown in Exhibit 3.3 that PivotTable users will find familiar.

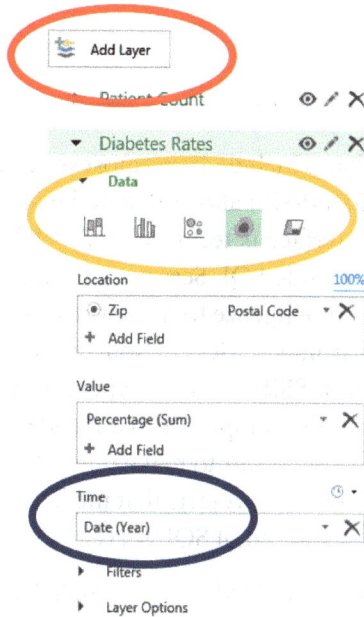

EXHIBIT 3.3 EXCEL: 3D MAP

The field list shows that you can add layers (circled in red) to a map. One layer may show new patients and a second layer could show referring physicians or clinic location. There are five different varieties of maps (circled in yellow), each of which offers distinctive features to better communicate a message. For example, the selected option will display a heat map, where "hotter" and "colder" areas have different colors. Other options allow categories such as locations or physician specialties to be plotted on the map. The field list also has a time section (circled in blue). The clever thing about adding a time dimension to a 3D Map is that Excel can animate the mapped data to show a geographic change over time.

Excel allows you to save different maps as Scenes and combine those Scenes into a Tour. You can save animations of data changing over time, and those animations can be saved as videos. The videos can show either data changing over time or the cumulative effect of data growing over time. Combining geography and time, added to the ability to save animations as videos, offers a unique and insightful way to analyze data.

SSIS AND SSAS

SSRS isn't the only tool that is included with most versions of SQL Server. SQL Server Integration Services (SSIS) allows data to be imported to or exported from SQL Server. The interface is technical and will likely require IT help. If the practice has data outside SQL Server and wants to take advantage of the some of the Business Intelligence tools that require SQL Server, SSIS can help. SSIS imports data from a variety of sources, such as other databases, spreadsheets, and csv files. SSIS can also export data from SQL Server to spreadsheets and csv files. For example, SSIS can send upcoming appointment information to a third-party vendor to make reminder calls. Appendix 2 has screen captures and examples of projects that medical practices have created with SSIS to move data in and out of SQL Server.

SQL Server Analysis Services (SSAS) is also included at no charge with most versions of SQL Server. SSAS can build cubes, which are an efficient, compact way to store a very large amount of data. If you are a large practice and want to see the detail of every charge for more than a couple of years, cubes may be a good solution. SSAS can also be used for data mining projects. The data mining project described in more detail in Appendix 2 gathered several years of appointment data to look for patterns and predict which patients were more likely to not show for their appointment. Data mining projects with SSAS are probably not the first place to start Business Intelligence for most practices, but can be very useful for practices that have more advanced needs.

For most practices, especially those starting in Business Intelligence, begin with PivotTables and then move to SSRS. The majority of examples in this book use those two tools. PivotTables are the analysis tool. SSRS is the tool to communicate critical messages throughout the practice. With these chapters as a foundation, Part 2 of the book has example after example of how practices around America are implementing and leveraging Business Intelligence. Part 2 also discusses how to know which Business Intelligence tool to use.

PART 2

HOW PRACTICES SEE
THEIR DATA

T his is the fun part of the book. It takes work to build an organizational culture conducive to Business Intelligence, and even more work to gather data, create datasets, learn BI tools, and get started with your first report, email, or dashboard. With that background and foundation, there are plenty of ideas in Part 2 to apply to your unique practice situation. But Business Intelligence isn't a cut-and-paste effort. What has worked and is working for these practices will give you ideas at best, but the real power is in tweaking, combining, and rearranging these examples to make a significant difference for your practice. If the first three rules in real estate are location, location, and location, the first three words of this section are customize, customize, and customize.

You will see examples throughout Part 2 that build on concepts introduced in *Better Data, Better Decisions*, including plenty of PivotTables. If you are not familiar with PivotTables, please refer to the first book in this series, *Better Data, Better Decisions: Using Business Intelligence in the Medical Practice*. If an example in either book is presented as a PivotTable, it may work better in your environment as an SSRS dashboard or as weekly email. The reverse may be equally true. A practice example that uses SSRS to consume data does not prevent a PivotTable from being a solution for your practice.

WHICH BI TOOL TO USE

There is no guaranteed right answer to the question of which BI tool is best for a report. For practices starting in Business Intelligence, a general rule is to pull practice data into datasets in SQL Server and then to connect the datasets to Excel as a PivotTable. The PivotTable format gives end users a lot of flexibility to design their own reports and to create very powerful analyses. Once end users have a report they like, it's easy to save a copy of the report as a new spreadsheet for future use. The new spreadsheet can also refresh with new data each time the file is opened. As PivotTables help identify critical trends, metrics, and indicators, an SSRS report can push that information on a regularly scheduled basis. Rather than relying on end users to remember to open spreadsheets or run reports and thereby "pull" the data, SSRS can "push" the data via email as often as users need to see it. An automatic email to end users also saves staff from having to answer the same questions and rerun the same reports over and over.

Spreadsheets are a more flexible, easy-to-learn environment. Staff education and consistent encouragement to learn to use your reporting tools are essential to getting a return on investment. After you have selected a tool, continue to provide training and support as staff members gain familiarity and confidence with the tool. Managers should regularly assess whether their staff have mastered the tools they use. Again, there are hundreds of free videos at mooresolutionsinc.com on using Excel in a medical practice setting. Each video is only four to five minutes. Watching one video a day can quickly bring staff members up to speed with Excel.

PivotTables make it easy to change the analysis to focus on providers, locations, procedure codes, referring physicians, or any other data available in the PivotTable. Filters in Excel, either in PivotTables or in (normal) Tables, are usually much faster than canned reports in practice management systems since Excel does not have to re-query the data to respond to the filter. The downside of Excel is that users must remember to open the spreadsheet to get the data. Users, especially inexperienced users, can also break formulas and inadvertently change Excel logic.

SSRS provides a more controlled reporting environment. If you need to run a regulatory, compliance, or tax related report consider SSRS or even a canned report. End users typically don't have access or the knowledge to change an SSRS report and the inability to make changes tends to make SSRS reports more stable and more accurate over time than the average spreadsheet. As previously discussed, the ability of SSRS to deliver reports via email is another big advantage. Reports can be embedded in the email or they can be attached as a PDF file or spreadsheet. Embedding in an email or storing in a PDF file makes it difficult for end users to accidentally change the data. SSRS reports can also use complex SQL code to add features to reports with functionality that is difficult to replicate in Excel. The downside of SSRS is that it's less flexible and easy to use than Excel. If you want to save a slightly different Excel spreadsheet, you can use "Save as." If you want to save a slightly different SSRS report, you or your IT team need to be familiar with a tool like Report Builder to save it.

Ultimately, choose the reporting tool that meets the needs of your end users. If the end users are Excel-savvy and want to analyze and manipulate the data, use PivotTables or Excel Tables. If end users are not very familiar with Excel, SSRS may better meet their needs. If the ability to push data to end users is important, SSRS is an easy choice.

AS WE BEGIN

Many of the reports in Part 2 are complex and will require someone versed in SQL Server and in the specific PM or EHR system to write the code for the underlying dataset. Some internal IT departments are staffed and capable of writing the code. Most IT teams are generalists maintaining the network, servers, and computers as opposed to specialists in supporting specific PM or EHR software packages. Some PM and EHR vendors offer support and custom reports, but most of those are one-time canned reports as opposed to a dataset that can be reused on multiple occasions. Your IT group is a good place to start looking for the technical help to get started. If your IT group cannot help, find an outside vendor who can get access your data.

The data in the sample reports in Part 2 are masked, adjusted, or made up entirely so as not to indicate actual charges or payments received for specific procedures by specific providers. The graphics are intended as examples of reports that can be created, not actual practice numbers to be relied upon in any way.

CHAPTER 4

PAYER CONTRACTING

M any practices are at or close to capacity on their most important resource: provider time. As costs increase, payer contracting can help a practice survive and thrive by adding value directly to the bottom line. The place to start with payer contracting is with the actual contracts. Gather those contracts, use the concepts in Chapter 2 to get your team on board, and begin.

This chapter is a broad view of payer contracting, from comparing contracts to negotiating rates to evaluating paid claims to ensure they are adjudicated in accordance with those contracts. Sometimes the hardest part of the entire process is getting contracts from payers. Challenges run from getting all the data needed to make decisions to getting data in a format you can use. Start with your major payers. Get started even if you do not have all the data you need from your small payers.

Payer contracting can be tough. It takes time and effort and many practice managers struggle to find adequate time to devote to payer contracting. A January 2017 poll of MGMA members shown in Exhibit 4.1 revealed that over half of the respondents did not compare reimbursement with contracted payer rates daily, monthly, or quarterly. Clearly more needs to be done to make payer contracting, especially reviewing reimbursement, easier for practice managers.

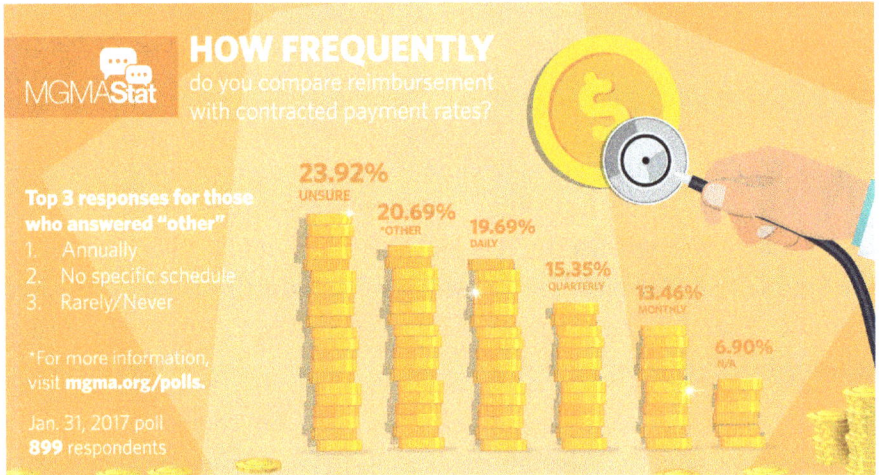

Exhibit 4.1 MGMA Stat: January 2017 Poll

A Contract Analysis Spreadsheet summarizes a practice's major payer contracts with the most common and highest dollar procedure codes for a practice. The spreadsheet is helpful as an analysis tool to compare reimbursement by code by payer. The spreadsheet can also be used as the foundation for more complex analyses, such as a patient balance estimator. Estimating patient balances before or at the time of service can increase cash flow and decrease bad debts.

Practices can also analyze what rates payers have allowed on procedures historically to spot trends and potential underpayments. Excel Tables are a very useful tool to compare allowed amounts over time. The Contract Payment Manager example takes the allowed analysis to a higher level by analyzing claims as they are adjudicated rather than as a historical analysis. To use the Contract Payment Manager tool, practices need to have an in-depth knowledge of their contracted rates for procedure codes (with and without modifiers) and the payers' rules. This in-depth knowledge of payer contracts pays off when practices can ensure that payers are paying claims appropriately.

This chapter contains tools that help prioritize and manage denials and track successful appeals. Tracking trends in denials and underpayments over time will provide insight into why claims are not being paid appropriately. Include tools to help staff appeal the most important denials quickly. This approach to managing denials and appeals often takes changing the way billing staff work. Managers may need to re-align work routines to prioritize appeals based on payer deadlines as well as the amount of the charge that was denied. Staff may need to enter information into the PM system so that appeals can be tracked and appeals without a timely response can be escalated. Identifying denials and pursuing successful appeals can dramatically increase a practice's bottom line.

Part of the trick throughout this chapter is to identify patterns among underpaid claims. If the practice can identify patterns, billing staff can more easily find other procedure codes by provider or location that need to be reviewed. Train staff to look for patterns instead of simply finding underpayments or denials a code at a time.

The chapter next considers a resource to compare what other practices in the area charge for services. Analyzing competitors' charges can help validate a fee schedule, especially as healthcare pricing becomes more transparent. The fee schedule analysis, like several tools in this chapter, takes IT support to get started. But, once again, after the data is available in a format staff can work with, IT's work is mostly finished and practice managers can use familiar tools to analyze and act on data.

The chapter concludes with a discussion of the future of payer contracting. As fee-for-service evolves into performance-based measures, tracking performance against payer incentives becomes the next obstacle to overcome. Especially in the initial stages of this transition, payers' performance measures vary widely. An example from a small primary care practice showing how they monitor Medicare Advantage plans gives insight into where payer contracting is heading.

CONTRACT ANALYSIS SPREADSHEET

Once you have payer contracts, creating a master contract analysis spreadsheet in Excel will greatly assist you. The spreadsheet might look something like Exhibit 4.2, with procedure codes and descriptions in the first two columns, followed by the billed charge and the annual volume (number of times billed), work RVU values, and a column with reimbursement rates for each major contract.

EXHIBIT 4.2 MASTER CONTRACT ANALYSIS SPREADSHEET SAMPLE

	A	B	C	D	E	F	G	H	I	J
1							Contracted Amounts			
2	Code	Description	Charge	Volume	Work RVU	Payer A	Payer B	Payer C	Payer D	Payer E
3	27447	Total Knee	$ 7,100	3,102	20.72	$ 1,700	$ 1,400	$ 3,200	$ 3,800	$ 2,100
4	27130	Total Hip	$ 6,500	1,165	20.72	$ 1,800	$ 1,300	$ 3,900	$ 3,500	$ 2,000
5	99203	New Patient Level 3	$ 270	18,120	1.42	$ 130	$ 160	$ 70	$ 90	$ 110
6	99214	Est Patient Level 4	$ 240	21,107	1.50	$ 130	$ 200	$ 60	$ 70	$ 110
7	99213	Est Patient Level 3	$ 180	42,108	1.02	$ 90	$ 140	$ 40	$ 50	$ 70

This spreadsheet can be used in several different ways. First, you can compare reimbursement by procedure code from payer to payer. Having the annual volume in the contracting spreadsheet makes it easy to compare the most frequently used codes and to calculate a weighted average reimbursement across contracts. One approach might be to take the top 20 procedure codes for the top five or six payers, plus Medicare as a reference or benchmark.

Another approach would be to calculate dollars per work Relative Value Unit (wRVU) as shown in Exhibit 4.3 below. The following steps modify Exhibit 4.3 to calculate dollars per wRVU for Payer A.

- Add a column (K) to multiply the contracted rate (F) by the expected annual volume (D) to determine the expected revenue from each of these codes.

- In a second added Excel column (L), multiply the wRVUs expended (E) by the expected volume (D) of each procedure to calculate the total wRVUs per code.

- In a third added Excel column (M), divide the expected revenue (K) by total wRVUs (L) and compare that value across payer contracts. In theory, carriers that have more volume in the practice should have a lower dollars-per-wRVU value. Payers with less volume should have a higher rate per wRVU value. That theory does not hold with government payers. As markets differ in terms of size, competition, and payer structure, the dollars per RVU calculation will vary. If all other factors are equal, contracts with a higher dollar value per RVU are better contracts for the practice.

EXHIBIT 4.3 DOLLAR CALCULATIONS VIA wRVUs SPREADSHEET SAMPLE

	A	B	C	D	E	F	G	H	I	J	K	L	M
1							Contracted Amounts					Payer A	
2	Code	Description	Charge	Volume	Work RVU	Payer A	Payer B	Payer C	Payer D	Payer E	Revenue	Work RVU	$/RVU
3	27447	Total Knee	$ 7,100	3,102	20.72	$ 1,700	$ 1,400	$ 3,200	$ 3,800	$ 2,100	$ 5,273,400	64,273	$ 82.05
4	27130	Total Hip	$ 6,500	1,165	20.72	$ 1,800	$ 1,300	$ 3,900	$ 3,500	$ 2,000	$ 2,097,000	24,139	$ 86.87
5	99203	New Patient Level 3	$ 270	18,120	1.42	$ 130	$ 160	$ 70	$ 90	$ 110	$ 2,355,600	25,730	$ 91.55
6	99214	Est Patient Level 4	$ 240	21,107	1.50	$ 130	$ 200	$ 60	$ 70	$ 110	$ 2,743,910	31,661	$ 86.67
7	99213	Est Patient Level 3	$ 180	42,108	1.02	$ 90	$ 140	$ 40	$ 50	$ 70	$ 3,789,720	42,950	$ 88.24

Some practices will choose to use wRVUs in this calculation while other practices prefer total RVUs depending upon the physicians' specialty, procedure code mix, compensation formulas, and other factors unique to each market. Practices can look at this data on a procedure code basis to compare reimbursement by code across payers. Another option is to compare the total contract to other payer contracts for an overall sense of which payers have better contracts for the practice.

PATIENT BALANCE ESTIMATOR

With the advent of high deductible plans, proactive practices can leverage a contract analysis spreadsheet to create a patient balance estimation tool. Exhibit 4.4 is a tool created by a group that offers physical therapy.

EXHIBIT 4.4 EXCEL: PATIENT BALANCE ESTIMATOR TOOL SAMPLE

Insurance: *Medicare Traditional Part B*

Discount or Co-insurance % (if needed):

CPT Code	Allowable
97012	$12.75
97001	$76.08
97112	$34.17
Subtotal	$123.00

Copay to Collect

Less pre-collect (HDHP)

| Total | $123.00 |

Cash Received

Change to give

The front desk team can choose an insurance carrier from a drop-down list (like Medicare Traditional Part B, shown) and enter the procedure codes that the patient will receive that day. The spreadsheet uses Excel's VLOOKUP feature to populate the allowable column with the appropriate contracted amount. (For more information about using VLOOKUP, please see the VLOOKUP Excel Mastery page at mooresolutionsinc.com/em-vlookup/.) This spreadsheet even calculates change for front desk staff to make reconciling cash a little easier at the end of the day.

This example may not look like big dollars, but physical therapy has a high volume of these types of claims. Collecting at the time of service is important for cash flow, but it also helps minimize billing expenses after the fact. Even if you know all your contracted amounts, payers use a variety of processing rules that affect reimbursement. The issue in this physical therapy example is multiple procedure discounts. Multiple procedure discounts reduce payments for codes billed together on the same claim. In this practice, the first code is paid at 100% of the allowed amount and subsequent codes are paid at a lower percentage. The difficulty is that some payers rank the codes by the allowable amount and other payers rank the codes by RVUs. To make an accurate tool requires logic and calculations to implement the specific payer rules and the order of those rules behind the scenes. This spreadsheet ranks the codes based on the method used by the carrier selected and calculates the allowable amounts accordingly. The advantage of doing these calculations in Excel is that Excel has functions like VLOOKUP and RANK.EQ to do the math. Practices can create a tool like this to handle common codes and payers. Practices can also enter the deductible, copay, and coinsurance amounts on the spreadsheet to further refine the patient estimate. You do not need to have all payers and codes to achieve a lot of return on the investment in this tool. Do not let perfecting all the contracting nuances be the enemy of at least starting to collect from patients.

BE CAREFUL TO PROTECT SPREADSHEETS LIKE THIS WITH COMPLEX CALCULATIONS. ONE ACCIDENTAL TYPING OF "25" OVER THE CALCULATION IN THE ALLOWABLE COLUMN COULD MAKE THE ALLOWABLE $25 FOR ALL CODES FOR MONTHS UNTIL THE ERROR IS FOUND.

TO PROTECT A WORKSHEET, FIRST RIGHT-CLICK THE CELLS THAT YOU WANT STAFF TO HAVE ACCESS TO EDIT. IF THE CELLS ARE CONTIGUOUS (NEXT TO EACH OTHER), YOU CAN SELECT A GROUP OF CELLS AT ONCE. HOLDING DOWN THE CTRL KEY WILL ALLOW YOU TO SELECT NON-CONTIGUOUS CELLS. FROM THE MENU THAT APPEARS, SELECT FORMAT CELLS, AS SHOWN IN EXHIBIT 4.5.

EXHIBIT 4.5 PROTECT SPREADSHEETS: FORMAT CELLS

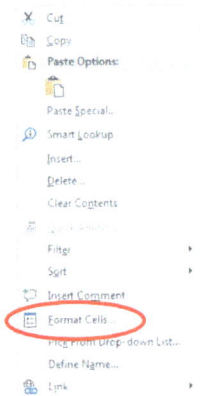

FROM THE FORMAT CELLS WINDOW, CHOOSE THE PROTECTION TAB AND UNCHECK THE LOCKED BOX, AS SHOWN IN EXHIBIT 4.6.

EXHIBIT 4.6 PROTECT SPREADSHEETS: LOCKED CELLS

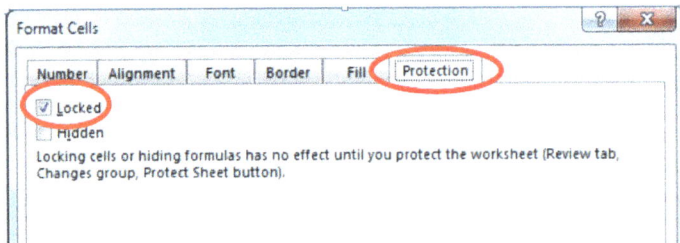

UNCHECKING THE LOCKED BOX ALLOWS USERS TO EDIT THE CELL ONCE THE SPREADSHEET IS PROTECTED. TO PROTECT THE SPREADSHEET, FROM THE REVIEW TAB, CHOOSE PROTECT SHEET AND ENTER A PASSWORD TO UNPROTECT THE SHEET, AS SHOWN IN EXHIBIT 4.7. THE PASSWORD PROTECTION DESCRIBED IS DESIGNED TO KEEP USERS FROM INADVERTENTLY MODIFYING FORMULAS IN A COMPLEX SPREADSHEET. DO NOT RELY ON PROTECTING WORKSHEETS TO SAFEGUARD CONFIDENTIAL MATERIAL LIKE PROTECTED HEALTH INFORMATION OR PAYROLL TRANSACTIONS.

EXHIBIT 4.7 PROTECT SPREADSHEETS: PASSWORD PROTECTED

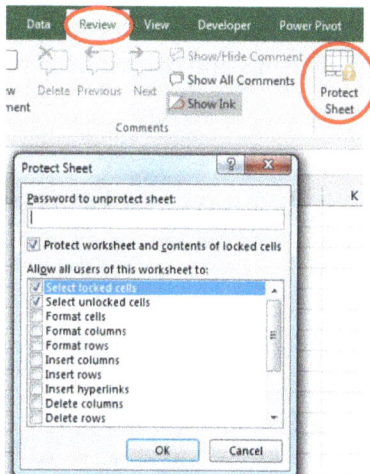

PAYER CONTRACT RATE SPREADSHEETS

One way to monitor payer reimbursement rates is to capture the allowed amount by procedure code by payer and compare those allowed amounts, looking for discrepancies. Initially search for inconsistent allowed amounts as opposed to explicitly comparing the allowed amounts to the contracts described above. This approach is especially helpful if the practice is struggling to get contracted amounts from payers. Exhibit 4.8 is an example based on a surgical center and Exhibit 4.9 is based on what a practice might see.

In the surgical center example there is a Paid and an Allowed column. For purposes of this analysis, the Allowed column is more important than the Paid column. This analysis is attempting to ensure that the allowed amount is in accordance with the contract. Whether the practice collects the allowed amount is a very important question, but is not a payer contracting question.

In this example, the Excel Table has been filtered to one procedure code for one plan. Based on the preponderance of the claims, $4,201 appears to be the contracted amount. After confirming the $4,201 with the contract, the real question is why so many other claims were adjudicated with a lower allowed amount. Two claims in the middle of the table have no payments but $4,201 allowed. Those claims may be the result of high deductible plans and should certainly be followed up on, but the focus here is on the allowed amount. The table is designed to provide billing staff with enough information to quickly identify potential underpayments and contact the payer to appeal.

EXHIBIT 4.8 PAYER CONTRACT RATE SPREADSHEET: SURGICAL CENTER SAMPLE

DOS	Visit Number	Insurance	CPT Code	Mod1	Mod2	Charge	Paid	Allowed	Surgeon	Specialty	Units	Claim Date
8/8/2017	398323	Payer A	50590 Lithotripsy	LT		$ 10,100.00	$ 4,201.00	$ 4,201.00	Smith	Urology	1	8/11/2016
8/8/2017	330873	Payer A	50590 Lithotripsy	RT		$ 10,100.00	$ 4,201.00	$ 4,201.00	Young	Urology	1	8/11/2016
7/25/2017	332816	Payer A	50590 Lithotripsy	LT		$ 10,100.00	$ 4,201.00	$ 4,201.00	Young	Urology	1	7/27/2016
7/25/2017	383160	Payer A	50590 Lithotripsy	LT		$ 10,100.00	$ 4,201.00	$ 4,201.00	Smith	Urology	1	8/7/2016
5/2/2017	320248	Payer A	50590 Lithotripsy	LT		$ 10,100.00	$ 4,201.00	$ 4,201.00	Young	Urology	1	5/9/2016
4/18/2017	361877	Payer A	50590 Lithotripsy	LT		$ 10,100.00	$ 605.10	$ 605.10	Smith	Urology	1	4/21/2016
4/18/2017	328439	Payer A	50590 Lithotripsy	LT		$ 10,100.00	$ 4,501.00	$ 4,501.00	Young	Urology	1	4/27/2016
4/4/2017	368317	Payer A	50590 Lithotripsy	RT		$ 10,100.00	$ 4,201.00	$ 4,201.00	Young	Urology	1	4/8/2016
2/4/2017	302439	Payer A	50590 Lithotripsy	LT		$ 10,100.00	$ -	$ 4,201.00	Young	Urology	1	8/25/2016
1/5/2017	346846	Payer A	50590 Lithotripsy	RT		$ 10,100.00	$ -	$ 4,201.00	Smith	Urology	1	8/25/2016
12/27/2016	399973	Payer A	50590 Lithotripsy	RT		$ 10,100.00	$ 4,201.00	$ 4,201.00	Smith	Urology	1	1/11/2016
12/27/2016	301096	Payer A	50590 Lithotripsy	RT		$ 10,100.00	$ 4,201.00	$ 4,201.00	Young	Urology	1	1/4/2016
11/29/2016	340245	Payer A	50590 Lithotripsy	LT		$ 10,100.00	$ 4,201.00	$ 4,201.00	Young	Urology	1	12/7/2015
11/15/2016	357506	Payer A	50590 Lithotripsy	RT		$ 10,100.00	$ 4,110.50	$ 4,110.50	Smith	Urology	1	11/19/2015
11/15/2016	349476	Payer A	50590 Lithotripsy	LT		$ 10,100.00	$ 4,201.00	$ 4,201.00	Young	Urology	1	11/19/2015
11/15/2016	309335	Payer A	50590 Lithotripsy	RT		$ 10,100.00	$ 4,201.00	$ 4,201.00	Young	Urology	1	11/19/2015
10/4/2016	386776	Payer A	50590 Lithotripsy	RT		$ 10,100.00	$ 4,201.00	$ 4,201.00	Young	Urology	1	10/7/2015
9/20/2016	360719	Payer A	50590 Lithotripsy	RT		$ 10,100.00	$ 4,201.00	$ 4,201.00	Young	Urology	1	9/27/2015
8/9/2016	333719	Payer A	50590 Lithotripsy	RT		$ 10,100.00	$ 3,254.00	$ 3,254.00	Young	Urology	1	8/18/2015
6/14/2016	367278	Payer A	50590 Lithotripsy	LT		$ 10,100.00	$ 4,010.00	$ 4,010.00	Smith	Urology	1	6/22/2015
3/22/2016	334924	Payer A	50590 Lithotripsy	RT		$ 10,100.00	$ 4,010.00	$ 4,010.00	Young	Urology	1	3/31/2015
3/22/2016	399887	Payer A	50590 Lithotripsy	RT		$ 10,100.00	$ 4,010.00	$ 4,010.00	Young	Urology	1	3/31/2015
3/8/2016	310810	Payer A	50590 Lithotripsy	RT		$ 10,100.00	$ 3,608.17	$ 3,608.17	Young	Urology	1	3/17/2015

In Exhibit 4.9 another practice approaches the question differently but uses similar logic in creating a Business Intelligence tool to monitor payer contract rates. The exhibit is also filtered for one procedure code for one payer. This practice has sorted the allowed amount in ascending order so that the biggest offenders rise to the top of the list. There are three claims that were completely denied, and three other claims allow less than what appears to be the contracted rate. In this situation, the practice has included the place of service (POS) and additional modifiers that may affect reimbursement. This practice also includes the location and the provider in the analysis. As tools become more sophisticated, staff will need more training to appreciate the nuances that modifiers, places of service and other factors have on contracted rates. Make sure that staff members are fully educated on how to use this powerful tool.

EXHIBIT 4.9 PAYER CONTRACT RATE SPREADSHEET: MEDICAL PRACTICE SAMPLE

Encounter	Financial Class	Payer Name	CPT Code	Mod1	Mod2	Mod3	Mod4	Units	Charge	Allowed	POS	DOS	Entry Date	Location	Rendering
1918366	Fin Class 7	Plan 104	45385	33				1	$ 1,500.00	$ -	24	7/21/2017	8/22/2017	North Endoscopy Center	Carlson MD, Wilhemina
1618819	Fin Class 7	Plan 104	45385	33				1	$ 1,500.00	$ -	24	6/5/2017	7/17/2017	Park Endoscopy	Javier MD, Gertie L.
1723310	Fin Class 7	Plan 104	45385	33				1	$ 1,500.00	$ -	24	8/14/2017	9/7/2017	North Endoscopy Center	Seavey MD, Marni B
1835874	Fin Class 7	Plan 104	45385	59				1	$ 1,500.00	$ 243.96	24	1/3/2017	2/8/2017	North Endoscopy Center	Bisbee MD, Dario C.
1515695	Fin Class 7	Plan 104	45385					1	$ 1,500.00	$ 431.13	24	1/17/2017	2/22/2017	Park Endoscopy	Deshong MD, Lilly
1945252	Fin Class 7	Plan 104	45385	33				1	$ 1,500.00	$ 431.13	24	1/25/2017	3/1/2017	Hamilton Endoscopy Center	Ringgold MD, Jarod D.
1740777	Fin Class 7	Plan 104	45385	33				1	$ 1,500.00	$ 449.54	24	3/24/2017	5/1/2017	Main Endoscopy	Urbanski MD, Chante
1754299	Fin Class 7	Plan 104	45385	33				1	$ 1,500.00	$ 449.54	22	6/20/2017	7/31/2017	St. Francis Hospital	Deshong MD, Lilly
1804609	Fin Class 7	Plan 104	45385	33				1	$ 1,500.00	$ 449.54	24	5/30/2017	7/17/2017	North Endoscopy Center	Deshong MD, Lilly
1804975	Fin Class 7	Plan 104	45385					1	$ 1,500.00	$ 449.54	24	4/13/2017	5/17/2017	North Endoscopy Center	Mckenzie MD, Carol D.
1785290	Fin Class 7	Plan 104	45385					1	$ 1,500.00	$ 449.54	24	4/20/2017	5/12/2017	Hamilton Endoscopy Center	Carlson MD, Wilhemina
1609960	Fin Class 7	Plan 104	45385	33				1	$ 1,500.00	$ 449.54	24	5/24/2017	7/4/2017	North Endoscopy Center	Seavey MD, Marni B
1687350	Fin Class 7	Plan 104	45385	33				1	$ 1,500.00	$ 449.54	24	3/20/2017	5/1/2017	Hamilton Endoscopy Center	Deshong MD, Lilly
1500109	Fin Class 7	Plan 104	45385	33				1	$ 1,500.00	$ 449.54	24	6/28/2017	7/31/2017	North Endoscopy Center	Carlson MD, Wilhemina
1564833	Fin Class 7	Plan 104	45385	33				1	$ 1,500.00	$ 449.54	24	7/17/2017	9/1/2017	Main Endoscopy	Mikell MD, Coralee F.
1609865	Fin Class 7	Plan 104	45385	33				1	$ 1,500.00	$ 449.54	24	3/13/2017	4/26/2017	Hamilton Endoscopy Center	Vickrey MD, Mathilda F
1837440	Fin Class 7	Plan 104	45385	33				1	$ 1,500.00	$ 449.54	22	5/18/2017	7/17/2017	St. Francis Hospital	Andres MD, Beau
1829772	Fin Class 7	Plan 104	45385	33				1	$ 1,500.00	$ 449.54	24	4/13/2017	5/12/2017	Hamilton Endoscopy Center	Carlson MD, Wilhemina
1627167	Fin Class 7	Plan 104	45385					1	$ 1,500.00	$ 449.54	24	7/12/2017	8/13/2017	North Endoscopy Center	Mathis MD, Reinaldo B.
1841681	Fin Class 7	Plan 104	45385	33				1	$ 1,500.00	$ 449.54	24	4/4/2017	5/12/2017	North Endoscopy Center	Andres MD, Beau
1789241	Fin Class 7	Plan 104	45385					1	$ 1,500.00	$ 449.54	24	6/20/2017	8/4/2017	Hamilton Endoscopy Center	Deshong MD, Lilly
1905712	Fin Class 7	Plan 104	45385	33				1	$ 1,500.00	$ 449.54	22	5/18/2017	7/17/2017	St. Francis Hospital	Andres MD, Beau
1610242	Fin Class 7	Plan 104	45385	33				1	$ 1,500.00	$ 449.54	24	3/6/2017	5/12/2017	Main Endoscopy	Keifer MD, Vinita
1619069	Fin Class 7	Plan 104	45385	33				1	$ 1,500.00	$ 449.54	24	1/30/2017	3/15/2017	Hamilton Endoscopy Center	Deshong MD, Lilly
1573027	Fin Class 7	Plan 104	45385	33				1	$ 1,500.00	$ 449.54	24	4/28/2017	5/31/2017	Hamilton Endoscopy Center	Deshong MD, Lilly
1876948	Fin Class 7	Plan 104	45385	33				1	$ 1,500.00	$ 449.54	24	3/13/2017	4/19/2017	North Endoscopy Center	Andres MD, Beau
1941072	Fin Class 7	Plan 104	45385	33				1	$ 1,500.00	$ 449.54	24	8/14/2017	9/7/2017	Hamilton Endoscopy Center	Keifer MD, Vinita
1897458	Fin Class 7	Plan 104	45385	33				1	$ 1,500.00	$ 449.54	24	4/19/2017	5/17/2017	Main Endoscopy	Deshong MD, Lilly

One caveat in some PM systems is calculating what the allowed amount is or validating the PM software's calculation. Generally, the allowed amount is the practice contracted to receive. If an allowed amount is reduced by other rules, such as a multiple procedure discount, those rules should be part of and in accordance with the contract. The only adjustments from the billed charge should be adjustments included in the contract that are outside the practice's control. For example, a timely filing denial may be justified based on the contract, but claims should still be filed in a timely manner. Failure to file a claim isn't an allowed issue or a contracting issue, it is a billing office issue or a provider documentation issue.

A practice in Texas tabulated all the adjustment codes over the prior two years and divided the codes into two groups, practice adjustments and payer adjustments. Practice adjustments are under the practice's control and should be reduced as much as possible. Errors in patient demographics, failure to pre-authorize a procedure, provider credentialing and timely filing are most often under the practice's control. Estimating and collecting patient balances at the time of service (see the example earlier in this chapter) is also under the practice's control and will reduce bad debt. Payer adjustments are adjustments due to the payer paying less than the contract specifies. The Texas group focused on trending and reducing practice adjustments.

It is important to recognize that allowed spreadsheets will have some variation in allowed amounts within the contract. Variations may be due to things like place of service differentials. Different providers contracting at different rates, such as physicians vs. advanced practitioners or specialists vs. primary care can also cause differences. Some modifiers clearly cause differences. Including the place of service, provider, and modifiers on the allowed spreadsheet can identify and resolve those variations. A harder variation to spot on the spreadsheet is multiple procedure discounts. Some codes may appropriately be paid less based on the way the payer ranks and applies the multiple procedure discount rules. Even then, the discount amount should be consistent. A practice may see the contracted amount and 50% of the contracted amount, for example. It may take an encounter-by-encounter review of several claims per payer to make sure the rules are being applied consistently and correctly over time.

In summary, an allowed spreadsheet is a good way to get a general feel for how accurately and consistently a payer follows the contract. Allowed spreadsheets are relatively simple and inexpensive to create and are a good measuring stick. The downside is that practices must continually search the spreadsheet for errors. Practices that want to automate the review process and take their contract review analysis to an advanced level can develop a contract payment management system.

CONTRACT PAYMENT MANAGER

The most advanced option to analyze contracts is a tool that builds on the first two concepts in this chapter, knowing your contracts and comparing allowed amounts. The goal is to design a system that audits the Electronic Remittance Advice (ERA) or Explanation of Benefits (EOB) data from each payer for each line item billed. Teach the system the appropriate payer rules to identify underpayments by comparing the allowed amount from the ERA (or hand keyed) data. The system is designed to process claims the way the contract requires the payer to adjudicate claims, so any rules employed by carriers need to be implemented. Ultimately practices need a system that will automatically flag any allowable amounts less than the contracted amount and help trend variances.

A tool like this requires storing contracted amounts for each procedure code in a data warehouse. Practices need to stay current with payer rates and rules, and update the data warehouse accordingly. Some contracts change frequently, such as quarterly changes for drug codes. Contracts also expire at various times. A process needs to be implemented to track these changes and keep the tool current. Added benefits would include tracking each payer's payment rules for each modifier, multiple procedure discounts, anesthesia policies, and so forth. An example of this tool was developed by a practice in a system they call Contract Payment Manager (CPM). Exhibit 4.10 is an example of daily CPM email, delivered daily through SSRS. Any claims paid less than a practice expected are reported on a daily email to billing office staff.

EXHIBIT 4.10 CPM: EXCEPTIONS AND VARIANCES DAILY EMAIL SAMPLE

CPM Dashboard as of 8/31/2017

Yesterday's Exceptions

Insurance Group	$ Variance	Count
Anthem BCBS 1103	$1,872.29	15
Medicare 1000	$294.72	20
Medicare Managed Care 1019	$128.80	1
Humana 1108	$111.40	1
Work Comp 1003	$72.88	2
Lutheran Preferred 1110	$54.93	2
Totals	$2,535.02	41

Open Exceptions

Insurance Group	$ Variance	Count
Anthem BCBS 1103	$30,586.62	207
Medicare Managed Care 1019	$11,023.77	153
HIP 1132	$9,797.91	131
Medicare 1000	$8,148.46	198
Work Comp 1003	$5,675.32	41
Misc Contracts 1123	$3,849.86	138
Lutheran Preferred 1110	$2,941.82	20
Cigna 1104	$2,746.52	25
Signature Care 1115	$1,802.48	21
Three Rivers Preferred TRMA 1118	$691.71	7
Aetna 1100	$546.43	15
Sagamore 1117	$198.31	5
Medicaid 1001	$135.61	4
Humana 1108	$111.40	1
Nursing Home 1000	$16.27	1
Totals	$78,272.49	967

Top 10 open exceptions by variance($)

CPT Code	Insurance Group	$ Variance	Count
27130	Work Comp 1003	$2,719.03	1
22558	Anthem BCBS 1103	$2,170.40	3
23430	Anthem BCBS 1103	$2,141.84	8
22633	Medicare Managed Care 1019	$1,723.75	5
27447	HIP 1132	$1,303.99	1
22845	HIP 1132	$1,218.14	3
23440	Anthem BCBS 1103	$1,097.48	4
38220	Anthem BCBS 1103	$1,094.05	5
27687	Anthem BCBS 1103	$1,069.26	6
29827	Medicare Managed Care 1019	$1,018.43	2
	Totals	$15,556.37	38

Top 10 open exceptions by count

CPT Code	Insurance Group	$ Variance	Count
99406	HIP 1132	$561.60	39
99213	Misc Contracts 1123	$558.16	37
64447	Anthem BCBS 1103	$676.71	21
64721	Medicare 1000	$370.75	20
99203	Misc Contracts 1123	$378.60	17
23472	Medicare 1000	$989.76	14
27447	Medicare Managed Care 1019	$305.58	14
27447	Medicare 1000	$697.31	13
29824	Medicare 1000	$889.17	12
99214	Misc Contracts 1123	$386.51	12
	Totals	$5,814.15	199

Expiring Contracts (Next 180 Days)

Carrier	End Date
Anthem	9/30/2017

The first section is *Yesterday's Exceptions.* This is obviously the most recent exceptions, sorted from highest to lowest variance. The key is that this practice has programmed CPM to wait one week before running the data. That interval gives the practice time to reconcile and correct any issues entering and reconciling remittances in the PM so that CPM is running off the most accurate information possible. Some practices may change the interval between entering remittances and starting CPM to meet their requirements.

Open Exceptions are summarized next. An open exception is an exception that has been identified by CPM but has not been worked by the billing staff. The billing staff members resolve open exceptions by reviewing the claim and the EOB in the PM system. If the CPM exception is valid, they file an appeal. Once an appeal has been filed, the exception is automatically removed from this list. The billing staff can also ignore the exception if an appeal was not warranted. Practices can and should run reports to see how many exceptions have been ignored. Ignored exceptions indicate either issues with CPM logic or potential exceptions that should have been appealed and were not. Practices can also set a threshold for CPM to identify exceptions. For example, practices can automatically ignore exceptions less than $1.

The bottom left section is a summary of any contracts loaded in CPM that are set to expire in the next 180 days. The 180-day window is built to give the practice time to negotiate, finalize, and then upload the contract into CPM. Practices typically start with a few major contracts and then add payers over time as the CPM logic is tested and the billing staff has time to appeal exceptions.

The right side of the CPM dashboard summarizes the *Top 10 Open Exceptions* by procedure code, first by the dollar amount of the variance and then by the count of procedure codes. This practice has been using CPM for some time and has managed the exceptions down to very reasonable levels based on the volume of claims processed through their system. The dashboard is emailed every morning to the team who work the appeals as well as to managers who supervise the staff.

Staff can run reports, upload contracts, and quickly prioritize their appeals. Exhibit 4.11 shows the exceptions screen, a sample view of the staff worklist. This is the main window for the appeals team to review exceptions. The screen makes it easy to filter all CPM exceptions to a specific payer.

Exhibit 4.11 CPM: Exceptions Report

	↓ Tickler	Patient	Ticket Number	Procedure Code	CPT code	CPT description	Service date
☐	163		3138475	27536	27536	27536-Open Tx Tibial...	05/31/2017
☐	163		3164103	64447	64447	64447-Injection Nerve...	07/05/2017
☐	163		3181297	64447R	64447	64447-Injection Nerve...	07/27/2017
☐	163		3174815	28120	28120	28120-Part Removal ...	08/01/2017
☐	163		3174815	27687	27687	27687-Gastrocnemius ...	08/01/2017
☐	163		3185976	27687	27687	27687-Gastrocnemius...	08/01/2017
☐	163		3185977	64447L	64447	64447-Injection Nerve...	08/01/2017
☐	163		3185943	26720L	26720	26720-Tx Phalangeal ...	08/09/2017
☐	163		3186745	28060	28060	28060-Partial Rem Fo...	08/03/2017
☐	163		3186752	64447L	64447	64447-Injection Nerve...	08/03/2017

Exhibit 4.12 shows the appeals window. The appeals window lists the status of all open appeals in CPM. Again, the appeals can be filtered by payer to make it simple for the billing office to follow up with a selected payer.

Exhibit 4.12 CPM: Exceptions Report - Filtered

	↓ Tickler	Ticket number	Service date	CPT code	Appeal amount	Current ins balance	Last appeal type
☐	148	3138453	05/30/2017	64636	$207.00		Appeal First Level Sent
☐	135	3159837	06/26/2017	64490	$348.00	$348.00	Appeal First Level Sent
☐	134	3152977	06/13/2017	29891	$516.55	$1545.75	Appeal First Level Sent
☐	127	3031519	12/16/2016	64636	$650.00		CC
☐	107	3146843	06/13/2017	99203	$9.00		Appeal First Level Sent
☐	100	3136918	05/21/2017	12035	$73.44	$73.44	Appeal First Level Sent
☐	80	3121270	04/25/2017	01402	$185.83	$187.50	Appeal First Level Sent
☐	80	3121270	04/25/2017	01402	$185.83	$187.50	Appeal First Level Sent
☐	49	3105143	03/31/2017	27590	$763.42	$763.42	Appeal First Level Sent
☐	49	3105144	03/31/2017	27590	$91.61	$91.61	Appeal First Level Sent

Since CPM knows all the contracted rates, the practice has built in a code lookup function so staff can quickly retrieve contracted information by procedure code. Exhibit 4.13 is an example of the code lookup window, and Exhibit 4.14 is an example of the results of the lookup.

EXHIBIT 4.13 CPM: CODE LOOKUP WINDOW SAMPLE

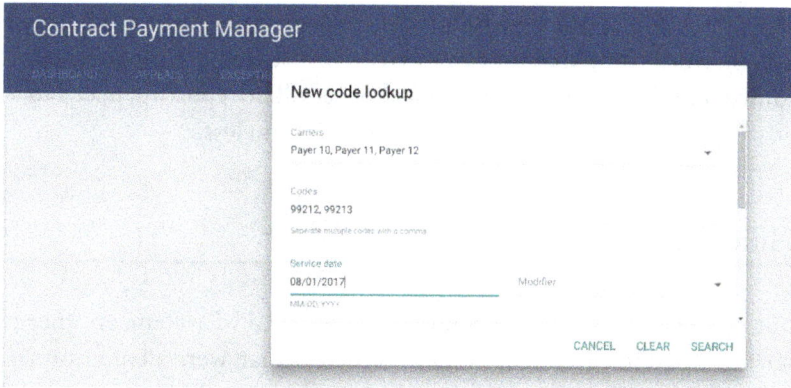

EXHIBIT 4.14 CPM: CODE LOOKUP RESULTS SAMPLE

Carrier	Code	Site of service	Doctor	Midlevel	Start	End
Payer 11	99212	OFF	$30.9	$23.17	02/01/2015	12/31/2099
Payer 11	99213	OFF	$51.99	$38.99	02/01/2015	12/31/2099
Payer 12	99212	OFF	$41.15	$34.98	01/01/2016	12/31/2016
Payer 12	99212	NOF	$24.34	$20.69	01/01/2016	12/31/2016
Payer 12	99213	OFF	$69.58	$59.14	01/01/2016	12/31/2016
Payer 12	99213	NOF	$49.47	$42.05	01/01/2016	12/31/2016
Payer 13	99212	OFF	$74.16	$59.74	11/01/2009	05/31/2017
Payer 13	99212	NOF	$43.83	$35.31	11/01/2009	05/31/2017
Payer 13	99213	OFF	$124.78	$100.51	11/01/2009	05/31/2017
Payer 13	99213	NOF	$89.1	$71.78	11/01/2009	05/31/2017

The practice could add the additional functionality because it has an internal IT department with the capability and experience to make it work. The CPM program is the most technically complex example in the book. A tool like CPM would definitely require IT help to implement, but again, the help does not have to be internal IT. There are other commercially available programs to validate reimbursement. Like any IT tool, the key is to ensure that the program is customizable enough that it can be tailored to meet your practice's unique needs. The tool needs to be cost effective without creating too much additional work compared to the return on investment. The logic needs to be customized to the requirements of local payers. The reporting needs to show exactly what the practice needs to see. No more, no less.

DENIED CLAIMS

If your practice isn't quite ready for a full-blown CPM system, another place to start is to capture all the procedure codes that were denied on EOBs. Denials can be captured without having to know or load contracts. Be careful to look for procedure codes where the carrier did not allow anything, as opposed to applying the balance to the patient's out-of-pocket deductible. PM systems track denied claims differently, but the objective is to capture as much information about the denial as possible (likely using a remittance code) so that the claim can be efficiently appealed.

Exhibit 4.15 is an example of how one practice captures and works denied claims.

Exhibit 4.15 Denied Claims Sample

Tickler	Ticket Number	Acct Num	VisitOwner	Visit Description	Insurance	Procedure Code
-3	2578608	725844	Unassigned	083017 ncd	Veterans Choice Program VACAA Tricare 16563	73562
-3	2578608	725844	Unassigned	083017 ncd	Veterans Choice Program VACAA Tricare 16563	99204
-3	3019351	744803	Case Complete-AR errors	called therapy	Medicare Trad** 4854 MCR	99213
-2	2955160	684304	Unassigned	091917 ncd ncd	Medicare AARP UHC 15104 ADV	63048
-2	2960746	10723474	Case Complete-Auth ERA	062217	HIP Anthem ** 15229 MCD	24300
-2	2993990	10725775	Outreach	081017 ncd Clone of visit	Medicare ChoiceCare Humana 14050	27759
-2	3009070	10232510	Unassigned	091117 ncd	Medicare AARP UHC 15104 ADV	63047
-2	3009070	10232510	Unassigned	091117 ncd	Medicare AARP UHC 15104 ADV	72100
-2	3039478	611916	Case Complete-Auth ERA	072417 ncd call md wise	HIP MDWise Excel Network 16815 MCD	73630
-2	3039478	611916	Case Complete-Auth ERA	072417 ncd call md wise	HIP MDWise Excel Network 16815 MCD	99213
-2	3039478	611916	Case Complete-Auth ERA	072417 ncd call md wise	HIP MDWise Excel Network 16815 MCD	L3030
-2	3058162	9224950	Unassigned	09.22.17 ncd	HIP MDWise Excel Network 16815 MCD	64493
-2	3058162	9224950	Unassigned	09.22.17 ncd	HIP MDWise Excel Network 16815 MCD	64494
-2	3068254	10731121	Unassigned	09/22/17 ncd	HIP MDWise Excel Network 16815 MCD	99232
-2	3085951	9791610	Case Complete-Auth ERA		HIP MDWise Excel Network 16815 MCD	20610
-2	3085951	9791610	Case Complete-Auth ERA		HIP MDWise Excel Network 16815 MCD	73140
-2	3085951	9791610	Case Complete-Auth ERA		HIP MDWise Excel Network 16815 MCD	99214
-2	3085951	9791610	Case Complete-Auth ERA		HIP MDWise Excel Network 16815 MCD	J0702
-2	3085951	9791610	Case Complete-Auth ERA		HIP MDWise Excel Network 16815 MCD	L3908
-2	3086700	10693962	Case Complete-Auth ERA	071717 ncd DME call md wise	HIP MDWise Excel Network 16815 MCD	L4360
-2	3088693	10719554	Case Complete-Auth ERA		HIP MDWise Excel Network 16815 MCD	L4360
-2	3100102	10734372	Case Complete-Auth ERA		HIP MDWise Excel Network 16815 MCD	99203
-2	3100102	10734372	Case Complete-Auth ERA		HIP MDWise Excel Network 16815 MCD	L4360
-2	3100853	10697901	Case Complete-Auth ERA	call md wise 99152 not on list	HIP MDWise Excel Network 16815 MCD	64479
-2	3102311	10650901	Case Complete-Auth ERA		HIP MDWise Excel Network 16815 MCD	L1820

Pay attention to the column in red at the far left. The column is called tickler and counts down the number of days remaining before a payer's deadline to appeal claims expires. The tickler column employs a formula that uses the timeframe for filing an appeal based on the payers' various contracts, with a built-in margin to allow for weekends, holidays, mail, etc. The margin gives the billing office a little leeway to work the claim. For example, an insurance carrier with a 90-day appeal deadline may be entered in the data warehouse with a deadline of 83 days. The Tickler column uses the appeal deadline to calculate the number of days remaining to appeal and turns red (using conditional formatting in Excel) when the deadline approaches.

The example above illustrates how Mona Reimers manages her staff by making it easier for them to do the right thing. The denial tickler report would prioritize an appeal for a $500 denial that expires next week ahead of a $5,000 denial that can still be appealed for six months. Sorting this spreadsheet by the tickler column and then the amount column prioritizes work to help staff appeal the most immediate denials first.

ADJUSTMENT REASON CODES

Another way to look at denials and underpayments in aggregate is to create a dataset with the adjustment group codes and reason codes from the EOB. Exhibits 4.16 and 4.17 are examples of how two different practices analyze these codes. In Exhibit 4.16, the practice focuses on a three-year trend of adjustment codes as well as the count of how often the adjustment codes are used on EOBs. The practice has filtered out some of the common codes, like CO-45, to focus more on adjustments that the practice can control. (CO-45 is a claim adjustment reason code indicating that charges exceed the contracted allowable amount.) The second code on the list, CO-87, had a big increase in 2015 for what appears to be a credentialing issue. The reason to run these reports is to persistently identify problems to solve. Continue running these reports to ensure that workflow changes and other measures designed to solve difficulties continue to be implemented so that the problem doesn't reoccur.

EXHIBIT 4.16 ADJUSTMENT REASON CODES: 3-YEAR TREND SAMPLE

Financial Class	(All)
Payer Name	(All)
Location	(All)
Rendering	(All)
EOB Date	(All)
Reason Subgroup	(All)

		Values	Years							Total Sum of Adj Amt	Total Count of Adj Amt
		Sum of Adj Amt			Count of Adj Amt						
Reason Code	Reason Code Desc	2015	2016	2017	2015	2016	2017				
CO253	Sequestration- Reduction In Federal Pmt	$64,012	$60,025	$36,178	33,461	30,699	17,739			$160,215	81,899
DA23	Payment adjusted because charges have...	$2,128,851	$2,178,438	$1,306,446	12,236	12,857	7,238			$5,613,735	32,331
CO59	Processed On Multiple Procedure Rule	$86,550	$109,054	$69,946	609	1,919	1,155			$265,550	3,683
CO87	Prov Not Elig For Proc On This DOS	$836,978	$2,285	$712	3,496	15	7			$839,975	3,518
0418	Duplicate claim/service.	$183,451	$178,305	$98,572	722	635	403			$460,329	1,760
CO223	Sequestration- Reduction In Federal Pmt	$2,620	$22		1,447	4				$2,643	1,451
CO97	Payment Is Included In the allowance ...	$109,641	$111,781	$147,312	370	400	603			$368,733	1,373
0422	Payment adjusted because this care ma...	$27,299	$73,609	$67,614	226	531	505			$168,522	1,262
0A813	Previously Paid Payment For This Claim H	$98,441	$133,991	$84,927	389	496	270			$316,959	1,155
CO237	Legislated/Regulatory Penalty		$1,768				1,042			$1,768	1,042
CO23	Payment adjusted because charges have...	$11,352	$20,532	$7,245	332	321	165			$39,130	818
CO151	Payment adjusted because the payer de...	$26,821	$51,692	$92,413	90	164	304			$170,926	558
CO18	Duplicate claim/service.	$10,397	$101,769	$21,916	42	392	72			$134,081	506
CO129	Payment denied - Prior processing inf...	($21,426)	($25,371)	($6,407)	165	242	99			($53,203)	506
CO29	The time limit for filing has expired.	$19,936	$29,093	$1,689	105	199	14			$50,698	318
P123	Payment adjusted because charges have...	$9,011	$4,304		237	59				$13,315	296
PI204	Service/equip No Covered Under Current B	$29,323	$11,201	$3,802	118	102	59			$44,326	279

The adjustments PivotTable example in Exhibit 4.17 only looks at the dollar amount of adjustments, but focus on the ways those adjustments can be filtered and analyzed. The list of fields, shown at the top of the exhibit, allow managers and staff to see adjustments by procedure code, financial class, location, rendering physician, adjustment type, month, and more. Note the number of duplicate claims in this exhibit. Managers may want to understand why there are so many duplicate claims being filed. As with any PivotTable, users can double-click any of the values to get details supporting the value. Being able to see a list of the duplicate claims will help find the underlying cause so that the practice can work to eliminate the holdup.

EXHIBIT 4.17 ADJUSTMENT REASON CODES: DOLLAR AMOUNTS

CPT Code	(All)	
Financial Class	(All)	
Location	(All)	
Rendering	(All)	
Type	(All)	
EOB Date	(All)	
Reason Subgroup	(All)	

| Sum of Adj Amt | | Years | | | |
Reason Code	Reason Code Desc	2016	2017	2018	Grand Total
CO45	Insurance Adjustment	$8,360,715	$14,862,317	$22,177,612	$45,400,644
OA23	Payment adjusted because charges have...	$1,862,568	$3,042,484	$3,220,932	$8,125,984
CO59	Charges are adjusted based on multipl...	$489,719	$846,741	$1,301,527	$2,637,987
OA18	Duplicate claim/service.	$324,936	$189,336	$1,122,543	$1,636,814
CO16	Claim/service lacks information which...	($8,140)	$32,515	$1,454,167	$1,478,542
CO18	Duplicate claim/service.	$263,715	$377,257	$743,803	$1,384,775
CO97	Payment is included in the allowance ...	$316,343	$184,581	$715,821	$1,216,745
CO96	Non-covered charge(s).	$194,390	$330,620	$656,795	$1,181,805
PR1	Deductible Amount	$369,666	$320,874	$397,774	$1,088,314
CO22	Payment adjusted because this care ma...	$35,623	$248,058	$76,008	$359,689
PR3	Co-payment Amount	$74,210	$127,755	$143,337	$345,301
CO23	Payment adjusted because charges have...	$12,968	$155,036	$96,216	$264,220
PR27	Expenses incurred after coverage term...	$15,357	$138,165	$90,147	$243,669
CO29	The time limit for filing has expired.	$14,849	$103,581	$102,730	$221,160
PR31	Claim denied as patient cannot be ide...	$6,522	$97,961	$104,989	$209,472
CO197	Payment denied/reduced for absence of...	$34,455	$9,165	$145,946	$189,566
CO151	Payment adjusted because the payer de...	$43,934	$4,757	$140,796	$189,487
CO104	Managed care withholding.	$43,172	$42,108	$100,380	$185,659

These two examples are both derived from EOB adjustments. Manual adjustments made to accounts for reasons other than those required on the remittance advice should also be analyzed. These adjustments are often stored in a different table in the PM system, meaning a different dataset may be required to capture these adjustments. The key element in this dataset would be the name of the person making the adjustment.

Tracking manual adjustments helps practices monitor write offs, bad debt, and staff productivity trends. Tracking the dollar value of manual adjustments that reduce patient balances by month and by user can also help practices monitor and protect against unnecessary write offs.

TRACKING SUCCESSFUL APPEALS

After going to the work of filing appeals, practices should track appeals made to make certain the payer responds and to keep track of wins and losses. Most PM systems do not have a useful built-in mechanism to track appeals. Practices can put a dummy transaction code on each procedure code they appeal, ensuring that the dummy code does not show up on electronic claims to insurance companies or paper statements to guarantors. At its most basic, the code is simply an indicator that the procedure code was appealed, and when it was appealed. Even that basic code contains several key pieces of information. It tells who appealed the claim (since PM systems store the login for each transaction entered), the specific procedure code, who the primary insurance was on the claim and who the rendering provider is. Now we have plenty of information to trend appeals. A good start is to use a PivotTable to analyze the number of appeals by staff, by month, by code, by primary insurance, and more. One practice uses different appeals codes for different types of appeals to analyze the data even further. For example, was the appeal simply a corrected claim, or was it a first level appeal, a second level appeal, or an administrative law judge appeal? With a little effort, appeal data can be in your system with enough detail to help you improve your bottom line. Follow up with payers to eliminate repeated issues. Work on the practice's internal issues that lead to appeals.

The next step can be harder, and may take either internal or external IT help in building the dataset. It's nice to know many appeals are being sent, but it's even nicer to know how many of those appeals were successful. One way to quantify successful appeals is to look for payments received after the date of the appeal. The calculation might best be represented by an example.

- Suppose a service was billed for $1,000 on August 1 and the primary insurance should have allowed $500.
- On August 22, the primary insurance allowed $200 and paid $160.
- An appeal is filed on September 4 for the remaining $300 ($500 - $200).
- After the appeal is sent, on September 8, the secondary insurance paid $40.
- On October 7, the primary insurance agrees with the appeal and allows an extra $300, paying $240.
- Finally, the secondary insurance pays the remaining $60 on November 7. The detail of this example is shown in Exhibit 5.18.

EXHIBIT 4.18 SUCCESSFUL APPEALS: TRACKING SAMPLE

Date	Action	Billed	Allowed	Should Have Allowed	Paid
8/1	Initial claim	$ 1,000			
8/22	Primary insurance		$ 200		$ 160
9/4	Appeal			$ 300	
9/8	Secondary insurance				$ 40
10/7	Primary insurance accepts appeal		$ 300		$ 240
11/7	Secondary insurance accepts appeal				$ 60

The amounts in red were received after the appeal was filed, while the amounts highlighted yellow are the payments that relate solely to the successful appeal. The $40 received on 9/8 was paid by the secondary insurance despite the appeal. Including the $40 artificially inflates the value of successful appeals.

On the other hand, assume the same facts with two changes:

- There is no secondary insurance.
- The patient did not pay those balances ($40 on 9/8 and $60 on 11/7).

Because the appeal is calculated based on payments received and the patient did not make any payments, the value of successful appeals would only be calculated as the $240 the primary insurance paid on October 7, circled in blue. The actual value of the successful appeal is $300, circled in red.

As complex as these problem examples are, they are relatively straightforward as far as appeals go. Some appeals have many lines of detail adding and subtracting to the balance as primary and secondary insurance respond to multiple appeals. Sorting through each line to calculate the correct amount of a successful appeal is doable if there only a few appeals; building rules to quantify successful appeals for thousands of claims is much harder.

Depending on the PM system, there are several ways to calculate the value of successful appeals. One approach is to look for the increase in allowed amount, such as the increase of $300 on 10/7 (circled in red) in our example. This can be difficult to track if the PM system does not store enough detail to recognize the increase in allowed amount due to the appeal. Another approach is to divide all payments received after the appeal into two parts: payments received from the primary insurance and all payments received. The logic is that the successful appeals are at least as much as the amounts received from the primary insurance after the date of the appeal, up to a maximum of the total payments received. In our example, the minimum amount of successful appeals is $240 (circled in blue), which was received from primary insurance. The maximum amount of successful appeals is all three payments in red font, or $340. The dollar amount of successful appeals is critical to the success of a payer contracting projects like this. Rather than let the perfect be the enemy of the good, at the very least apply a minimum and a maximum estimate of successful appeals and track this data. Exhibit 4.19 is a PivotTable analysis from a practice that uses the minimum/maximum approach to estimate successful appeals. The wide variation in appeals by staff member is a function of staff member responsibilities. Some staff members only appeal denied claims. Other staff members only do appeals infrequently. For this practice the difference between the minimum appeals (subsequent payments by primary insurance, labeled as Same Payer Payments in the example) and the maximum appeals (all subsequent payments, labeled as All Payer Payments in the example) isn't very significant.

EXHIBIT 4.19 SUCCESSFUL APPEALS: THE MINIMUM AND MAXIMUM SAMPLE

Procedure Code	(All)	
Provider	(All)	
Facility	(All)	
Appeal Type	(Multiple Items)	
Insurance Group	(All)	
Insurance Carrier	(All)	

Row Labels	Sum of Same Payer Payments	Sum of All Payer Payments
Billing	$496,240.75	$557,338.04
	$357,153.96	$386,657.97
Staff	$147,972.39	$162,664.75
	$554,210.17	$590,543.75
Members	$52,834.23	$60,092.60
Who	$730,958.46	$802,492.02
	$284,010.99	$315,904.11
Appealed	$478,017.33	$489,863.90
	$67,031.11	$67,576.97
the Claim	$75,519.67	$82,120.42
	$77,365.85	$78,239.92
	$55,326.37	$55,346.37
	$95,792.11	$95,792.11

If the billing staff tracks different levels of appeal (corrected claim vs. first level appeal, for example), another question the dataset can answer is which level of appeals are successful. In other words, for Payer A for a given procedure code, does it consistently take two appeals to be reimbursed? Are there codes that will never be successfully appealed? Which codes are most likely to be successfully appealed on the first try?

Exhibit 4.20 is a revised version of the previous example, Exhibit 4.19. Since the practice enters an adjustment code every time the staff takes any follow up action on a claim, the list is expanded to include requests for documentation, following up with payers, and other activities to show even bigger numbers. The take home message of this PivotTable is that it's well worth the practice's time to follow up and appeal claims.

EXHIBIT 4.20 SUCCESSFUL APPEALS: FOLLOW-UP

Procedure Code	(All)	
Provider	(All)	
Facility	(All)	
Insurance Group	(All)	
Insurance Carrier	(All)	

Row Labels	Sum of Same Payer Payments	Sum of All Payer Payments
ALJ	$889.15	$974.22
Appeal First Level Sent	$446,067.10	$486,082.41
Appeal Second Level Sent	$24,801.41	$30,276.97
CC	$387,814.05	$451,287.13
Provider Rep	$167,268.66	$175,663.85
Documentation	$1,633,754.52	$1,713,870.79
INS Follow Up Ph.Call	$449,709.30	$534,525.76
Documentation- Subsequent Submission	$66,146.92	$72,072.68
Appeal Verbal	$187,814.32	$207,371.08
WC- Follow Up	$434,056.51	$442,430.92
WCB	$38,277.87	$43,472.87
WC Request for Assistance	$45,696.49	$45,696.49
Grand Total	**$3,882,296.30**	**$4,203,725.17**

In summary, short of building a case to hire more staff, it does not do much good to identify denials and underpayments that the billing office does not have the resources to appeal. Building data like this can help a busy billing office overwhelmed with appeals prioritize work. The first priority for one practice may be big dollar appeals that have been successfully appealed in the past. A different practice may find that the first priority should be correcting claims. Proactive practices could take corrected claims a step further by identifying denials that result from issues the practice can control, such as lack of documentation or demographic errors. Reports that track who billed a claim that didn't have the required documentation or who checked in a patient without confirming demographics should reduce those types of appeals over time. If the front desk never knows there is a holdup, the problem isn't very likely to solve itself. The more a practice can change workflow to reduce the need to appeal, the more appeals the billing department will have time to address.

SETTING BILLED CHARGES

There are several ways to set billed charges in a practice. As transparency continues to pervade healthcare, defensible fee schedules become increasingly important. From the public's perspective, billed charges that are dramatically different (and especially higher) from competitors may be a source of concern. One way data can help inform better decisions is to use publicly available data to compare fee schedules in the market.

Many readers are aware that CMS annually releases a Medicare Physician Fee Schedule with allowed amounts for all procedures and services. CMS has also released public data on billed charges by procedure by National Provider Identifier (NPI) number. The CMS data includes NPI information, geographic information, and average charge information for procedures billed to Medicare. An example analysis is shown in Exhibit 4.21.

EXHIBIT 4.21 CMS DATA: AVERAGE BILLED CHARGES TO MEDICARE BY NPI SAMPLE

Average of Avg Charge	Column Labels				
Row Labels	99211	99212	99213	99214	99215
Addiction Medicine				$110.94	$149.27
Allergy/Immunology	$49.81	$73.43	$106.58	$162.74	$219.52
Anesthesiology	$56.31	$126.89	$176.37	$255.98	$344.17
Cardiac Electrophysiology	$54.11	$88.80	$149.85	$220.43	$302.14
Cardiac Surgery	$49.89	$85.03	$138.07	$207.05	$247.99
Cardiology	$47.74	$84.03	$139.53	$206.96	$283.78
Certified Clinical Nurse Specialist	$29.00	$83.27	$131.76	$194.43	$310.35
Certified Nurse Midwife			$112.44		
Chiropractic			$85.00		
Colorectal Surgery (formerly proctology)	$37.26	$87.46	$138.77	$199.32	$279.77
Critical Care (Intensivists)	$48.33	$77.25	$122.44	$186.27	$246.03
Dermatology	$39.48	$70.10	$112.12	$160.98	$230.78
Diagnostic Radiology	$35.87	$94.38	$170.61	$186.92	$346.00
Emergency Medicine	$46.73	$80.64	$125.64	$191.81	$274.22
Endocrinology	$45.21	$75.99	$130.45	$196.99	$266.42
Family Practice	$40.79	$75.87	$119.02	$175.32	$234.46
Gastroenterology	$43.17	$81.42	$125.90	$187.20	$259.31
General Practice	$36.83	$67.96	$107.66	$154.41	$222.28
General Surgery	$53.15	$86.99	$135.71	$201.44	$285.11
Geriatric Medicine	$44.79	$77.72	$134.86	$203.01	$284.39
Geriatric Psychiatry		$44.88	$86.69	$119.40	
Gynecological/Oncology	$67.00	$90.14	$144.96	$228.72	$369.72
Hand Surgery	$47.21	$86.25	$165.39	$215.42	$273.00
Hematology	$65.00	$91.46	$150.82	$228.92	$315.72
Hematology/Oncology	$62.37	$87.81	$148.70	$224.87	$331.20
Hospice and Palliative Care		$80.00	$121.90	$195.57	$344.52
Infectious Disease	$55.82	$85.39	$136.00	$200.22	$301.44
Internal Medicine	$41.21	$75.65	$121.07	$179.53	$247.59
Interventional Pain Management	$54.37	$117.14	$170.94	$227.08	$273.48
Interventional Radiology	$79.20	$111.33	$208.58	$223.04	$300.00
Maxillofacial Surgery	$44.00	$72.25	$115.43	$187.67	$155.00

This example highlights established patient visits billed by Texas providers in 2014. Any time you have this type of detailed data for analysis, start with a PivotTable. The PivotTable quickly shows average billed charges to Medicare by NPI specialty. Pay attention to the example circled in red at the bottom of Exhibit 4.21. The average billed charge for code 99214 is actually more than the average billed charge for 99215, a more complex code. The PivotTable makes further analysis easier by drilling down on the detail. It turns out that the provider who billed the 99215 charges did not bill 99214 charges. The detailed data showed three practices with a total of 64 charges made up the 99214 total, while the 99215 total was only one practice with 16 total charges. To protect patient privacy, CMS only includes data from practices billing procedures to at least 11 unique patients. Some of the maxillofacial practices that billed 99214 may have billed 99215 as well, but did not have at least 11 unique patients.

Practices can apply filters to see data by city or zip code. Both fields are included in the CMS data. For example, 797 general surgery practices in Texas were included in the data for procedure code 99213, a very common established patient visit code. 92 of those practices were based in Houston. The average charge for code 99213 in Houston is $155, with a median of $134, a high of $575 and a low of $63. That type of information at a very detailed level can give practices insight into market rates and confidence in a fee schedule strategy. The detail goes down to NPI number, so if you know a provider's NPI number, which is publicly available, you can get historical fee schedule information. This same CMS provider utilization data is also discussed in Chapter 5 as it relates to attracting patients and visualizing where services are being rendered in a market.

Part of the reason to include this example is to emphasize that practices are not limited to their internal data as the only source of Business Intelligence. Just because the data is publicly available does not mean competitors are using the data and reacting to the data in a timely manner. The Texas maxillofacial surgery provider billing 99215 for less than a competitor billed 99214 may be an example. The CMS data is over nine million rows in size and cannot be analyzed with traditional Excel, but Power Pivot can manage nine million rows. With a little IT help to configure the data in PowerPivot, a practice can focus on what is critically important to their market and their competition.

THE FUTURE OF PAYER CONTRACTING

The entire reimbursement model is in transition. Major payers, particularly CMS, have indicated a desire to change the fee-for-service model to paying for results. Payer contracting and monitoring the results of payer contracting will only become more important as payment models evolve. Proactive practices may move from after-the-fact monitoring (did the payer pay according to contract?) to monitoring ongoing practice operations to ensure that the practice will meet objectives defined in the contract.

Exhibit 4.22 is an example from a small primary care practice. There are several payers in their market who offer incentives for annual wellness visits, tracking patients, and completing forms for Medicare Advantage plans. The practice administrator calculated the value of the incentive payments available, the reimbursement for the visit, and the additional services rendered because of that visit. The total was worth $800 - $900 per patient in additional revenue to the practice. That translates to a potential revenue increase of over $100,000 per primary care physician. (The practice is in a sunny climate with a high percentage of Medicare patients and a high Medicare Advantage penetration.) The Medicare Advantage plans and Accountable Care Organizations in this market are the payers with the $800 - $900 of incentives. To quote the practice, "This is a huge amount of revenue to a primary care physician who uses the right tools to jump through these hoops in an organized, strategic manner. It really just takes opening their minds to earning money in a different manner."

The incentive programs got the practice's attention, but each payer required different information in a different format to qualify for the incentives. Each payer also had a different way of providing the census information reporting which patients could qualify for each incentive. The practice needed a tracking mechanism to know which patients were assigned to each payer program and which patients met the requirements for each incentive. Practices may complain that too many of the incentives for meeting meaningful use went to software instead of to the practices complying with meaningful use. This practice took a different approach.

Exhibit 4.22 Payer Contracting: Tracking Incentive Programs and Requirements

Patient Name	Last Name	DOB	Lookup	Sex	Age	Tel. No	Acct Num	Insurance	PCP	Last AWV	Next AWV
Batres, Emmanuel	Batres	12/6/1935	BatresX13124	M	81	555-280-653	C264615	Payer C	Rodriguez		
Saldana, Oneida	Saldana	7/16/1929	SaldanaX10790	F	88	555-706-368	C323853	Payer B	Anderson	1/9/2016	2/25/2017
Houlihan, Anton	Houlihan	7/12/1942	HoulihanX15534	M	75	555-872-198	C797516	Payer C	Martinez		
Byron, Hank	Byron	1/10/1943	ByronX15716	M	74	555-179-918	C747764	Payer A	Garcia	4/24/2016	
Scarbrough, Madie	Scarbrough	11/14/1934	ScarbroughX12737	F	82	555-983-599	C692070		Anderson	2/2/2016	4/24/2017
Cahn, Henry	Cahn	8/31/1935	CahnX13027	M	81	555-785-927	C716682		Garcia	11/30/2016	12/14/2017
Noone, Francisco	Noone	7/25/1925	NooneX9338	M	92	555-172-958	C802894	Payer A	Wilson	12/26/2016	
Sauls, Carlton	Sauls	6/13/1926	SaulsX9661	M	91	555-608-643	C839818	ACO	Wilson	1/30/2016	4/5/2017
Kraemer, Mitchell	Kraemer	9/16/1941	KraemerX15235	M	75	555-290-859	C784758	Payer C	Garcia	5/10/2016	10/24/2017
Wingfield, Loni	Wingfield	3/12/1931	WingfieldX11394	F	86	555-237-928	C738317	Payer B	Wilson		
Weise, Charissa	Weise	3/22/1949	WeiseX17979	F	68	555-511-269	C194514	ACO	Wilson	4/18/2016	5/29/2017
Stack, Chung	Stack	7/30/1948	StackX17744	M	69	555-406-779	C649791	ACO	Anderson	9/25/2016	10/14/2017
Gaddy, Micki	Gaddy	5/3/1927	GaddyX9985	F	90	555-907-736	C225646		Martinez		
Blakeslee, Elroy	Blakeslee	8/29/1942	BlakesleeX15582	M	75	555-650-143	C927570	Payer A	Anderson		
Canton, Eneida	Canton	12/2/1929	CantonX10929	F	87	555-472-238	C258155	ACO	Rodriguez		
Kipp, Porter	Kipp	4/15/1936	KippX13255	M	81	555-353-480	C908236		Anderson	5/27/2016	
Hetrick, Ayako	Hetrick	7/24/1950	HetrickX18468	F	67	555-112-324	C529771	Payer A	Rodriguez		
Trainer, Elissa	Trainer	5/30/1930	TrainerX11108	F	87	555-448-119	C722352	ACO	Rodriguez		
Berliner, Elisabeth	Berliner	4/14/1939	BerlinerX14349	F	78	555-181-685	C277250	Payer A	Rodriguez	7/19/2016	
Smithers, Isela	Smithers	3/17/1935	SmithersX12860	F	82	555-817-859	C440613	Payer C	Garcia		
Vannatta, Alva	Vannatta	8/12/1930	VannattaX11182	M	87	555-235-197	C714909	Payer B	Martinez	3/31/2016	4/23/2017
Breazeale, Bill	Breazeale	8/20/1926	BreazealeX9729	M	91	555-155-044	C319965	Payer A	Martinez		
Truex, Gregory	Truex	2/13/1926	TruexX9541	M	91	555-609-242	C939043	ACO	Garcia	4/30/2016	5/26/2017
Brafford, Rick	Brafford	11/14/1948	BraffordX17851	M	68	555-726-667	C932458	Payer B	Garcia	11/1/2016	

Each patient over age 65 in the PM system is listed in Exhibit 4.22, above (patient data listed isn't actual patient data). The main demographic and contact information makes managing the data easy for the staff member assigned to oversee all the incentive programs. Focus on the columns after the patient demographic information.

The Insurance column shows which incentive program the patient is assigned to. Staff can confirm this column to make sure each patient is enrolled and qualifies for their respective program. To determine which patients are in which plan, the practice downloads a census or plan roster from each payer monthly. Each payer gathers and reports different data in a different order using different reporting periods, so the practice built a process to simplify importing the data into the spreadsheet. That import process used to be very labor-intensive, taking about 10 hours just to get data from the payers. The process has been optimized and simplified so that the entire import process now takes minutes.

The primary care physician is tracked, as are dates of the last and next annual wellness visit. At a minimum, the practice wants each patient over 65 to have an annual wellness visit. Columns further to the right (not shown) can track which patients have qualified for that payer's incentives. The practice can also build a tracking mechanism into the spreadsheet to ensure that the practice receives the incentive payment for each patient who qualifies.

Some of the incentive programs require a minimum percentage of patients in the program to qualify for an incentive payment. Other payers award higher incentives as more enrolled patients meet objectives. To manage each plan, the practice created a separate spreadsheet tab for each incentive program. An example is shown in Exhibit 4.23.

EXHIBIT 4.23 PAYER CONTRACTING: TRACKING INCENTIVE PROGRAMS INDIVIDUALLY

Lookup	Not in PM	PCP Name	Member Name	Last Name	DOB	Attestation	Measure 1	Measure 2	Measure 3	Sex	Age
ByronX15716		Garcia	Byron, Hank	Byron	1/10/1943		Met	Not Met	Met	M	74
NooneX9338		Wilson	Noone, Francisco	Noone	7/25/1925		Not Met	Not Met	Not Met	M	91
BlakesleeX15582		Anderson	Blakeslee, Elroy	Blakeslee	8/29/1942		Not Met	Not Met	Not Met	M	74
DelgadoX16637	Not in PM	Wilson	Delgado, Jenny	Delgado	7/19/1945		Not Met	Met	Met	F	71
HetrickX18468		Rodriguez	Hetrick, Ayako	Hetrick	7/24/1950		Met	Met	Met	F	66
BerlinerX14349		Rodriguez	Berliner, Elisabeth	Berliner	4/14/1939		Not Met	Met	Met	F	77
BreazealeX9729		Martinez	Breazeale, Bill	Breazeale	8/20/1926		Not Met	Met	Met	M	90
LathanX11221		Rodriguez	Lathan, Shaquana	Lathan	9/20/1930		Not Met	Met	Met	F	86
MullicanX12462		Martinez	Mullican, Jc	Mullican	2/12/1934		Met	Met	Met	M	82
BradberryX15239		Garcia	Bradberry, Eldon	Bradberry	9/20/1941		Not Met	Not Met	Not Met	M	75
RiosX16303	Not in PM	Anderson	Rios, Sonia	Rios	8/19/1944		Not Met	Not Met	Met	F	72
StanleyX11867	Not in PM	Martinez	Stanley, Misty	Stanley	6/27/1932		Met	Met	Met	F	84
BrakefieldX14578		Wilson	Brakefield, Yer	Brakefield	11/29/1939		Not Met	Not Met	Met	F	77
WhitsettX11913		Anderson	Whitsett, Aaron	Whitsett	8/12/1932		Not Met	Not Met	Not Met	M	84
KnisleyX13880		Garcia	Knisley, Tarsha	Knisley	12/31/1937		Met	Met	Met	F	79
MeunierX14651		Garcia	Meunier, Foster	Meunier	2/10/1940		Met	Met	Met	M	76
FreelX12943		Martinez	Freel, Walter	Freel	6/8/1935		Not Met	Met	Not Met	M	81
BarnettX16129	Not in PM	Wilson	Barnett, Claire	Barnett	2/27/1944		Not Met	Not Met	Met		72
BruckX14521		Rodriguez	Bruck, Jefferey	Bruck	10/3/1939		Not Met	Met	Met	M	77
ScherrX12621		Martinez	Scherr, Corrine	Scherr	7/21/1934		Not Met	Met	Met	F	82

One of the key columns in this spreadsheet is the third column, "Not in PM." The spreadsheet compares each patient on the payer tab to the patient registry tab in Exhibit 4.22. Any patient on the payer census but not in the PM system is a patient the practice has not seen and needs to contact. The comparison is done with an Excel VLOOKUP formula. The patient registry tab also uses several VLOOKUP formulas to combine each group of payer data into a one-page summary. The obstacle is that the payers all have different identification numbers for patients and those identifiers are not in the PM system. Instead, the practice uses the patient last name and date of birth to look up each patient in the PM data. (VLOOKUP will only search for one field, so the search field is a combination of the patients' last name and date of birth, separated by an X. An example lookup column is in the column labeled "Lookup" in Exhibit 4.23.) Any patients not found in the patient registry tab are highlighted using conditional formatting and researched. (For more information about using VLOOKUP, please see the VLOOKUP Excel Mastery page at mooresolutionsinc.com/em-vlookup/)

This example tracks three measures that the payer uses to incentivize the practice. The Excel Table format makes it easy to count which measures have been met and which patients need to meet measures. Tables are a very effective way to manage detailed data in Excel, and are a key component in the practice's cost-effective strategy for tracking incentive programs. (For more information about using Tables, please see the Tables Excel Mastery page at mooresolutionsinc.com/em-tables/)

CHAPTER 5

ATTRACTING PATIENTS

Patients, particularly new patients, are the life blood of a practice. Trends in new patients are critical to monitor and appropriately address over time. This chapter looks at some traditional ways to analyze new patients in a practice by collecting data, analyzing existing data, and using outside data sources to estimate a practice's market share of patients.

Referral sources and referring physicians are a fruitful place to begin to understand the source of new patients. For many practices, a new patient visit isn't enough. It becomes very important to track how many new procedures are generated each month. Examples of practices performing these tasks appear throughout this chapter.

Another way to evaluate new patients is to pull patients' zip codes from the demographic data and use Excel's new mapping tools to create a geographic analysis of new patients or procedures, or both. Practices can use these maps to determine where to market for new patients, where to open a new clinic location or where to better schedule providers. The ability to map patient data makes geographic data much easier to visualize.

In addition to knowing where patients live and how they are referred to your practice, understanding patient loyalty to a given location or a given physician can also help strategize and manage practice resources. The loyalty analysis in this chapter was developed for a practice opening a new location. Combining mapped data with this loyalty data helped determine the new location for a practice and which providers are optimal candidates to staff the new location.

This chapter includes publicly available data that can be used in a variety of ways to attract patients. Several practices have used the data to estimate their market share of referrals from a physician. If the practice only uses internal data, estimating market share can be very difficult. Estimating market share is doable and quite interesting once publicly available data is combined with the practice's data. For example, what percentage of patients does a local family practice send to our practice compared to our competitors? Other practices have used the public data to estimate their market share of procedures in a market. For example, what percentage of hip replacements do our physicians perform in this city compared to the competition? Using publicly available data dramatically increases the amount of competitive information available to a savvy practice manager.

Finally, examples below reveal how payers influence market share, new patients, and physician productivity in a market. With the advent of the Affordable Care Act and the narrowing of networks and patient choice, payers can influence market share more than in the past, especially in markets with reduced numbers of insurance carriers. This practice used their analysis to look at ways to proactively schedule providers more frequently at hospitals in networks supported by the remaining payers.

REFERRAL SOURCES

Practices apply different metrics to evaluate the flow of new patients to the practice. Primary care practices generally have a harder task identifying the source of new patients compared to specialty practices. Referring physician information for specialty practices is part of the CMS-1500 data and stored in the PM system. Primary care and other practices that do not typically have referring physicians need to make a concerted effort to track where patients are coming from. Some PM programs have a field to store the source of new patients, but that brings up another hurdle. The referral source field is often a free text field where users can enter whatever they want as opposed to a list of referring physicians that populates the referring physician field. A free text field means that a new patient who came to the practice based on a neighbor friend's recommendation could have a referral source as neighbor, friend, or other (or even misspellings of those words). This data entry inconsistency can make the data difficult to analyze.

THE FIRST SOLUTION TO DILEMMAS LIKE THESE IS OFTEN *NOT* TO RUN MORE REPORTS. THE FIRST SOLUTION IS TO FIND WAYS TO WORK WITHIN THE SYSTEM TO CLEAN UP THE DATA TO MAKE THE EVENTUAL REPORTS MORE USEFUL. FOR EXAMPLE, SOME PM SYSTEMS WILL ALLOW FIELDS TO BE DESIGNATED AS REQUIRED TO COMPLETE A FORM OR EXIT A SCREEN. MAKING THE REFERRAL SOURCE FIELD REQUIRED IS ONE WAY TO GET DATA INTO THE SYSTEM. IF THE PM SYSTEM WILL NOT REQUIRE THE REFERRAL SOURCE TO BE ENTERED, THEN A REPORT CAN BE GENERATED TO SEE WHICH STAFF MEMBER LAST MODIFIED THE PATIENT'S DEMOGRAPHIC INFORMATION. MANY PM SYSTEMS TRACK THE LAST LOGIN TO MODIFY PATIENT INFORMATION. A REPORT LIKE EXHIBIT 5.1 COULD BE GENERATED TO TREND MISSING REFERRAL SOURCES BY THE NAME OF THE PERSON WHO CHECKED IN THE PATIENT.

EXHIBIT 5.1 MISSING REFERRAL SOURCE REPORT

Sum of Missing Demographics	2018			
Front Desk Staff	Feb	Mar	Apr	Grand Total
aknaus	14	10	8	32
akuehne	18	3	4	25
bmagallon	18	13	2	33
cahlstrom	8	10	2	20
cstegner	9	9	0	18
cwhitlow	5	11	8	24
emolina	17	1	4	22
gducker	5	4	10	19
gschnitzer	16	4	5	25
ldarwin	4	10	2	16
mbrighton	16	6	9	31
mheffelfinger	4	15	0	19
mmcelveen	8	2	3	13
npewitt	19	6	8	33
prathbone	8	11	8	27
tfarrior	11	4	7	22
tmcdavid	20	9	4	33
Grand Total	200	128	84	412

THESE NUMBERS COULD ALSO BE SHOWN AS A PERCENTAGE OF THE PATIENTS CHECKED IN. IN THIS EXAMPLE, ALL THE FRONT DESK STAFF WORK SIMILAR SHIFTS AT SIMILAR LOCATIONS. IF ANDREA KNAUS (THE PERSON AT THE TOP OF THE PIVOTTABLE) ONLY WORKED TWO DAYS A WEEK, THE PERCENTAGE OF HER ERRORS WOULD BE MUCH HIGHER THAN THE OTHER, FULL-TIME STAFF. CUSTOMIZE YOUR ANALYSIS TO MEET THE NEEDS OF YOUR PRACTICE.

If the PM system does not have a field for referral source data, practices have found other fields in the PM system to track this information. Completely unrelated fields like dental information have been used by medical practices to record referral source information. The difficulty with using unrelated fields is that the field is often on a different tab or in a different area of the PM system that requires extra staff effort to remember to use and extra clicks to navigate to.

To work around the free text field difficulty, one option is to write code to include multiple choices in one category. To use the neighbor, friend, neigbor example earlier, code in SQL Server can include all three options in a category called "friend." That solution probably requires IT help to write SQL code. Another way to solve the free text field problem is to group data in a PivotTable. The advantage of the PivotTable solution is that end users can group data in PivotTables without IT support.

FOR REFERENCE, HERE IS A BRIEF EXPLANATION OF HOW TO GROUP DATA IN A PIVOTTABLE.

ASSUME YOUR DATA LOOKS LIKE THE DATA IN THE PIVOTTABLE IN EXHIBIT 5.2.

EXHIBIT 5.2 PIVOTTABLE: SAMPLE DATA

Row Labels	Sum of Count
ER	6
Friend	25
Hospital Outreach	12
Neigbor	1
Neighbor	10
Social Media	22
Grand Total	**76**

HOLD DOWN THE **CTRL** KEY TO SELECT CELLS A5, A7, AND A8 SO YOUR
SCREEN LOOKS LIKE **EXHIBIT 5.3**

EXHIBIT 5.3 PIVOTTABLE: GROUPING DATA

3	Row Labels	Sum of Count
4	ER	6
5	Friend	25
6	Hospital Outreach	12
7	Neigbor	1
8	Neighbor	10
9	Social Media	22
10	**Grand Total**	**76**

RIGHT-CLICK THE SELECTED CELLS AND CHOOSE **GROUP** FROM THE MENU
THAT APPEARS, AS CIRCLED IN RED IN **EXHIBIT 5.4**

EXHIBIT 5.4 PIVOTTABLE: GROUPING DROPDOWN

3	Row Labels	Sum of Count
4	ER	
5	Friend	25
6	Hospital C	12
7	Neigbor	1
8	Neighbor	10
9	Social Me	22
10	Grand To	76
11		
12		
13		
14		
15		

Calibri · 11 · A A $ · % ·
B I ☰ ◇ · A · ⊞ · ⁀⁰⁰ ⁰⁰⁰ ✦

- Copy
- Format Cells...
- Refresh
- Sort ►
- Filter ►
- ✓ Subtotal "Referral Source"
- Expand/Collapse ►
- Group...
- Ungroup...
- Move ►
- ✕ Remove "Referral Source"
- Field Settings...
- PivotTable Options...
- Hide Field List

For reference, instead of right-clicking the selected cells, you can also choose Group from the PivotTable Tools Analyze menu, as shown in Exhibit 5.5. (Microsoft has renamed this menu in prior versions of Excel. This screen capture was taken with Excel 2016.)

Exhibit 5.5 PivotTable: Group Selection in the Toolbar

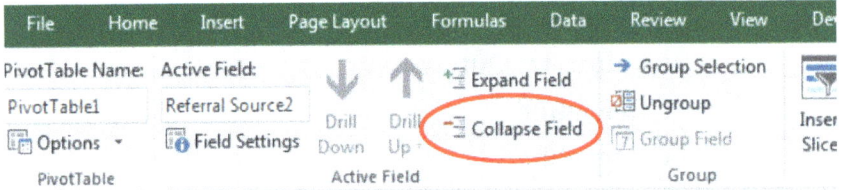

With either approach, Excel groups the data as shown in Exhibit 5.6.

Exhibit 5.6 PivotTable: PivotTable: Grouping Results

	Row Labels	Sum of Count
3		
4	☐ **ER**	
5	ER	6
6	☐ **Group1**	
7	Friend	25
8	Neigbor	1
9	Neighbor	10
10	☐ **Hospital Outreach**	
11	Hospital Outreach	12
12	☐ **Social Media**	
13	Social Media	22
14	**Grand Total**	**76**

Notice Group1 in cell A6. Simply select cell A6 and type a new name for the group to replace "Group 1." In Exhibit 5.7, the new group is named "Friends."

Exhibit 5.7 PivotTable: Changing Group Names

	Row Labels	Sum of Count
3	Row Labels	Sum of Count
4	⊟ ER	
5	ER	6
6	⊟ **Friends**	
7	Friend	25
8	Neigbor	1
9	Neighbor	10
10	⊟ **Hospital Outreach**	
11	Hospital Outreach	12
12	⊟ **Social Media**	
13	Social Media	22
14	**Grand Total**	**76**

Now collapse the groups from the PivotTable Tools Analyze menu as shown in Exhibit 5.8.

Exhibit 5.8 PivotTable: Analyze Menu

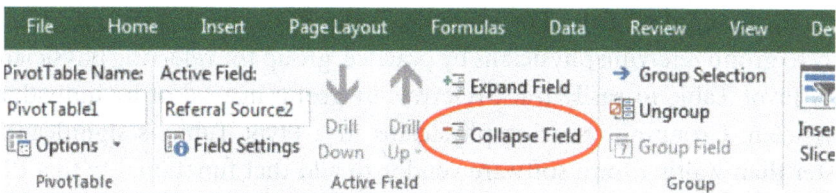

THE NEW GROUPED, COLLAPSED PIVOTTABLE THAT COMBINES FRIEND, NEIGHBOR, AND NEIGBOR IS SHOWN IN EXHIBIT 5.9.

EXHIBIT 5.9 PIVOTTABLE: COLLAPSED GROUPS

	Row Labels	Sum of Count
3		
4	± ER	6
5	± Friends	36
6	± Hospital Outreach	12
7	± Social Media	22
8	Grand Total	76

FOR MORE INFORMATION ABOUT GROUPING AND OTHER PIVOTTABLE FEATURES, WATCH THE SERIES OF FREE EXCEL VIDEOS AT MOORESOLUTIONSINC. COM.

Once referral source data is available, PivotTables are a productive way to trend sources of patients. The ability to group and otherwise manipulate data inside a PivotTable without IT support is a major advantage of PivotTables. The same grouping process can combine data to create information that isn't in the original data. For example, if the PM system does not offer a way to group referring physicians by practice, group the referring physicians in a Pivot Table to easily track referrals by group instead of by individual physician. Grouping referring physicians in a Pivot Table is significantly faster than waiting for a software vendor to add that functionality to a PM system.

Grouping data is a solid way to quickly analyze information. If this grouping is a one-time project, the problem is solved. The downside is that the grouping is only available in the PivotTable where the grouping was created. A new spreadsheet analyzing referring physicians from a different dataset would have to group the physicians again, with the potential for error. There is also the potential that when Dr. Jones changes practices one spreadsheet has her with her old practice and another spreadsheet has her with the new practice. One way to solve this problem is to use the same spreadsheet with the grouping for all referring physician analyses. This solution might work well for a smaller practice. Two possible solutions for larger practices are to do the physician grouping in the data warehouse instead of in the PivotTable (which requires IT help to create and maintain the list) or use the new Excel Data Model described in Chapter 3. Like a data warehouse, the Excel Data Model is also designed to keep one source of truth in one place and have all spreadsheets use that data.

TRENDING REFERRING PHYSICIANS

When practices begin to mine data, there is often a data quality issue with referring physicians. If the data was not being used in reports in the past or the data was not even available to be reported on, the referring physician data may be inaccurate or incomplete. Sometimes the referring physician data points to other providers in a group practice instead of an outside referring physician. Data governance is important here. It's well worth the time to carefully define what the practice will store as a referring physician, where the information will be stored, and when it's appropriate to change referring physician information.

For practices whose patients are referred by referring physicians, there are several ways to trend the data. A surgical practice looks at referring physicians as part of a dashboard this way:

EXHIBIT 5.10 REFERRING PHYSICIANS: TRACKING DATA

Locations: ALL Providers: ALL
Procedure Classes: ALL Plan Classes: ALL
Departments: ALL POS: ALL

New Patient Trends for the Top 20 Groups and Physicians

Referring Physician	Current 6	Last 6	Var	Combined Referring Groups	6 Mo	Var
	9.7	8.3	16.0%	Combined	1,564	-0.4%
Referring	6.7	5.8	14.3%		661	-6.8%
	6.5	4.5	44.4%		219	0.5%
	5.2	2.3	121.4%	Groups Here	106	-10.9%
Physicians	4.7	6.2	-24.3%	Referring Group	6 Mo	Var
	4.5	3.3	35.0%		420	59.7%
Listed	4.5	5.7	-20.6%	Referring	269	0.4%
	4.5	4.0	12.5%		198	11.2%
	4.3	6.0	-27.8%		178	2.9%
Here	4.3	3.2	36.8%	Groups	139	-6.1%
	4.3	4.7	-7.1%		134	7.2%
	4.0	4.3	-7.7%	Listed	133	7.3%
	3.8	4.5	-14.8%		106	-14.5%
	3.8	4.0	-4.2%		98	-4.9%
	3.7	2.5	46.7%	Here	97	21.3%
	3.7	4.5	-18.5%		94	20.5%
	3.5	2.7	31.3%		84	5.0%
	3.3	2.8	17.6%		81	-8.0%

This dashboard has changed over time. When it was originally designed, this portion of the dashboard included a section tracking the date of the last new patient referral. For some surgical practices, the last new patient referral can be an important indicator. A surgeon may think she just did surgery on a patient from a referring physician, so that referring physician is still referring patients. If that patient had pre-authorization problems or had trouble qualifying for surgery clinically, it may have been months since the last new patient referral. By the time a physician realizes the referrals have stopped, a new referral pattern to a competing surgeon could be in place. In this practice's situation, the variance between new patients in the current six-month period compared to the prior six-month period was more meaningful, so they made the change. Good dashboards evolve over time to meet the needs of a practice, and this dashboard is no exception.

In a world of practices consolidating and being acquired by hospital systems, knowing referrals by practice group can be very important. If a competing system acquires an entire practice, the impact on new patient referrals could suddenly become very important. The right side of the dashboard in Exhibit 5.10 groups referring physician groups two ways, an overall combined network grouping and by referring physician group.

Two more things to notice about the dashboard in Exhibit 5.10. The colors in the column displaying the current six months (Current 6) and the column displaying the variance (Var) change from green (up) to red (down) as trends fluctuate. This feature is called conditional formatting in an Excel spreadsheet and is very flexible in SSRS. SSRS also allows users to interact with and add filters to a dashboard using parameters. The Locations, Providers, Procedure Classes, Plan Classes, Departments, and POS filters at the top of Exhibit 5.10 are parameters that allow the end user to quickly filter data. For example, a practice manager could see new bariatric Medicare patients at the North location.

Exhibit 5.11 is the way a gastrointestinal practice looks at referring physician data. The data does not have to be limited to new patients. This analysis factors in referrals for colonoscopies and for new patients. You can quickly see that some referrals send far more colonoscopies than new patients. Some of the reason may be clinical, such as how frequently the patient needs a colonoscopy. Other reasons may be how long the relationship has been established with the referring physician. A physician who has been referring for 20 years will have more repeat colonoscopy procedure referrals than a physician who just started last year.

EXHIBIT 5.11 REFERRING PHYSICIANS: SAMPLE DATA

Provider	Colonoscopy	New Pt	Grand Total
	447	139	586
Referring	308	211	519
	306	188	494
Physicians	251	197	448
	273	149	422
	314	105	419
Listed	282	131	413
	286	108	394
Here	230	149	379
	285	92	377
	255	109	364
	247	116	363
	237	123	360
	242	107	349
	262	83	345
	251	94	345
	269	74	343
	220	118	338

Physicians could have also slowed down significantly in new patient referrals while prior referrals continue to return for regularly scheduled colonoscopies. That is one reason to consider including the date of a last new patient referral on a report like this. Another approach would be to only report distinct patients so that the count of colonoscopies or other procedures does not double count patients receiving multiple colonoscopies. Selecting distinct patients is easily done in SQL Server, though practices without IT help could use Excel's Remove Duplicates feature to make this calculation.

Another way to customize the procedure and new patient analysis is to trend referrals by year. Practices can also analyze what kinds of patients the referring physicians send. Questions practices might want to ask include:

- Does one referral source send more Medicare patients?

- Does another referral source generate a higher percentage of Medicaid patients?
- Is one location or provider more likely to get better-paying referrals?
- Which physicians are more likely to obtain referrals?

PivotTables are a productive way to interactively study referral questions like these to better understand and capitalize on referral patterns Exhibit 5.12 is an example of a three-year trend based on a PivotTable.

EXHIBIT 5.12 REFERRING PHYSICIANS: PATTERNS

Referring Physicians	Colonoscopy			Colonoscopy Total	New Pt			New Pt Tot	Grand Total
	2015	2016	2017		2015	2016	2017		
	432	1,311	313	2,056	290	419	135	844	2,900
Sort by	680	562	359	1,601	257	234	126	617	2,218
	638	552	469	1,659	63	82	53	198	1,857
	530	420	318	1,268	192	202	123	517	1,785
Major	547	435	242	1,224	226	202	123	551	1,775
	517	431	324	1,272	170	172	60	402	1,674
	379	268	272	919	294	229	141	664	1,583
Referring	543	461	193	1,197	148	151	83	382	1,579
	497	351	242	1,090	206	169	112	487	1,577
	485	402	251	1,138	204	151	80	435	1,573
Physicians	460	430	298	1,188	145	154	76	375	1,563
	454	349	273	1,076	189	159	110	458	1,534
	372	315	322	1,009	192	165	111	468	1,477
Here	439	325	244	1,008	152	170	79	401	1,409
	303	296	220	819	135	144	89	368	1,187
	357	326	2	685	62	55	1	118	803
	30	103	114	247	28	96	63	187	434
	1	16	145	162	1	17	124	142	304
	53	50	40	143	58	47	41	146	289

Another practice analyzed a conversion rate by calculating the number of procedures per 100 new patients. The practice wanted to understand why some of the new patients did not result in procedures. Is it an insurance issue? Do the patients not qualify for the procedure? Are the patients getting a competing procedure from a different provider? These questions again require information that is often not readily available in a PM system. It may take some detective work, conversations with nurses, and reviewing prior authorizations to understand why some patients were not treated. Practices may have to take a representative sample of new patients instead of reviewing all new patients. If the study results in a better understanding of the practice's patients that helps the practice better serve and retain patients, the detective work will be well worth the effort.

A different practice, this one specializing in neurosurgery, calculated the time from initial visit to procedure by doctor. Neurosurgery is a very pre-authorization intensive specialty where documenting conservative care and qualifying for procedures is work intensive. Analyzing time to surgery by provider and by payer helped the practice see which providers had the most efficient processes to get patients qualified for surgery. The data can help a clinic develop best practices by payer to get procedures approved. The data may also be helpful in predicting how insurers view the practice in terms of quality of care.

ZIP CODES AND MAPPING

Another way to analyze new patients or specific procedures regardless of whether a practice relies on referrals is to review the zip codes stored in a patients' demographics. This approach has drawbacks for practices in southern locations who see an influx of seasonal patients, but most practices can benefit from a zip code analysis. A dataset of new patients could be defined by evaluation and management codes, or for this analysis some practices could define a new patient as a one who has not been to the practice in a certain number of months (or years). While this approach works for new patient visits, use caution when defining a procedure code-based dataset. Many procedures are billed with multiple procedure codes. Be sure to count patient visits or encounters, not procedure codes, or you may end up double counting procedures.

Once you have a dataset, you can use Excel (2013 or earlier) to map data. The examples in Exhibit 5.13 were generated in Excel by a Texas practice considering a new location. The first maps highlight regions with patients based on zip codes. The map uses shades of orange, purple, and blue to indicate the relative density of patients who currently visit one of the practice's existing three locations. Darker shades of orange, purple and blue indicate more patients, while lighter shades indicate fewer patients.

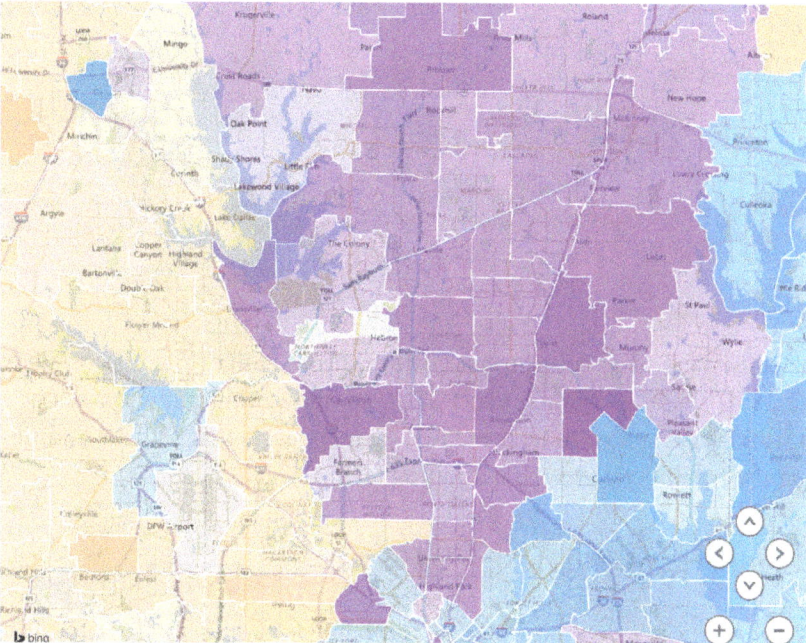

Once the practice understood which locations patients were currently visiting, the marketing team created this map to track overall patient population density regardless of which current practice location the patient was visiting. Again, darker shades indicate a higher density of patients.

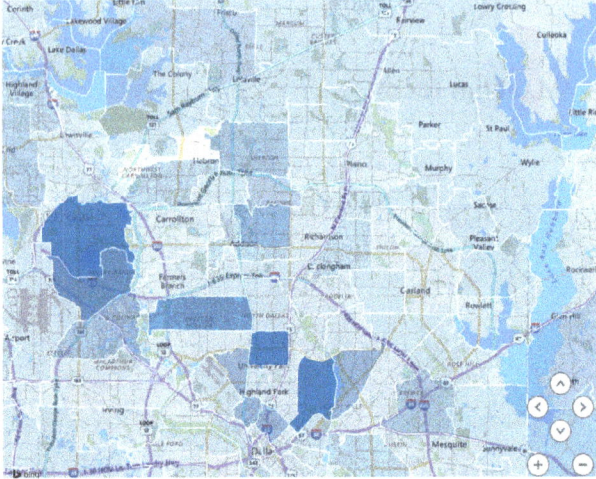

The third map used column height to indicate patient population density instead of shading regions. Excel 3D Map allows multiple ways to see the data, and the display can be presented on map layers that provide additional insights and direction to the marketing team.

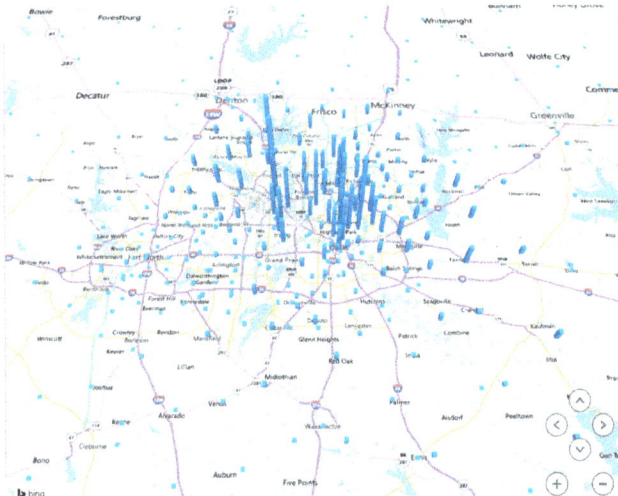

Zip code mapping is very useful when considering locations for a new clinic location. Use maps to determine where new patients live, which referring physicians would be key to support a new location, and which existing locations could be cannibalized by a new location. As with the colonoscopy example above, it doesn't just have to be new patients. Mapping procedures can be just as useful.

LOCATION LOYALTY AND PROVIDER LOYALTY

As part of analyzing the extent to which a new location may cannibalize an existing location, one practice took the analysis a step further. The marketing team wanted to analyze how loyal patients were to a given location. Here is a redacted version of the analysis:

EXHIBIT 5.16 LOCATION LOYALTY

LOCATION LOYALTY
Patient seen in the current year or prior 2 years

Row Labels	Sum of SameLocation	Sum of DifferentLocation	Sum of %
	18,939	12,309	60.6%
	22,692	7,273	75.7%
	35,837	10,531	77.3%
Grand Total	**77,468**	**30,113**	**72.0%**

The three closest locations to a proposed new location site were selected and then the following analysis was performed in SQL Server. First, the logic determined the first location a patient visited. Then the logic filtered out patients who had not visited those locations at least three times in the current year or prior two years. The PivotTable above in Exhibit 5.16 shows the percentage of subsequent visits that were at the same location compared to visits to a different practice location. Patients are much less loyal to the first location on the table as compared to the following two locations (60.6%

at the first location compared to 75.7% and 77.3% at the other locations). Patients closer to the first location may be more likely to change to support a new practice location. Clearly each of these variables is very practice-specific. A different practice might require more patient visits, more recent patient visits, or any of several other filters. The key is that an analysis like this can be done and can be customized to meet the specific needs of a practice. The dataset behind this analysis probably takes IT help, but it's likely more of a one-time analysis than an ongoing report.

Exhibit 5.17 is another way to think about patient loyalty.

EXHIBIT 5.17 PROVIDER LOYALTY

PROVIDER LOYALTY
Patient seen in the current year or prior 5 years

Row Labels	Sum of SameProvider	Sum of DifferentProvider	Sum of %
Provider 1	3,648	721	83.5%
Team A	52,772	13,056	80.2%
Team B	38,714	10,050	79.4%
Provider 2	3,114	1,674	65.0%
Provider 3	8,573	3,897	68.7%
Provider 4	16,047	7,494	68.2%
Team C	45,657	10,618	81.1%
Grand Total	**168,525**	**47,510**	**78.0%**

Using logic like the Location Loyalty analysis in Exhibit 5.16, this test examined how likely patients were to see the same provider they initially visited when they returned to the practice. The difference between Location Loyalty and Provider Loyalty is that providers may be a physician or an advanced practitioner who works with the physician. In the redacted analysis, some of the providers are shown as teams, meaning the provider or the advanced practitioner. Many factors are involved in how loyal patients are to a specific provider. One factor practices may have more control over is how hard it is to get into see that provider. Chapter 6 has several examples of measuring physician availability and ideas on how to improve patient access to the physician of their choice.

CMS DATA

Savvy practices can use data outside of their computer systems to analyze patient referral patterns. One source of data to consider is that provided by CMS. In response to a Freedom of Information Act request, CMS released data relating to providers who provide services to common patients. If two providers bill services to the same patient within 30 days, 60 days, 90 days, or 180 days, those two providers' NPI numbers are linked in the data. The data assumes a shared relationship between the first provider and the second provider if the two providers submit claims within those four date intervals. The data shows five columns:

- The first NPI number to render services
- The second NPI number to render services
- The number of visits
- The number of unique common patients, and
- The number of patients treated on the same day.

Exhibit 5.18 shows an example of the presumed shared relationship data.

EXHIBIT 5.18 NPI LINKED DATA FOR PROVIDERS' SHARED PATIENTS

FromNPI	ToNPI	Referrals	Beneficiaries	SameDay
1000000004	1548295421	25	11	8
1000000004	1790775229	60	22	30
1000026017	1598773715	35	15	18
1003000126	1003888777	32	12	0
1003000126	1003951625	147	78	27
1003000126	1003975400	51	28	1
1003000126	1013051119	24	15	1
1003000126	1013902600	45	25	3
1003000126	1023027109	29	21	3
1003000126	1023029964	42	23	0
1003000126	1033187000	119	34	2
1003000126	1033469317	33	19	3
1003000126	1043265804	68	26	34
1003000126	1053306746	94	47	41

The trick is to use the CMS data as a proxy for patient referrals. For example, if 45 patients saw Provider A and then saw Provider B, there is a good chance that at least some of those 45 patients were referred by Provider A to Provider B. By carefully analyzing the referral proxy data, practices can get an estimate of their share of referrals in a given market. Using the same example, if Provider A also had a relationship with Provider C that shared 90 patients, Provider B could estimate that she is getting about one-third (45 / (45 + 90)) of the patients referred by Provider A. Exhibit 5.19 groups all referrals to a practice in one column and referrals outside a practice separately in a PivotTable analyzing the CMS data.

EXHIBIT 5.19 GROUPED REFERRALS: REFERRED PATIENTS VS. NOT REFERRED PATIENTS

Group Name	(All)	
Referred By Zip	(All)	
Specialty	(All)	
Referred By County	(All)	
Hospital or Provider	Provider	

Row Labels	Sum of Referred	Sum of NOTReferred	Sum of %
+ Espino MD, Joey V.	437	219	66.6%
+ Petrillo MD, Eugenie	418		100.0%
+ Marciniak MD, Shayne A.	407	520	43.9%
+ Dash MD, Robert	365	385	48.7%
+ Gunther MD, Micah D.	332	277	54.5%
+ Disanto MD, Carletta E.	286	211	57.5%
+ Handy MD, Berta S.	261	130	66.8%
+ Rimer MD, Sharyn O.	245	234	51.1%
+ Fields MD, Grisel K.	237	261	47.6%
+ Dimauro MD, Rueben G.	233	134	63.5%
+ Loveland MD, Loura	223	114	66.2%
+ Dull MD, Janee	213	281	43.1%
+ Mayne MD, Francesca V.	204	109	65.2%
+ Mclendon MD, Ruthanne	201	76	72.6%

There are some issues to be aware of when using the CMS data. Though CMS releases four sets of data based on the interval between Provider A and Provider B (30, 60, 90 and 180 days), the 30-day data tends to have the least amount of noise in it. The longer the time between seeing Provider A and seeing Provider B, the higher the odds that something besides a referral is driving the shared patient relationship.

CMS considers a wide range of providers when creating this data. Ambulances and labs are very commonly added. To give some feel for the scope of this, the 2014 full-year data with a 30-day shared interval is over 55 million rows. The same data with a 180-day interval is over *138 million rows*. To even download that much data takes a tool much more powerful than Excel. SQL Server is the typical go to, but specialized statistical software packages are also used. Once the data is downloaded, practices may find can look for specific NPI numbers in the data. One approach would be to identify an important referral source to search for as the first provider in the data. Then, look for referral patterns from that source. Since the CMS data only includes NPI numbers, it is helpful to download an NPI database and cross-reference the NPI numbers. The NPI data will include a business mailing address and one practice address. Having only one address limits the ability to map data to see where referrals are coming from when providers practice at more than one location. The NPI data also includes multiple taxonomy codes which can be used to estimate provider specialties. Exhibits 5.20 and 5.21 use the NPI practice location zip code data to map presumed referrals using Excel's 3D Maps feature.

EXHIBIT 5.20 NPI 3D MAPPING: PART 1

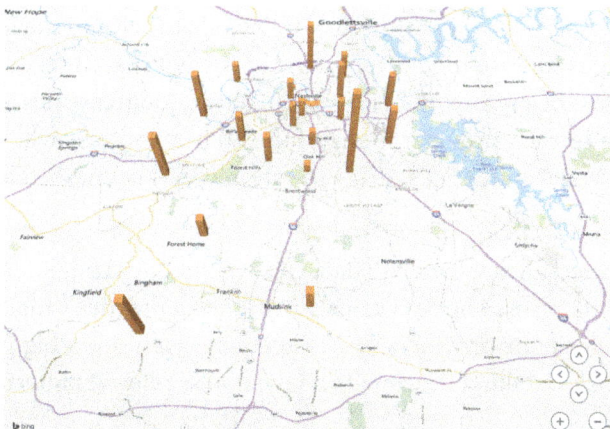

Exhibit 5.21 NPI 3D Mapping: Part 2

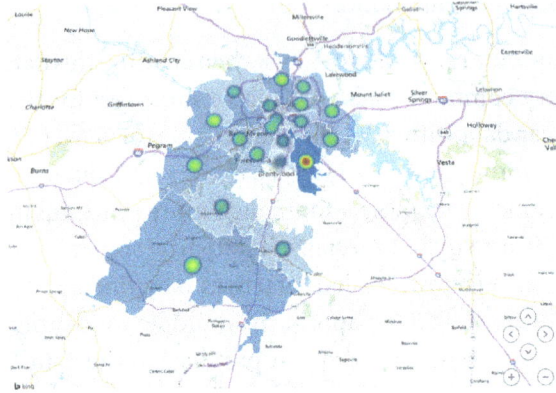

Using the taxonomy codes and a practice's general knowledge of their market helps filter out providers that are unlikely sources of referrals. By applying several levels of filtering, the massive amount of CMS data available can be made more manageable and thereby more useful.

Another complication with the NPI numbers is that the CMS data reflects how the claim was billed. If the claim is billed under a different NPI number than the practice is expecting, the data may not reflect the underlying referral patterns. If the NPI relates to a group or organization instead of an individual provider, it can be more difficult to determine the sources of referrals or how many referrals a provider might be making to competing practices.

CMS has also filtered the data to protect patient privacy. Relationships between Provider A and Provider B with fewer 11 than unique beneficiaries are excluded from the data. If a referral source has a shared relationship with eight providers in a group practice and the referral source sends 10 Medicare beneficiaries to each provider, none of the 80 beneficiaries will be included in the data. Major potential sources of referrals can be masked by the fewer than 11 beneficiaries rule.

Even with these caveats, the CMS data can give practices unparalleled insight into referral patterns. The data can also estimate a practice's market share of referrals from major providers. If Medicare referrals are a big part of your practice, consider taking the time to analyze your referral patterns.

118

CMS PROVIDER UTILIZATION DATA

Another potential source of outside data that can help practices attract patients is the Medicare Provider Utilization and Payment Data. This is another large dataset (2014 data was over nine million rows) that summarizes utilization and payment data by provider and procedure code. This dataset contains more identifying information than just the provider's NPI number, including zip code and specialty. The data also shows the number of times a procedure was billed to CMS, the number of unique beneficiaries, and the average charge by procedure code. The data has the same 11-beneficiary caveat as the other CMS dataset.

Practices familiar with procedure codes can group the codes into categories and analyze the data accordingly. Exhibit 5.22 is the way general surgery procedures could be studied by zip code using Excel.

EXHIBIT 5.22 PROCEDURE CODE MAPPING SAMPLE

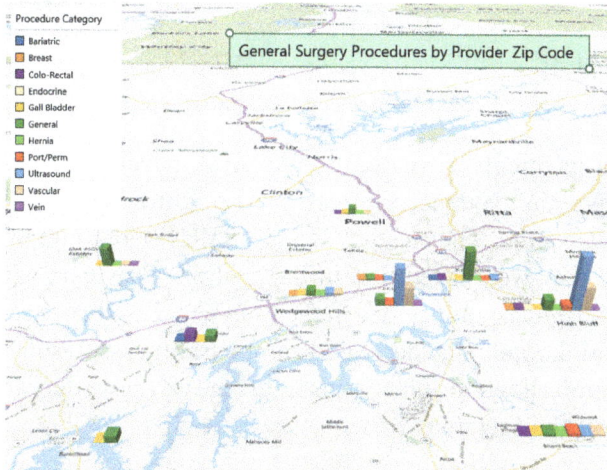

Keeping in mind the 11-beneficiary rule and the fact the data only includes Medicare patients, the provider utilization data could be used to estimate how many procedures are being done at a given location or by a competitor. Practices could estimate their market share by region for a given specialty or subspecialty using this data.

PAYERS

Payers in a market can impact efforts to attract patients. One practice noticed a change in payer mix because of the Accountable Care Act (ACA). As payers adjusted to the ACA and tailored networks accordingly, this practice's payer mix and market share changed. Providers who traditionally practiced in a hospital that was not in one of the narrow networks saw volumes decrease. To analyze the change in volumes and payer mix, the practice created the following analysis, first for the practice overall, and then for each individual provider.

EXHIBIT 5.23 wRVU PAYER VOLUME CHANGES

Financial Class	Sum of wRVU				Sum of Charge				Sum of Payments			
	2014	2015	2016	2017	2014	2015	2016	2017	2014	2015	2016	2017
ACA Payer	26,132	28,828	33,247	18,493	15.69%	16.64%	17.85%	15.74%	21.71%	24.41%	25.96%	22.82%
Non ACA Payer	22,035	22,675	22,962	14,933	14.94%	15.88%	15.04%	15.45%	17.13%	17.07%	17.09%	17.25%
Medicare	35,961	37,581	39,351	24,287	22.23%	21.64%	21.88%	21.50%	15.48%	14.34%	14.23%	14.00%
Payer C	10,701	11,123	12,315	7,922	6.33%	5.65%	6.72%	7.72%	7.69%	6.69%	8.04%	9.95%
Medicare HMO	21,380	22,373	24,070	14,762	12.78%	12.50%	12.72%	12.42%	8.81%	8.21%	7.52%	7.10%
Payer D	6,953	7,764	9,635	6,824	4.49%	4.82%	5.79%	6.30%	4.48%	4.93%	5.88%	6.17%
Payer E	5,106	5,384	7,325	4,477	3.35%	3.33%	4.43%	4.38%	3.55%	3.52%	5.26%	6.13%
Payer F	7,332	8,616	1,706	361	4.68%	5.04%	0.93%	0.32%	6.52%	7.33%	2.13%	0.56%
Payer G	5,818	6,060	7,107	4,922	3.59%	3.61%	4.11%	4.53%	3.56%	3.39%	3.86%	4.44%

Charges and payments increased for the ACA payer while the non-ACA payer's charges and payments decreased. Also notice the related changes in the work RVU values. The changes in work RVUs were so important to this practice that they were listed first in the analysis. Providers who primarily practiced at hospitals not included in the ACA payer's network saw decreased work RVUs and potentially decreased compensation as a result. Monitoring this information allows the practice to adjust the way providers are scheduled to better attract and retain patients.

Be aware of one other feature in this PivotTable. The 2017 wRVU column (18,493 wRVUs for the ACA payer) is a year-to-date calculation, not a full year like 2014-2016. Year-to-date calculations are harder in traditional PivotTables. This is an example of where Power Pivot's ability to use time intelligence to create YTD calculations is helpful. Power Pivot is discussed in Chapter 3.

PRIMARY CARE PRACTICE PANEL SIZE

Attracting patients is fantastic, but having capacity to see those patients is even better—it's all about panel size. Exhibit 5.24 is from a primary care practice located in a university town. The physicians were concerned about maintaining an appropriate patient panel size to accommodate the patients in the community. One of the physicians researched optimal panel size for primary care physicians and compared the current panel size to national averages. The calculation uses the current panel size, the average number of daily appointments, and the available appointments per year. Available appointments vary based on physician work load (some of the providers work part time) and schedules. Expected patient visits per year factors in national averages and the way the physicians practice. Those calculations lead to an ideal panel size. The far right calculation compares the current panel size to the ideal panel size. Doctors Green and Adams have a much higher patient panel size than the calculation projects.

Exhibit 5.24 Patient Panel Size Sample

Panel Size Year	PCP	Panel Size	Avg Daily Visits	Avail Appts Per Year	Expected Patient Visits Per Year	Ideal Panel Size	Over Ideal
2017	Wright	681	11.5	2,208	2.40	920	(239)
2018	Wright	1,071	15.0	2,803	3.00	1,059	12
2017	King	1,640	18.0	3,456	3.06	1,128	512
2018	King	1,528	17.6	3,379	3.38	1,001	527
2017	Scott	705	11.3	2,170	2.88	754	(49)
2018	Scott	1,087	15.0	2,957	3.00	966	121
2017	Green	1,892	20.0	3,917	3.00	1,222	670
2018	Green	1,869	21.0	3,974	4.00	1,123	746
2017	Baker	1,392	19.0	3,571	3.00	1,133	259
2018	Baker	1,320	18.0	3,514	3.00	1,017	303
2017	Adams	1,959	18.0	3,456	3.00	1,159	800
2018	Adams	1,868	18.0	3,437	3.00	1,060	808
2017	Nelson	1,346	18.0	3,475	3.00	1,186	160
2018	Nelson	1,313	18.0	3,398	3.00	1,007	306
2017	Hill	1,397	16.0	2,592	3.00	972	425
2018	Hill	1,297	16.0	2,458	3.00	821	476

This calculation is very labor-intensive, so after the practice did the initial calculation, they did not take the time to run the numbers again. What analyses in your practice are so time-consuming that you do not have the time to re-run the numbers?

The practice carefully reviewed the components of the calculation and added data to the data warehouse on physician workload and preferences to automate the calculation so it can be run on demand. Since the calculation is intensive, it can also be set to run monthly so that when the administrators want to review the numbers they do not have to wait for the code to run. Because the calculations run overnight, the numbers are available as soon as the spreadsheet opens. The data is displayed for two years. Because the data is stored in the data warehouse, ideal panel size can be trended over time to see if patient access is improving.

There are many more examples of evaluating patient access and how difficult it can be to get an appointment with a provider in Chapter 6.

CHAPTER 6

SEEING AND MANAGING THE FUTURE BY ANALYZING APPOINTMENTS

This is a long chapter for a reason. Appointment data is as close as practices can come to seeing the future. There are a wide variety of revenue-enhancing and cost-saving options available to groups who cleverly use appointment data to see upcoming opportunities. Mining appointments data is a solid way administrators can run their practice like a business. As lengthy as this chapter is, it's just the tip of the iceberg when it comes to leveraging appointment data.

Obviously, no one can truly see the future, but a careful analysis of scheduled patient appointments can come very close. Imagine what retailers would stock if they knew exactly how many customers planned to come to their store tomorrow. Imagine how precise a retailers' staffing schedule would be if they knew how many people would be in the store at any given time. A manufacturer who knew how many and which products would be ordered and sold tomorrow, next week, or next month would produce differently. Imagine what a restaurant would do if they knew what their customers would order tomorrow. Are they vegan or are they all preparing for a barbeque? Stores would stock, staff and manage to meet their customers' predicted expectations.

Coupling that knowledge of known patient arrivals tomorrow with the in-depth knowledge practices have about their patients is uniquely powerful. A restaurant might know about an upcoming dinner reservation, but how many restaurants would know that the customer isn't ordering broccoli under any circumstances? Think about the tremendous savings available to traditional businesses and the reduction of waste if those businesses had a crystal ball to predict how business would be next week or next month.

Prominent online retailers are getting better at knowing their customers, but those retailers do not have a detailed health history with their established patients. This chapter isn't an argument to use patient data to market to customers as traditional businesses might. Instead, it's about practices proactively serving patients better by knowing and anticipating their needs. Consider a practice that follows up on no shows and canceled appointments for patients with serious health concerns to make sure those patients are treated. And there are examples of other practices tracking canceled appointments regardless of health status to ensure patients who need to see a provider are rescheduled quickly, since experience has shown that many canceled patients end up being lost to the practice. The chapter also has examples that are on the leading edge of how a medical practice can manage the requirements of value-based healthcare contracting, using data to design lean, cost-efficient, and medically effective workflows.

This chapter includes examples of practices using appointment data to improve patient access to care. Improving access to care means having more of the right providers available to be scheduled. It means shorter wait times by managing unsold appointments, reducing no shows, and getting patients to the right provider faster. Watch for ways to measure patient access, such as the number of days to the third next available appointment and the average days to schedule an appointment.

There are financial implications to managing appointments. Clearly no-show patients are lost revenue, but patient appointments are also an excellent opportunity to collect from patients. Collecting copays reduces accounts receivable balances and the number of days in accounts receivable. Patient appointments are also an opportune time to collect old patient balances. These topics are also discussed in Chapter 7.

This chapter reveals how practices measure the duration of patient appointments from check in through check out. One practice used scheduling data to optimize front desk staff and see more patients without hiring more front desk employees. Another used patient appointments to save money by reducing the need to buy expensive equipment.

There are also clinical implications to managing appointments. Practices can see where providers are scheduled and adjust clinical staff schedules to better serve patients and providers. Seeing upcoming open surgery appointments can help patients waiting for a procedure get treated sooner. Schedules can also be reviewed to make certain that the necessary pathology or lab test results are available before the patient arrives. Using clinical information to better serve patients with upcoming appointments has become even more important for many practices.

Several times each year, I visit Ortho NorthEast in Fort Wayne, Indiana. I fly out of Salt Lake City, and the best way for me to fly to Fort Wayne is through Detroit. One afternoon on my way to the Fort Wayne airport to catch a flight home, I got a text message from Delta saying the flight was delayed. One delay led to another and eventually the flight was about six hours delayed. By the time the flight left for Detroit, everyone from Fort Wayne who needed to be in Detroit had either made the two-and-a-half-hour drive to Detroit or had changed their travel plans. My flight from Fort Wayne to Detroit that night looked like this:

EXHIBIT 6.1 EMPTY DELTA FLIGHT TO DETROIT

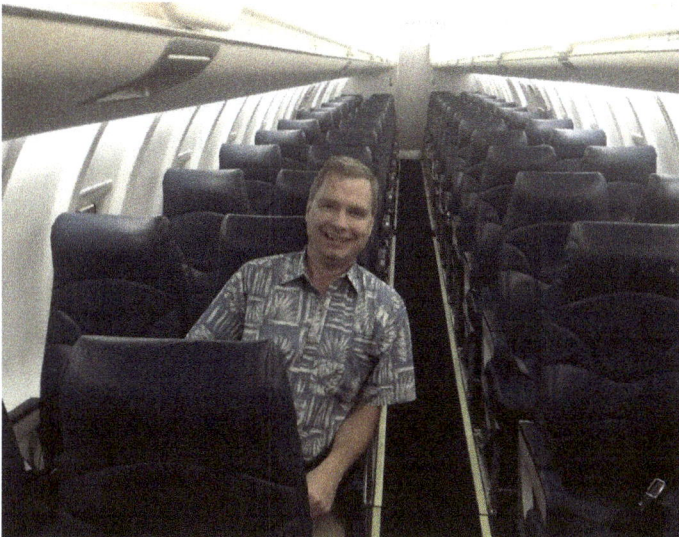

The flight left with two pilots, a flight attendant, and me. Delta clearly lost money on that flight, but the plane needed to be in Detroit to go further north in Michigan later that night. Airlines and medical practices are both concerned about using their resources as efficiently as possible. The bottom line for many practices is that provider time is a precious resource and analyzing appointments provides many opportunities to manage and leverage that resource.

Unsold appointments are like that Delta flight. Once the time of the appointment is past, the opportunity to sell that appointment is past. Managing capacity and reducing unsold appointments is a major topic of this chapter.

UNSOLD APPOINTMENTS

There are 10 different examples of unsold appointments in this section, and there could have been even more examples. But each tool that follows is customized to meet each practice's needs in the way the practice needed help.

UNSOLD APPOINTMENTS PIVOTTABLE

Depending on the PM system, unsold appointments can be difficult to quantify. PM systems track and store kept appointments, but to save space some PM systems do not store unsold appointments or the template data to determine unsold appointments. For example, GE's Centricity™ PM software only stores historical template data for 30 days. To track unsold appointments, practices need to calculate unsold appointments and store the data before the template data is purged. To work around this limitation, practices can preserve unsold appointment data in a data warehouse. It might help to store the date, location, provider, appointment type, or other relevant information about the unsold appointment to make tracking and trending unsold appointments easier in the future. Exhibit 6.2 is an example from a practice that tracks unsold appointments.

EXHIBIT 6.2 UNSOLD APPOINTMENTS: TRACKING

UNSOLD APPOINTMENTS

Years	2017
ApptStart	(All)
New Est Test	(All)
Provider Category	(All)
Facility	(All)

Count of Facility	Colu								
Row Labels	Jan	Feb	Mar	Apr	May	Jun	Jul	Aug	Grand Total
Bingaman FNP-C, Beth	35	26	33	22	37	58	19	19	249
Bowman MD, Michael H	24	26	21	60	71	71	42	21	336
Boyce MD, Leslie H	76	73	61	76	163	118	51	61	679
Carnes MD, Kenneth M	25	26	14	38	28	15	17	10	173
Carnes MD, Paul	11	16	16	10	9	16	17	13	108
Carroll ANP, Stacey	44	42	45	39	88	62	42	31	393
Cato PA-C, Kelsie	65	9	116	34	23	105	67	56	475
Dunne PA, Laurie	56	60	63	40	72	44	15	23	373
EEG Room 1	12	12	18	18	17	13	19	12	121
EEG Room 1 Durham	40	39	48	40	64	46	38	40	355
EEG Room 2	21	17	15	16	29	14	14	15	141
EEG Room 3	13	11	17	11	30	16	12	12	122
EEG Room 4	25	23	31	30	36	30	27	18	220
EEG Room 5	42	42	48	39	66	61	36	33	367
Ferrell MD, William G	21	16	42	19	42	36	18	15	209

This first example is a PivotTable that allows the practice to see unsold appointments by provider, provider category, date, facility, and appointment type. The top provider in the PivotTable went from 22 unsold appointments in April to 37 unsold appointments in May to 58 unsold appointments in June. To use the airplane analogy, this flight was taking off with fewer and fewer passengers. The PivotTable made it easy to look for trends underlying the increase. The PivotTable also made it easy to drill down to see the actual unsold appointment slots. One of the things the practice learned is that the PM system was treating no-show appointments as unsold appointment slots. An unsold appointment slot that was never filled is different problem than an unsold appointment slot that was "sold" to a patient who did not show up for the appointment. That insight helped the practice focus on reducing no-show appointments.

UNSOLD APPOINTMENTS PIVOT TABLE WITH NO SHOWS

A different medical group analyzed unsold appointments using a different PivotTable, as shown in Exhibit 6.3.

EXHIBIT 6.3 UNSOLD APPOINTMENTS: WITH NO SHOWS

Months	(All)	
ApptStart	(All)	
Years	2017	
Provider	(All)	
Facility	(Multiple Items)	

Count of Facility	Column Labels			
Row Labels	Canceled	No Show/Short Notice	Unsold	Grand Total
Providers and Other Appointment Resources Listed Here	650	1,138	1,821	3,609
			3,173	3,173
	787	1,369	738	2,894
	63	107	1,724	1,894
	176	83	557	816
	236	83	324	643
	68	97	447	612
	11		454	465
	103	116	197	416
	94	62	30	186
	44	18	71	133
	1	5	125	131
	44	56	22	122
	44	73	4	121
	15	3	42	60
			41	41
	10	3	25	38
	11	22		33
	7	5	20	32

Instead of having one unsold appointments bucket, this practice separated no-show patients into another category. As they continued to analyze the data, the practice administrator and managers realized that, for this practice, canceling an appointment within 24 hours was much like not showing up for the appointment since it was hard to fill appointment slots in that short time frame. When unsold appointments still seemed high, the administrator asked for a third category, appointments that were canceled more than 24 hours before the appointment time (the "canceled" column in Exhibit 6.3). Now the practice has three separate sections of unsold appointments to reduce.

An unsold appointment that resulted from a cancellation more than 24 hours before the appointment time needs more attention from the scheduling department. No-show appointments can be addressed differently and are a topic later in this chapter. Appointments that were never sold are a different problem. This practice is analyzing templates to see if certain appointment days of the week, locations, or appointment types are consistently hard to fill. Appointment templates, locations, or schedules may need to be adjusted to meet changing patient demands.

Some practices may find their templates are too rigorous and need to be more flexible. For example, if a provider has lots of unsold established patient appointments but it takes five weeks for a new patient to see the provider, the appointment template might need more new patient slots. The appointment template may also need more flexible appointment slots that allow one new patient or two established patients to book the slot.

UNSOLD APPOINTMENTS AS A PERCENTAGE OF SOLD APPOINTMENTS

A Rocky Mountain practice looked at unsold appointments as a percentage of sold appointments. Exhibit 6.4 shows that on many days, every appointment was sold. On other days, however, there were a significant number of unsold appointments. The PivotTable analysis makes it easy to understand whether the days with unsold appointments differed in terms of location, appointment type, time of day, or other factors.

EXHIBIT 6.4 UNSOLD APPOINTMENTS: A PERCENTAGE OF SOLD APPOINTMENTS

Row Labels	Unsold Count	%	Sold Count	%	Total Count	Total %
Aug	25	6.2%	377	93.8%	402	100.0%
1-Aug	3	16.7%	15	83.3%	18	100.0%
2-Aug	1	3.8%	25	96.2%	26	100.0%
3-Aug		0.0%	2	100.0%	2	100.0%
4-Aug		0.0%	24	100.0%	24	100.0%
7-Aug	1	3.8%	25	96.2%	26	100.0%
8-Aug		0.0%	2	100.0%	2	100.0%
9-Aug	1	4.3%	22	95.7%	23	100.0%
10-Aug		0.0%	3	100.0%	3	100.0%
11-Aug	3	12.5%	21	87.5%	24	100.0%
14-Aug	2	7.4%	25	92.6%	27	100.0%
15-Aug		0.0%	23	100.0%	23	100.0%
16-Aug		0.0%	22	100.0%	22	100.0%
17-Aug		0.0%	1	100.0%	1	100.0%
18-Aug	1	3.3%	29	96.7%	30	100.0%
21-Aug		0.0%	3	100.0%	3	100.0%
22-Aug		0.0%	2	100.0%	2	100.0%
23-Aug	3	10.7%	25	89.3%	28	100.0%
24-Aug	6	30.0%	14	70.0%	20	100.0%
25-Aug	2	7.7%	24	92.3%	26	100.0%
28-Aug		0.0%	26	100.0%	26	100.0%
29-Aug	1	5.3%	18	94.7%	19	100.0%
30-Aug	1	3.7%	26	96.3%	27	100.0%
Grand Total	25	6.2%	377	93.8%	402	100.0%

UNSOLD APPOINTMENTS FOR A NEW PROVIDER

The practice in Exhibit 6.5 focuses on appointments for procedures by tracking those appointment types in a separate SSRS email. The practice also had a brand-new provider whose schedule was important to fill. Procedure appointments for that new provider are the main component of this daily email. The status column lists all open appointment slots.

EXHIBIT 6.5 UNSOLD APPOINTMENTS: APPOINTMENTS BY PROCEDURE TYPES

Open Procedure Appointments as of 8/31/20

Provider	Appt Date	Appt Time	Loc	Status
	8/31/2017	3:00PM	PL	Open
	9/1/2017	11:00AM	ND	Open
	9/1/2017	3:30PM	ND	Open
	9/4/2017	8:00AM	LC	Open
	9/4/2017	9:00AM	LC	Open
	9/4/2017	10:00AM	LC	Open
	9/4/2017	11:00AM	ND	Open
	9/4/2017	11:00AM	BA	Open
	9/4/2017	11:00AM	ND	Open
	9/4/2017	11:00AM	LC	Open
	9/4/2017	11:00AM	BA	Open
	9/4/2017	11:15AM	ND	Open
	9/4/2017	11:15AM	LC	Open
	9/4/2017	11:15AM	PL	Open
	9/4/2017	11:15AM	ND	Open
	9/4/2017	1:30PM	LC	Open
	9/4/2017	2:30PM	LC	Open

UNSOLD APPOINTMENTS SSRS TRIAGE TOOL

The Southwest practice in Exhibit 6.6 has a different problem. Most PM software does a reasonably good job of displaying open appointments across locations by provider. This practice needed a better tool to display the five next open appointment slots by appointment type by location by provider to support a triage nurse who is also answering calls and scheduling appointments. An online dashboard built with SSRS has filtering parameters at the top to show the practice what they needed to see to book appointments more efficiently than the PM software would allow. Employees can refresh this dashboard on demand throughout the day.

Exhibit 6.6 Unsold Appointments: SSRS Triage Tool

Open Appointments as of 8/31/2017 02:36 PM

Provider						
Appt Category	ALL					
Location	ALL					
		1	**2**	**3**	**4**	**5**
		09/06/17 11:30 AM	09/13/17 11:30 AM	09/20/17 11:30 AM	09/27/17 11:30 AM	10/02/17 11:30 AM
	Established	09/12/17 08:45 AM	09/12/17 09:00 AM	09/12/17 09:15 AM	09/12/17 09:30 AM	09/12/17 09:45 AM
		09/04/17 01:30 PM	09/04/17 01:30 PM	09/04/17 01:45 PM	09/04/17 02:15 PM	09/04/17 02:15 PM
		09/04/17 08:00 AM	09/04/17 08:00 AM	09/04/17 08:15 AM	09/04/17 08:30 AM	09/04/17 08:45 AM
	New Patient	09/12/17 09:00 AM	09/12/17 09:45 AM	09/12/17 10:00 AM	09/12/17 10:30 AM	09/12/17 11:00 AM
		09/04/17 01:30 PM	09/04/17 01:45 PM	09/04/17 02:00 PM	09/04/17 02:30 PM	09/04/17 03:00 PM
		09/04/17 08:15 AM	09/04/17 08:30 AM	09/04/17 09:00 AM	09/04/17 09:15 AM	09/04/17 09:30 AM

UNSOLD APPOINTMENTS DATA-DRIVEN EMAIL

One way to address canceled appointments quickly is to use a data-driven email built with SSRS. Recall that a data-driven email only sends an email if there is data to report. Exhibit 6.7 is an example email from a practice with 10 providers. The email is sent to the scheduling department every 15 minutes if an appointment has been canceled in the last 15 minutes. The logic stores canceled appointments that have been reported so that cancellations only appear once on an email. The email includes conditional formatting logic to highlight appointments that the practice especially wants to fill, such as procedure appointments.

Exhibit 6.7 Unsold Appointments: Data Driven Email

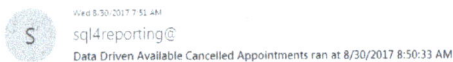

Wed 8/30/2017 7:51 AM

S sql4reporting@

Data Driven Available Cancelled Appointments ran at 8/30/2017 8:50:33 AM

To

Cc

This message was sent with High importance.
If there are problems with how this message is displayed, click here to view it in a web browser.

Recently Cancelled Appointments as of 8/30/2017 8:50 AM

Open Appointment	Loc	Acct Num
8/30/2017 1:30 PM		230787

There are trade-offs to data driven emails sent frequently during the day. The software needs to check for cancellations during normal business hours, which may slow down the system the rest of the practice is using to bill charges, record payments, and enter patient data. The emails can only come as often as the scheduling staff has time and resources to respond to the information. This practice was trying to solve a specific problem. Look at the chart in Exhibit 6.8.

EXHIBIT 6.8 UNSOLD APPOINTMENTS: NO SHOW TRACKING CHART 2011

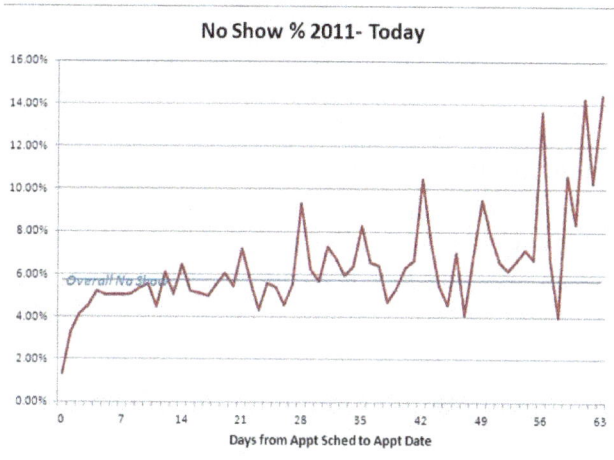

The practice tracked historical no-show rates going back several years. The key to the chart is the x-axis. The x-axis tracks the number of days from the date the appointment was created to the date of the actual appointment. After 2-3 days, the no-show rate doubles. The practice manager was concerned that if the scheduling department could not get a patient an appointment within that 2-3-day window that the patients would make the appointment and then try to get an earlier appointment with a competing provider. Patients who could get an earlier appointment with a competing provider would then either not show up or cancel their appointment right before the appointment time. The data-driven email allowed the scheduling department to quickly identify newly opened appointment slots and fill those slots. The practice had to make other workflow changes to make providers available sooner and to deal with patient eligibility and benefits issues. As the workflow changed, the 10-provider practice was able to fill 250 appointment slots in that 2-3-day window in one week. Not only is their airplane taking off full, but new customers are being added to the practice, resulting in procedures and opportunities for more appointments that the practice would not have had. The data-driven appointment email is a major success.

UNSOLD CANCELED APPOINTMENTS

If real-time data and a data-driven email isn't an option for your practice, Exhibit 6.9 has another example of tracking canceled appointments. This PM system stored the prior appointment information when the appointment slot became available, so that information was included in the daily email. In other words, the PM system knows that the open appointment slot on Monday at 8:45 used to be filled by Mrs. Jones, and that knowing the previous patient's name helped the scheduling staff, so Mrs. Jones' name is included in the email (in the masked, "Prior Patient" column). The yellow appointment categories are appointments that the practice was specifically interested in filling. SSRS automatically highlights those appointments based on logic built into the email.

EXHIBIT 6.9 UNSOLD APPOINTMENTS: CANCELED APPOINTMENTS

Available Cancelled Appointments as of 8/31/2017 3:08 PM

Open Appointment	Loc	Appt Category	Prior Acct	Prior Patient	Last Change Date
8/31/2017 4:30 PM		Procedure/Filler	3063187		8/31/2017 9:37:33 AM
9/1/2017 9:15 AM		Established	2340552		8/31/2017 1:12:00 PM
9/5/2017 7:45 AM		Established	3128928		8/31/2017 2:55:02 PM
9/6/2017 8:30 AM		MOHS Surgery	211286		8/29/2017 11:24:20 AM
9/6/2017 10:45 AM		Nurse Only	3157078		8/31/2017 11:36:27 AM
9/1/2017 10:00 AM		Established	5199		8/30/2017 1:50:20 PM
9/1/2017 10:15 AM		Established	3064967		8/30/2017 1:33:05 PM
9/1/2017 10:30 AM		Established	3174319		8/30/2017 11:27:00 AM
9/1/2017 10:30 AM		Established	3174319		8/30/2017 11:27:00 AM
9/1/2017 1:15 PM		Established	3067201		8/31/2017 1:45:03 PM

UNSOLD APPOINTMENTS CANCELED YESTERDAY

A neurology practice in Exhibit 6.10 looks at canceled appointments another way. This is a daily, early-morning email that goes to the call center. Every appointment that was canceled yesterday that is for an appointment date in the next 30 days is included in the email. The practice has a wait list, but the PM system doesn't have a straightforward way to help the call center fill canceled appointments from that wait list. The call center uses this email to match canceled appointment slots with waitlisted patients. The way this call center is structured, it makes the most sense to organize the email by provider category and then by provider. The data is sorted to display the soonest appointments first.

EXHIBIT 6.10 UNSOLD APPOINTMENTS: YESTERDAY'S CANCELED APPOINTMENTS

Yesterday's Cancelled Appointments as of 8/31/2017

Appt Start	Facility	Appt Type
9/5/2017 8:30:00 AM		Established Patient(P) - 15
9/27/2017 10:30:00 AM		New Patient (P) - 30
9/5/2017 9:40:00 AM		Botox (P) - 20
9/5/2017 3:00:00 PM		Established Patient(P) - 20
9/5/2017 3:00:00 PM		Established Patient(P) - 20
9/1/2017 1:00:00 PM		Established Patient(P) - 15
9/27/2017 9:15:00 AM		New Patient (P) - 45

UNSOLD APPOINTMENTS TODAY AND TOMORROW

Exhibit 6.11 is a different way to communicate open appointment slots. Exhibit 6.10 showed appointments canceled yesterday. This early-morning email shows all appointment slots for today and tomorrow regardless of why the slot is available. (Friday's email shows slots for Friday and the following

Monday.) Practices with fewer providers may be able to manage cancellations more easily, but this practice has over 70 providers and a large, centralized call center. The email helps ensure that appointments that can be filled are filled. A PM system with a faster, more effective way to waitlist patients may also change the frequency of these emails or the information included on the email.

EXHIBIT 6.11 UNSOLD APPOINTMENTS: OPEN APPOINTMENTS TODAY AND TOMORROW

Open Appointment Slots Today and Tomorrow as of 8/31/2017

Appt Start	Facility	Category	Type
8/31/2017 8:30:00 AM			WORK-IN (P) - 15
8/31/2017 3:15:00 PM			TRIAGE Work-In (P) - 45
8/31/2017 4:00:00 PM			TRIAGE Work-In (P) - 45
8/31/2017 8:30:00 AM			New Sleep Patient - 30
8/31/2017 11:15:00 AM			WORK-IN (P) - 15
9/1/2017 11:15:00 AM			WORK-IN (P) - 15
9/1/2017 3:15:00 PM			TRIAGE Work-In (P) - 45
9/1/2017 4:00:00 PM			TRIAGE Work-In (P) - 45
9/1/2017 1:00:00 PM			Established Patient(P) - 15

UNSOLD APPOINTMENTS INCLUDING ADD-IN APPOINTMENTS

A different example of analyzing unsold appointments is shown in Exhibit 6.12. This PivotTable looks at unsold appointments as a percentage of total appointments, with a twist. The practice is flexible enough to add-in patients to be seen on the same day. Creating add-in appointments makes the percentage of appointments sold look higher than it actually is, since the practice only creates add-in appointments that will be filled immediately. The PivotTable tracks those "Added and Sold" appointments separately. The PivotTable analyzes unsold appointments by provider, location, and day of the week to reduce the number of unsold appointments and better manage add-in appointments. Days with high numbers of add-in appointments and unsold appointments indicate opportunities to better manage scheduling templates to fill existing appointments and reduce add-in appointments.

EXHIBIT 6.12 UNSOLD APPOINTMENTS: A PERCENTAGE OF SOLD APPOINTMENTS WITH ADD IN APPOINTMENTS

SOLD VS UNSOLD APPOINTMENTS | AVERAGE TEMPLATE SLOTS/WEEK

	183
	209
	127
	125
	176
	48
Appt Category (Multiple Items)	128
Years (All)	130
Months (All)	122
Slot Date (All)	256

Count of Slot Status Column Labels

Row Labels	Sold	Added and Sold	Unsold	Sold	Added and Sold	Unsold	Sold	Added and Sold	Unsold	Grand Total
	92.81%	1.30%	5.89%	41.87% 87.54%	1.88% 10.58% 55.97%	98.01%	1.42% 0.57%	2.16%		100.00%
Monday	91.30%	1.27%	7.43%	92.37% 98.48%	1.52% 0.00% 6.80%	100.00%	0.00% 0.00%	0.83%		100.00%
Tuesday	98.48%	1.45%	0.06%	55.63% 88.03%	1.58% 10.38% 44.37%			0.00%		100.00%
Wednesday	90.89%	1.25%	7.86%	88.26% 98.25%	1.75% 0.00% 11.74%			0.00%		100.00%
Thursday				0.00% 87.82%	1.85% 10.33% 100.00%			0.00%		100.00%
Friday				0.00% 85.30%	2.08% 12.63% 100.00%			0.00%		100.00%
Saturday				0.00% 100.00%	0.00% 0.00% 10.63%	97.87%	1.52% 0.61%	89.37%		100.00%
				0.00% 87.51%	4.70% 7.79% 36.40%	86.63%	4.24% 9.13%	63.60%		100.00%
Monday				0.00% 88.39%	4.16% 7.45% 66.92%	87.06%	5.45% 7.49%	33.08%		100.00%
Tuesday				0.00% 87.06%	4.98% 7.96% 100.00%			0.00%		100.00%
Wednesday				0.00%		0.00% 88.08%	4.28% 7.64%	100.00%		100.00%
Thursday				0.00%		0.00% 90.35%	3.82% 5.83%	100.00%		100.00%
Friday				0.00%		0.00% 78.04%	4.31% 17.66%	100.00%		100.00%

SOURCE: *MGMA 2016 PRACTICE OPERATIONS REPORT: BASED ON 2015 SURVEY DATA*

AS YOUR PRACTICE CONSIDERS HOW TO REDUCE UNSOLD APPOINTMENT SLOTS AND MAXIMIZE PROVIDERS' TIME, CONSIDER THIS CHART FROM MGMA'S PRACTICE OPERATIONS REPORT. THESE MEDIAN APPOINTMENT SLOTS PER DAY PER PROVIDER BY SPECIALTY TYPE WILL GIVE YOU A GOOD SENSE OF WHAT OTHER PRACTICES ARE DOING.

EXHIBIT 6.13 MEDIAN APPOINTMENT SLOTS PER DAY PER PROVIDER

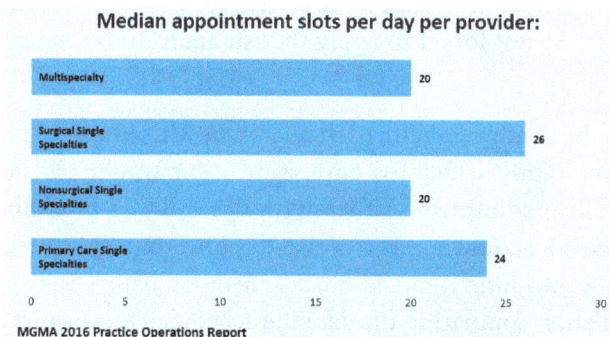

Median appointment slots per day per provider:

Multispecialty	20
Surgical Single Specialties	26
Nonsurgical Single Specialties	20
Primary Care Single Specialties	24

MGMA 2016 Practice Operations Report

BLOCKED APPOINTMENTS

Most systems will report on appointments, but reporting on appointment templates are a different question. PM systems handle blocked appointments differently, but the software offers functionality to prevent appointments from being scheduled at certain times or days. If an airline blocks a dozen seats on the plane, those seats are empty on every flight. Depending on the PM system, it can be difficult to get reports on how many appointments or how much time is blocked by provider by week or month. One example to consider is Exhibit 7.23 in Chapter 7 on resource utilization. There the question is productivity, or how much of a provider's overall schedule is being used by patient appointments. The numerator is the total number of hours or appointments booked. The denominator is the total number of hours or appointments available.

Comparing that denominator to other providers leads to analyzing how many hours a provider is available to see patients. The number of hours available can be complicated by weekly schedules (providers who take every other Friday off) or by vacation schedules.

When looking at how much availability a provider has, the practice needs to consider whether some providers allow their schedule to be double booked (booking more than one patient appointment in a time slot). This will complicate comparisons between providers. Comparing part-time to full-time providers is another issue. Call schedules may also complicate provider availability comparisons even further. The key is to find a calculation that makes sense in your practice environment that makes comparison to other providers straightforward. Once there is an agreed upon standard for blocked appointments, do not forget to apply that standard to resources other than providers.

A practice in the Southwest had a particular issue with advanced practitioners. On upcoming lightly scheduled days, a provider would ask staff to move existing patient appointments earlier in the day and then block the afternoon so that the provider could take rest of that day off. Some PM systems can solve this issue by controlling rights to block schedules. This practice designed a simple calculation comparing the date the schedule block was created to the date of the blocked schedule. An SSRS email to the practice administrator reported any recent blocks where the block date was too close to the schedule date. Blocking appointment templates just a few days out was a red flag for this practice that Exhibit 6.14 helped solve.

EXHIBIT 6.14 BLOCKED APPOINTMENTS: TRACKING

Provider	Appt Start	Appt Stop	Minutes	Description	Block Type	Action
	07/29/2016 12:00 AM	07/29/2016 11:59 PM	1439	PER DR	Block	Addition
	08/01/2016 12:00 AM	08/01/2016 11:30 AM	690		Block	Addition
	09/23/2016 12:00 AM	09/23/2016 11:59 PM	1439		Block	Addition
	07/29/2016 12:00 AM	07/29/2016 11:59 PM	1439		Block	Change

The email tracks the provider whose schedule was changed and the staff member who changed the block. The description column is the reason for the block as entered in the scheduling module. The circled change blocked the morning schedule to 11:30 for a provider. This may be a change to investigate, especially if it is part of a pattern. The bottom row is a change to a block. Those changes have been an issue for the practice, so changes are highlighted in the email.

HOLDING APPOINTMENTS SLOTS OPEN

Some practices will hold specific appointment types open in hopes of filling the appointment for a specific procedure, only releasing those appointment types as the date of the appointment gets closer. For example, a dermatology provider who wants to increase cosmetic business creates appointment slots specifically for cosmetic patients. If those appointment slots aren't filled 2-3 days before the appointment, the cosmetic slot can now be filled with other types of appointments. Pediatric and family practices might do something similar for sick patients and open those slots to other patients on the same day.

The key is to identify these flexible appointment slots in the schedule so that practices can evaluate whether the unsold flexible appointment rate is unacceptably high. Tracking these flexible appointment slots is important. If the workflow is to change the appointment type if the appointment is unfilled, the changing appointment type may be difficult to mine in PM data. To use the cosmetic patient example, if the cosmetic appointment is changed to a dermatology appointment two days before the appointment date and the slot goes unfilled, the data may look like an unsold dermatology appointment. As any medical provider knows, misdiagnosing the problem leads to the wrong solution.

A better solution includes several parts. Identify unsold flexible appointments earlier like the practice in Exhibit 6.14 earlier in this chapter. The notification may even be an automatic email like Exhibit 6.15. Maintain an easy to use waitlist for patients, which seems difficult in some PM systems. Make eligibility and benefits determinations as quickly as possible to get patients seen. Measure unsold flexible appointments and measure success in converting flexible appointments.

MGMA's 2016 Practice Operations Report gives a sense for how other practices manage same-day appointments:.

EXHIBIT 6.15 MEDIAN OF SAME DAY APPOINTMENTS

Median percentage of appointments that are same-day appointments:

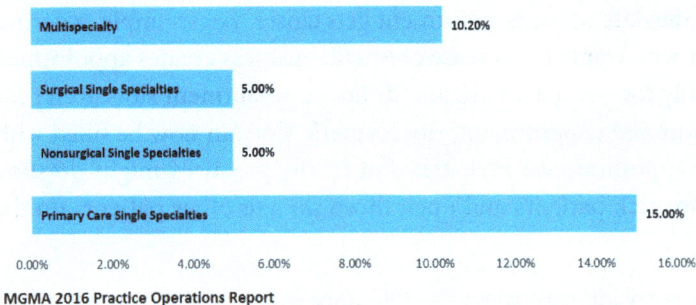

Specialty	Percentage
Multispecialty	10.20%
Surgical Single Specialties	5.00%
Nonsurgical Single Specialties	5.00%
Primary Care Single Specialties	15.00%

MGMA 2016 Practice Operations Report

OVERBOOKED APPOINTMENTS

Exhibit 6.16 is an example of how one practice tracks overbooked appointments using a daily email. Some practices' templates and schedule practices routinely build in overbooked appointment slots. Other practices limit overbooking to rare circumstances. This practice doesn't have many overbooked appointment slots and uses the email to alert front desk staff to plan accordingly.

EXHIBIT 6.16 OVERBOOKED APPOINTMENTS SLOTS

Overbooked Appointment Slots as of 8/31/2017

Start	Patient	Acct Number	Provider	Facility	Appt Type	Last Modified
9/8/2017		10347670			Recheck 15	8/22/2017
9/8/2017		10681133			Recheck 15	8/22/2017
9/8/2017		645547			Recheck 15	8/22/2017
9/8/2017		10463000			New Patient 15	8/22/2017
9/8/2017		10105040			Recheck 15	8/22/2017
9/8/2017		717120			Aftertest 15	8/22/2017
9/11/2017		9859850			New Patient 30	8/22/2017
9/11/2017		10655520			Recheck 15	8/25/2017
9/11/2017					ASC	8/30/2017
9/11/2017		10742806			New Patient 15	8/31/2017
9/11/2017		824960			New Patient 15	8/31/2017
9/11/2017		10742797			New Patient 15	8/31/2017
9/11/2017					EMG 30 - one extremity only	8/30/2017

Other practices have similar notification reports for physicians whose schedule starts earlier than the rest of clinic or to notify front desk staff about an evening clinic scheduled for that day. If there is scheduling outside the normal, SSRS is an easy way to alert the staff.

THIS EMAIL CONTAINS A COLUMN FOR THE PATIENT NAME. SOME PRACTICES CHOSE TO ONLY USE AN INTERNAL ACCOUNT NUMBER, ESPECIALLY FOR A NOTIFICATION-TYPE EMAIL THAT MAY GO TO STAFF MEMBERS' ELECTRONIC DEVICES. OTHER PRACTICES ONLY ALLOW WORK EMAIL TO BE RETRIEVED AFTER LOGGING INTO THE NETWORK SECURELY. SSRS MAKES REPORTING VERY CONVENIENT, BUT MAKE SURE THAT SSRS EMAIL COMPLIES WITH THE PRACTICE'S PRIVACY POLICIES AND PROCEDURES.

NO SHOWS

Reducing no shows is a challenge for many practices. A patient who doesn't show up for an appointment is an empty seat as the plane takes off. Airline customers pay in advance and unused tickets are often nonrefundable. Medical practices do not operate in that way. The first step to reducing no shows is to understand how many no-show appointments happen and to look for common characteristics of those no-show appointments. Exhibit 6.17 is just the Report Filter area in No Show PivotTable. The filters are an example of a variety of ways one practice analyzes no shows.

EXHIBIT 6.17 PIVOTTABLE: NO SHOW FILTERS SAMPLE

Company	(All)
Referral Source	(All)
Years	(All)
Months	(All)
Weekday	(All)
Probable Primary Insurance Group	(All)
Appt Start Hour	(All)
Days	(All)
Doctor	(All)
Facility	(All)
Appt Type	(All)
Days Since Appt Scheduled	(All)

The dataset supporting the PivotTable includes the current year and the prior two years' appointments. With those filters and that much data, there are over 750,000 appointments to analyze and look for trends. PivotTables are the ideal tool to get started. For example, the trend in no shows in Exhibit 6.18 is clearly trending up.

EXHIBIT 6.18 PIVOTTABLE: NO SHOW TRENDS

Row Labels	No Show
⊟ 2015	
Jan	4.21%
Feb	3.38%
Mar	3.68%
Apr	4.08%
May	4.05%
Jun	4.56%
Jul	4.92%
Aug	4.56%
Sep	4.33%
Oct	4.60%
Nov	4.77%
Dec	4.50%
⊟ 2016	
Jan	4.59%
Feb	4.29%
Mar	4.26%
Apr	4.46%
May	4.31%
Jun	4.42%
Jul	4.80%
Aug	4.56%
Sep	4.64%
Oct	4.51%
Nov	4.43%
Dec	4.30%
⊟ 2017	
Jan	4.64%
Feb	4.11%
Mar	4.23%
Apr	4.26%
May	4.46%
Jun	4.84%
Jul	5.00%
Aug	3.44%

Simply rearranging the date fields make it easy to see monthly trends by year, as shown in Exhibit 6.19.

EXHIBIT 6.19 PIVOTTABLE: NO SHOW TRENDS - FILTERED

Row Labels	No Show
Jan	
2015	4.21%
2016	4.59%
2017	4.64%
Feb	
2015	3.38%
2016	4.29%
2017	4.11%
Mar	
2015	3.68%
2016	4.26%
2017	4.23%
Apr	
2015	4.08%
2016	4.46%
2017	4.26%
May	
2015	4.05%
2016	4.31%
2017	4.46%
Jun	
2015	4.56%
2016	4.42%
2017	4.84%
Jul	
2015	4.92%
2016	4.80%
2017	5.00%
Aug	
2015	4.56%
2016	4.56%
2017	3.44%
Sep	
2015	4.33%
2016	4.64%
Oct	
2015	4.60%
2016	4.51%
Nov	
2015	4.77%
2016	4.43%
Dec	
2015	4.50%
2016	4.30%

Comparing 2016 no-show rates to 2017 shows that early in the year, 2017 no show rates were lower than 2016. From May through July, 2017 no-show rates increased from 2016 levels.

148

Further analysis showed that no-show rates increased every day of the week except Wednesdays in 2017. The no-show rate on Saturday, when the practice has a small fraction of the weekday appointments, has dramatically reduced since 2015. The 2016 reduction continued into 2017. Part of solving no-show rates is making sure the problem stays solved.

Sometimes a visual representation of the no-show problem can be more helpful than a long table of numbers and rates. Like the earlier example in chapter, the analysis in Exhibit 6.20 focuses on the number of days between the date the appointment was scheduled and the date of the actual appointment. The red line is the no-show rate for all providers in the practice. The blue line is the no-show rate for one specific provider. The provider's no-show rate roughly compares to the practice no-show rate until the appointment has been scheduled for more than three weeks. At that point, the provider's no-show rates doubles compared to the rest of the practice.

EXHIBIT 6.20 NO SHOW TRACKING CHART 2014

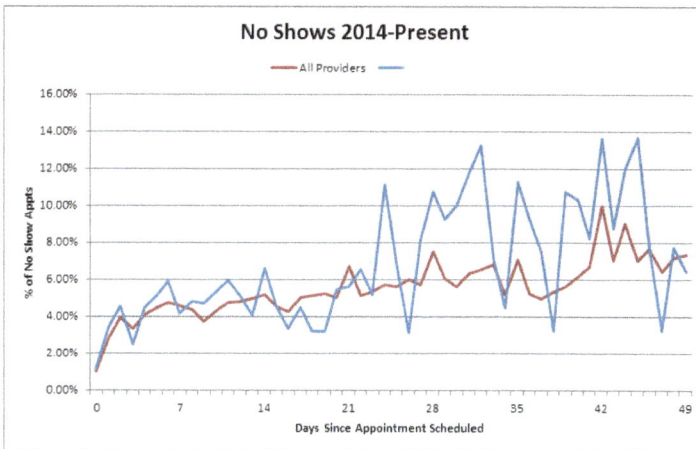

Comparing one provider to other providers in a practice can be a powerful way to influence physician behavior. In this example, the problem could be that appointments are made for all patients, but the patient leaves with the impression to only come back if their condition persists. Part of the concern may be physician availability. Does the patient (or the front desk) feel the need to schedule the appointment so far in advance to ensure there will be an appointment slot if the patient needs to be seen? The interesting thing about this example is that the chart did not come about through playing with the data. The scheduling staff had a hunch that this situation was occurring, and the data served to validate the suspicion. Rather than go to the physician with a vague feeling, the chart provided documentation. The PivotTable allowed staff to drill down and see specific patients who did not show up for appointments made more than three weeks previous.

Exhibit 6.21 is an example from a different practice that makes a similar analysis.

EXHIBIT 6.21 NO SHOWS: ESTABLISHED VS. NEW PATIENTS – BY YEAR

	No Show ▾	
Row Labels ▾	**2016**	**2017**
Established	2.7%	3.1%
New	2.8%	3.2%
Grand Total	**2.7%**	**3.1%**

To start with, the overall no-show rate is very low for both new and established patient office visits. The increase from 2016 to 2017 could be a sign of concern. This practice also looked at no-show rates by weekday, as shown in Exhibit 6.22.

EXHIBIT 6.22 No Shows: Established vs. New Patient – by Day of the Week

Row Labels	No Show 2016	2017
⊟ Established	2.7%	3.1%
Monday	2.8%	3.6%
Tuesday	2.9%	3.3%
Wednesday	2.7%	3.0%
Thursday	2.5%	2.9%
Friday	2.7%	2.9%
⊟ New	2.8%	3.2%
Monday	3.1%	3.6%
Tuesday	3.1%	3.1%
Wednesday	2.6%	3.3%
Thursday	2.7%	3.1%
Friday	2.3%	2.7%
Grand Total	2.7%	3.1%

Established patients on Mondays and new patients on Wednesdays were two areas of concern. The practice dug further into the data. Two big groups of patient appointments for this group are adult providers and pediatric providers. Exhibit 6.23 shows the same data by adult and pediatrics.

EXHIBIT 6.23 NO SHOWS: ESTABLISHED VS. NEW PATIENTS – BY
PROVIDER

	No Show	
Row Labels	2016	2017
─ Adult	2.1%	2.8%
─ Established	1.6%	2.4%
Monday	1.6%	2.6%
Tuesday	1.6%	2.5%
Wednesday	1.5%	2.1%
Thursday	1.5%	2.3%
Friday	1.6%	2.3%
─ New	2.7%	3.2%
Monday	3.0%	3.7%
Tuesday	2.9%	3.1%
Wednesday	2.9%	3.3%
Thursday	2.5%	3.2%
Friday	2.0%	2.8%
─ Pediatrics	3.6%	3.6%
─ Established	3.7%	4.0%
Monday	4.2%	5.1%
Tuesday	4.0%	3.8%
Wednesday	3.7%	4.2%
Thursday	3.2%	3.0%
Friday	3.6%	3.8%
─ New	3.5%	3.2%
Monday	4.4%	4.7%
Tuesday	4.1%	3.1%
Wednesday	2.6%	3.3%
Thursday	2.9%	2.5%
Friday	3.4%	2.3%
Grand Total	2.9%	3.2%

The grand totals of Exhibits 6.22 and 6.23 are not the same, since Exhibit 6.23 is a subset of Exhibit 6.22. The pediatric group has a higher no-show rate than the adult group. In 2016, the pediatric no-show rate was almost double the adult no-show rate (3.7% to 2.0%), but in 2017 the adult rate has increased while the pediatric rate has stayed close to 2016 rate. New patients are a bigger problem in the adult group, but established patients are a bigger issue in pediatrics. This analysis could be taken further to analyze specific providers, facilities, appointment types, and more. The PivotTable makes it very time-efficient to do that analysis. Whether a practice chooses to implement a no-show charge, double-book some appointment slots, or better educate patients about their appointments, the PivotTable helps providers make a more educated decision. Armed with better information, the practice can keep more patients on the plane for takeoff.

MGMA's Practice Operations Report provides good insight here. Multispecialty groups have the highest no-show rate. How does your practice compare to the MGMA benchmark? What can your practice do to reduce your no-show rate?

Exhibit 6.24 Median No Show Rate

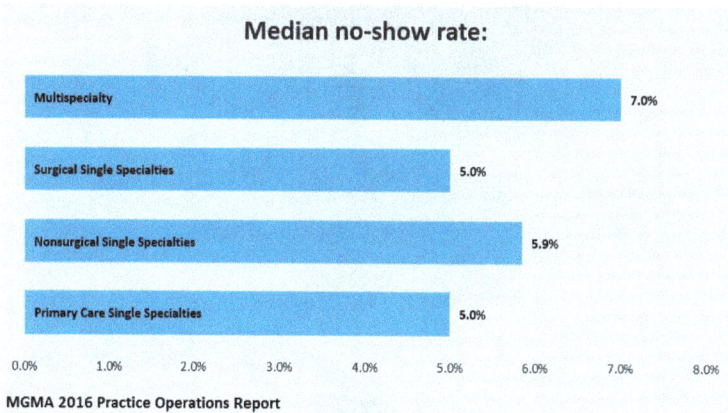

Median no-show rate:

Category	Rate
Multispecialty	7.0%
Surgical Single Specialties	5.0%
Nonsurgical Single Specialties	5.9%
Primary Care Single Specialties	5.0%

MGMA 2016 Practice Operations Report

Source: MGMA 2016 Practice Operations Report: Based on 2015 Survey Data

CANCELED APPOINTMENTS

Nobody looks forward to a colonoscopy. This gastro-intestinal practice was concerned about no shows, but it was also concerned about canceled appointments. If the patient cancels too close to the date of the appointment, that appointment slot can be challenging to fill—short-notice cancellations are essentially no shows. Therefore, the practice pulled three years of appointment cancellation data, tracked the number of days before the appointment that the appointment was canceled, and discovered the trend, as revealed in Exhibit 6.25.

EXHIBIT 6.25 CANCELED APPOINTMENT TRACKING

Referring Doctor	(All)
Appt DateTime	(All)
Appt Cancellation Reason	(All)
Appt Status	Cancelled
Appointment Type	(All)
Location Description	(All)
Appt Category	(Multiple Items)
Resource	(All)

| Count of Patient | Year | | | |
Days Before Appointment	2016	2017	2018	Grand Total
0	368	370	404	1,142
1	525	648	586	1,759
2	299	347	351	997
3	303	287	263	853
4	212	228	229	669
5	218	173	160	551
6	213	213	221	647
7	252	208	234	694
8	186	164	162	512
9	108	145	123	376
10	110	109	110	329
11	92	85	112	289
12	74	107	81	262
13	124	101	139	364
14	117	160	148	425
15	104	127	107	338
16	62	105	95	262
17	66	92	67	225
18	71	59	62	192
19	59	64	58	181
20	70	76	91	237

The largest number of appointment cancellations occurred the day of the appointment (Day 0) and especially the day before the appointment. The PivotTable can filter this data to trend by location, appointment type, appointment resource (provider), day of the week, and more. Equipped with this information, the practice manager can consider policies like those just discussed for no shows, including booking extra appointments, better education to prepare patients for appointments, or charging for short-notice cancellations.

RESCHEDULED CANCELED APPOINTMENTS

The following practice looked at canceled appointments in a unique way, because it tracked appointment cancellation reasons. The reasons were grouped into two categories, canceled by patient and canceled by provider. Exhibit 6.26 analyzes the how many canceled appointments were rescheduled within two, three, and four weeks of the original appointment date.

EXHIBIT 6.26 RESCHEDULED CANCELED APPOINTMENT TRACKING

All Providers

Canceled By	Rescheduled 2 Weeks	Rescheduled 3 Weeks	Rescheduled 4 Weeks
Overall	27.8%	34.4%	40.0%
Patient	20.5%	27.1%	32.3%
Doctor	43.2%	50.1%	56.6%

Pain Providers Only

Canceled By	Rescheduled 2 Weeks	Rescheduled 3 Weeks	Rescheduled 4 Weeks
Overall	27.8%	34.0%	39.9%
Patient	25.3%	32.1%	38.9%
Doctor	31.9%	37.2%	41.6%

All Non-Pain Providers

Canceled By	Rescheduled 2 Weeks	Rescheduled 3 Weeks	Rescheduled 4 Weeks
Overall	27.7%	34.6%	40.1%
Patient	18.9%	25.4%	30.0%
Doctor	49.1%	56.9%	64.4%

The top section, "All Providers" shows that if an appointment is canceled, there is a 27.8% chance that the patient will be rescheduled in two weeks. That chance goes up to 40% if the window to reschedule the appointment increases to four weeks. Staying with the Rescheduled in 4 Weeks column, if a patient cancels the appointment the chance of reschedule is 32.3%. If the doctor cancels the appointment, the chance of reschedule is significantly higher at 56.6%. The better way to look at that 56.6% number is that if a doctor cancels an appointment, 43.4% of the time the patient doesn't come back to see the provider in four weeks. In this practice environment, that patient could well be lost. Doctor cancellations are much more under the control of the practice than patient cancellations are.

The revenue cycle team suspected that patients seeing providers for pain might have a different patient profile than non-pain patients. Business Intelligence reports like this are a powerful way to use data to confirm a hunch or a suspicion. Looking at the Rescheduled in 4 Weeks column, the reschedule rate for pain providers is similar between patient cancellations (38.9%) and doctor cancellations (41.6%). However, the reschedule rates diverge dramatically for non-pain providers. Only 30% of patient cancellations reschedule in four weeks. For this practice, that means 70% of the patients who cancel appointments may have gone to a competitor. The practice also lost over a third of non-pain provider canceled appointments. After all the work the practice went to in Chapter 5 to attract patients, the last thing a practice wants to do is to lose patients to factors under its control.

WHICH PROVIDER TO SCHEDULE A PATIENT WITH

The Exhibit 6.27 spreadsheet was built for a practice that had difficulties with the scheduling functionality built into their PM system. The orthopedic practice has multiple locations and through a simple survey determined that about one-third of patients seeking an appointment failed to request a specific provider. The PM system did not do a good job of simultaneously searching across multiple appointment categories to show available appointments, so this spreadsheet read the schedule to find all open appointments by provider by location. The spreadsheet also knows which providers specialize in which body part. Schedulers who decide which provider to schedule a patient with must first determine the location where the patient would like to be seen. The spreadsheet then shows open appointments by body part. The spreadsheet allows for additional logic to favor new providers, partners, or to consider other factors in sorting and displaying open appointments. Exhibit 6.27 is an example of the scheduling spreadsheet for one location.

EXHIBIT 6.27 PROVIDER SPECIFIC SCHEDULING

Hip		NP	EST
Diaz	3/20	0	6
McMurray	3/20	0	2
Diaz	3/21	2	9
Blair	3/22	2	2
Diaz	3/22	5	8
Lawson	3/22	5	5
Moore	3/22	0	2
Schmidt	3/22	0	2
Watson	3/22	1	0
Blair	3/23	7	6
McMurray	3/23	0	1
Moore	3/23	0	14
Diaz	3/24	6	7
Lawson	3/24	9	9
Diaz	3/27	4	6

Knee		NP	EST
Diaz	3/20	0	6
McMurray	3/20	0	2
Diaz	3/21	2	9
Blair	3/22	2	2
Diaz	3/22	5	8
Lawson	3/22	5	5
Moore	3/22	0	2
Schmidt	3/22	0	2
Watson	3/22	1	0
Blair	3/23	7	6
McMurray	3/23	0	1
Moore	3/23	0	14
Diaz	3/24	6	7
Lawson	3/24	9	9
Diaz	3/27	4	6

Foot		NP	EST
Diaz	3/20	0	6
McMurray	3/20	0	2
Diaz	3/21	2	9
Blair	3/22	2	2
Diaz	3/22	5	8
Lawson	3/22	5	5
Moore	3/22	0	2
Smith	3/22	0	2
Watson	3/22	1	0
Blair	3/23	7	6
McMurray	3/23	0	1
Moore	3/23	0	14
Smith	3/23	0	1
Diaz	3/24	6	7
Lawson	3/24	9	9

Ankle		NP	EST
Diaz	3/20	0	6
McMurray	3/20	0	2
Diaz	3/21	2	9
Blair	3/22	2	2
Diaz	3/22	5	8
Lawson	3/22	5	5
Moore	3/22	0	2
Smith	3/22	0	2
Watson	3/22	1	0
Blair	3/23	7	6
McMurray	3/23	0	1
Moore	3/23	0	14
Smith	3/23	0	1
Diaz	3/24	6	7
Lawson	3/24	9	9

Shoulder		NP	EST
Diaz	3/20	0	6
McMurray	3/20	0	2
Diaz	3/21	2	9
Harrison	3/21	1	0
Blair	3/22	2	2
Diaz	3/22	5	8
Lawson	3/22	5	5
Moore	3/22	0	2
Watson	3/22	1	0
Blair	3/23	7	6
McMurray	3/23	0	1
Moore	3/23	0	14
Diaz	3/24	6	7
Lawson	3/24	9	9
Diaz	3/27	4	6

Elbow		NP	EST
Diaz	3/20	0	6
McMurray	3/20	0	2
Diaz	3/21	2	9
Harrison	3/21	1	0
Blair	3/22	2	2
Diaz	3/22	5	8
Lawson	3/22	5	5
Moore	3/22	0	2
Watson	3/22	1	0
Blair	3/23	7	6
McMurray	3/23	0	1
Moore	3/23	0	14
Diaz	3/24	6	7
Lawson	3/24	9	9
Diaz	3/27	4	6

Hand		NP	EST
Diaz	3/20	0	6
McMurray	3/20	0	2
Diaz	3/21	2	9
Harrison	3/21	1	0
Blair	3/22	2	2
Diaz	3/22	5	8
Lawson	3/22	5	5
Moore	3/22	0	2
Watson	3/22	1	0
Blair	3/23	7	6
McMurray	3/23	0	1
Moore	3/23	0	14
Diaz	3/24	6	7
Lawson	3/24	9	9
Diaz	3/27	4	6

Spine/Neck		NP	EST
McMurray	3/20	0	2
Moore	3/22	0	2
J Smith	3/23	2	9
McMurray	3/23	0	1
Moore	3/23	0	14
J Smith	3/24	0	1
McMurray	3/27	7	2
J Smith	3/28	0	8
Moore	3/28	0	11
Blair	3/29	6	10
J Smith	3/30	5	3
McMurray	3/30	0	9
Moore	3/30	4	19
J Smith	3/31	10	14
McMurray	4/3	9	5

There is a column for new patient appointments (NP) and one for established patient appointments (EST). The practice's chief operations officer describes the two columns as follows: "I think this is where the second 'value add' comes in since these columns empower the schedulers to override the rules in the PM system to ensure the physician's schedule is properly maximized. Again, this goes back to the limitation that the PM system doesn't allow for searching across multiple appointment categories. Maximizing the physician's schedule despite the PM system's limitations is the key that will resonate with other practices."

TRIAGE SCHEDULING

Exhibit 6.28 is a very customized form developed internally by an orthopedic practice. The form is designed to be used by call center staff with limited medical training. The objective is for those staff members to schedule a new patient appointment with the right provider the first time.

EXHIBIT 6.28 SPECIALIZED PROVIDER SPECIFIC SCHEDULING FORM

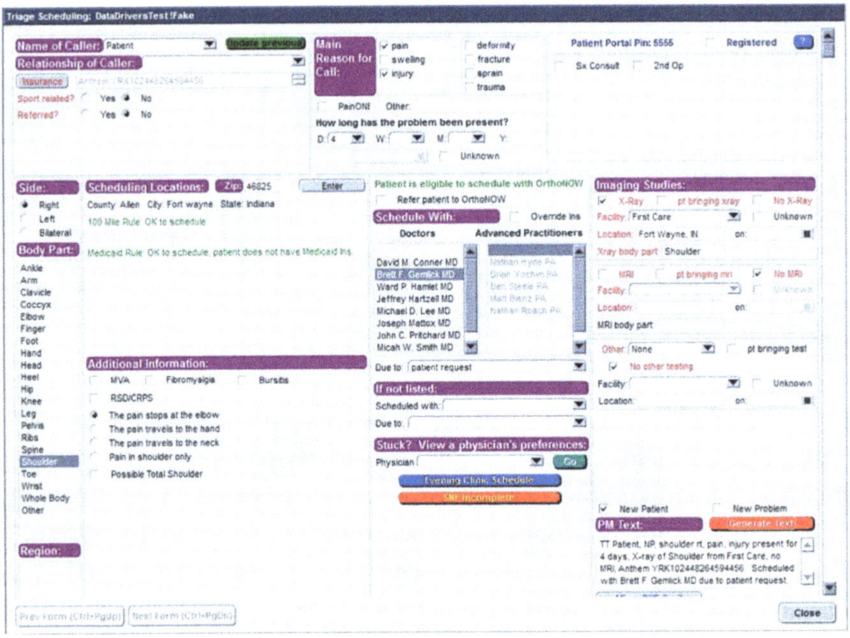

There is a ton of custom, practice-specific logic going on behind the scenes here. Based on the body part, the main reason for the call, and the additional information supplied, non-clinical phone staff can accurately schedule patients with the appropriate provider. Physician preferences are built in so the providers see the patients that are most suitable for their specialization. The information captured during the initial call is also saved, which has two advantages. First, the information is available to providers as part of the medical record. Second, the data can be used to improve the triage form. If a provider sees a new patient who he or she shouldn't have seen despite the form, the form logic can be improved so that the next new patient is routed correctly.

OPEN PROCEDURE SLOTS

Exhibit 6.29 is an example of how a Midwest practice reports open procedure slots to the scheduling team. Some of this information is available through the PM system, but this practice was looking for a one-page summary of the next five open procedure slots when insurance requires a patient to be treated in a specific facility type or network. This go-to list helps the surgery scheduling department decide where to schedule a procedure. The report is a daily email sent each morning, so as the day progresses the data becomes less accurate. An advantage of SSRS is that once the email is built, the same underlying report can be available on an internal web page if the scheduling staff needed to see more updated data during the day.

EXHIBIT 6.29 OPEN PROCEDURE SLOTS SAMPLE

Next 5 Pain Surgery Open Appt Slots

Provider	Facility	1	2	3	4	5
		10/05	10/12	10/19	10/26	11/02
		10/18	10/30	11/15	11/27	12/13
		10/06	10/11	10/18	10/26	11/01
		9/06	9/26	9/27	9/29	10/03
		9/15	9/21	10/13	10/19	11/10
		9/26	10/03	10/10	10/17	10/24
		9/01	9/29	10/27	12/22	1/19
		10/20	11/17	12/15	1/12	
		9/08	9/11	9/18	9/22	9/25
		9/13	9/20	9/27	10/04	10/11
		9/18	9/20	9/25	10/02	10/04
		10/11	11/08	12/06	1/03	1/31
		9/27	10/04	10/18	10/25	11/01
		9/06	9/07	9/11	9/13	9/14
		9/08	9/15	9/22	9/28	9/29
		9/13	9/20	10/11	10/18	

Exhibit 6.30 is another example of unfilled procedure slots. The pain surgery slots in the earlier example represented more standard time slots. This practice has surgery appointment slots that are much more variable. The scheduling staff use this report to find slots based on provider, location, and available time. For example, to schedule a one-hour surgery for the top provider in the top location in Exhibit 6.30, the second next available slot is the first suitable slot with sufficient time for the procedure.

EXHIBIT 6.30 OPEN PROCEDURE SLOTS SAMPLE – VARIABLE TIME SLOTS

Next 5 Unfilled Provider Surgery Schedules as of 9/1/2017

Provider	Location	1	2	3	4	5
		10/5/17 9:45 AM (15 min)	10/5/17 10:15 AM (75 min)	10/12/17 7:30 AM (30 min)	10/12/17 8:30 AM (15 min)	10/12/17 9:30 AM (90 min)
		10/6/17 7:45 AM (255 min)	10/11/17 7:45 AM (255 min)	10/18/17 1:00 PM (240 min)	10/26/17 1:00 PM (240 min)	11/1/17 8:00 AM (240 min)
		10/18/17 7:45 AM (30 min)	10/18/17 8:45 AM (150 min)	10/30/17 7:30 AM (240 min)	11/15/17 7:15 AM (240 min)	11/27/17 7:30 AM (240 min)
		9/26/17 9:00 AM (15 min)	9/27/17 4:15 PM (15 min)	9/29/17 7:45 AM (15 min)	9/29/17 8:15 AM (90 min)	9/29/17 10:15 AM (30 min)
		9/15/17 4:00 PM (60 min)	9/21/17 8:45 AM (135 min)	10/13/17 1:00 PM (240 min)	10/19/17 8:30 AM (180 min)	11/10/17 1:00 PM (240 min)
		9/13/17 11:15 AM (15 min)	9/20/17 8:45 AM (15 min)	9/20/17 9:15 AM (15 min)	9/20/17 10:15 AM (15 min)	9/20/17 10:45 AM (15 min)
		9/26/17 2:15 PM (165 min)	10/3/17 2:15 PM (165 min)	10/10/17 1:15 PM (225 min)	10/17/17 1:00 PM (240 min)	10/24/17 1:00 PM (240 min)
		10/20/17 8:45 AM (195 min)	11/17/17 8:30 AM (210 min)	12/15/17 8:30 AM (210 min)	1/12/18 8:30 AM (210 min)	
		9/1/17 10:15 AM (105 min)	9/29/17 11:30 AM (30 min)	10/27/17 8:30 AM (210 min)	12/22/17 8:30 AM (210 min)	1/19/18 8:30 AM (210 min)
		9/8/17 11:00 AM (15 min)	9/8/17 12:00 PM (60 min)	9/8/17 3:00 PM (60 min)	9/11/17 10:15 AM (165 min)	9/11/17 1:00 PM (240 min)

DAYS TO THIRD NEXT AVAILABLE APPOINTMENT

Scheduling algorithms are wonderful if providers have available appointment slots to schedule. One way to measure patient access is to try to set an appointment with each provider and to find the third next available appointment slot. Looking for the third next available slot (days to third) instead of the first or second next available appointment slot smooths out fluctuations that may be caused by last minute cancellations. Some practices do this calculation manually by paying a staff member to try to make an appointment for a dummy patient with each provider in the practice. As the manual calculation is error prone, practices have built logic algorithms to do the calculation automatically. Exhibit 6.31 is from *Better Data, Better Decisions: Using Business Intelligence in the Medical Practice.*

EXHIBIT 6.31 OLD DAYS TO THIRD NEXT APPOINTMENT CALCULATIONS

Exhibit 6.6 Days to Third Next Appointment

As of October 1, 2014

Provider	New	Follow Up
Dr. A. Simon	8	2
Dr. Cannon	6	6
Dr. Dawson	12	33
Dr. Fleming	15	25
Dr. Gibson	11	15
Dr. Gutierrez	55	55
Dr. Hardy	19	13
Dr. Hudson	8	26
Dr. King	21	21
Dr. Lynch	4	1
Dr. Medina	18	11
Dr. S. Simon	2	2
Dr. Vasquez	3	3
Dr. Walker	5	5
Dr. White	4	1

Compare that version to a more recent analysis in Exhibit 6.32.

EXHIBIT 6.32 NEW DAYS TO THIRD NEXT APPOINTMENT CALCULATIONS

Row Labels	New 2011	2012	2013	2014	2015	2016	2017	New Total	Recheck 2011	2012	2013	2014	2015	2016	2017	Recheck Total
+Foot&Ankle	10.13	5.38	5.78	10.87	11.32	12.10	13.48	9.62	16.20	5.85	7.40	10.40	10.23	9.63	8.91	8.75
+General	4.60	2.75	2.51	3.30	3.94	4.06	3.67	3.36	4.30	2.98	2.61	2.98	3.02	2.79	3.18	2.92
+Hand	27.70	4.68	3.17	4.86	6.10	6.95	7.22	5.48	9.80	4.20	4.20	5.19	5.78	5.85	5.11	5.07
+Pain	19.20	16.13	14.82	9.98	11.49	15.27	14.80	13.71	13.90	11.54	11.90	3.96	4.71	6.62	2.84	7.18
+Spine	11.87	8.56	6.12	4.29	8.86	14.42	7.24	8.39	8.07	7.65	6.92	4.40	6.79	8.57	5.80	6.68
+Sport	16.55	10.80	10.28	10.81	11.28	12.22	12.24	11.33	21.75	11.02	9.65	10.51	10.75	11.01	10.52	10.62
+Total	15.10	8.35	8.39	6.34	11.12	15.82	24.46	11.76	22.80	19.74	12.80	12.68	15.60	20.69	23.73	17.22
+Trauma	14.50	18.28	14.92	16.09	16.38	20.86	17.99	17.46	11.00	9.29	9.95	12.81	14.05	17.99	13.88	13.06

The two main differences are that the providers are grouped by subspecialty and that the data is available to trend over time. This additional detail allows for insights like the significant difficulty getting a new patient appointment with a total joint specialist now than in the past. If the practice is looking to expand, hiring total joint specialists is a good place to start.

THE LARGER POINT FROM THE COMPARISON OF THESE TWO EXAMPLES IS THAT A SAVVY PRACTICE IS NEVER "DONE" WITH BUSINESS INTELLIGENCE. YOU CAN'T JUST CHECK A BOX AND NEVER LOOK AT BUSINESS INTELLIGENCE AGAIN. THAT BEING SAID, THE DIFFERENCES ARE NOT LIFE CHANGING OR SUPER DIFFICULT TO GRASP, EITHER. THE UNDERLYING DATASET SIMPLY GROUPED THE PHYSICIANS BY SUBSPECIALTY AND STORED THE DATA NIGHTLY OVER THE COURSE OF SEVERAL YEARS.

This data must be calculated and stored nightly because of all the appointment changes that go on in a busy medical practice. The PM system doesn't keep enough data to go back in time and calculate the days to the third next available appointment last month or last year. The challenge is that the third next available appointment analysis needs to be stored nightly to be trended over time. Start storing data now so that over time trends become apparent.

A GOOD BENCHMARK TO COMPARE YOUR PROVIDERS' AVAILABILITY IS THIS CHART FROM MGMA'S PRACTICE OPERATIONS REPORT. THE DATA SHOWS THAT IT GENERALLY TAKES LONGER FOR A NEW PATIENT TO BE SEEN BY A PROVIDER THAN IT DOES FOR AN ESTABLISHED PATIENT TO BE SEEN. THE HARDER IT IS FOR A NEW PATIENT TO BE SEEN, THE HARDER IT IS FOR A PRACTICE TO GROW. PRIMARY CARE PROVIDERS MAY NOT BE INCLINED TO REFER TO SPECIALISTS WHO TAKE TOO LONG TO SEE A NEW PATIENT. MGMA'S DATA IS BASED ON BUSINESS DAYS. THE EXAMPLE IN EXHIBIT 6.33 IS BASED ON CALENDAR DAYS.

EXHIBIT 6.33 MEDIAN OF DAYS TO THIRD NEXT APPOINTMENT

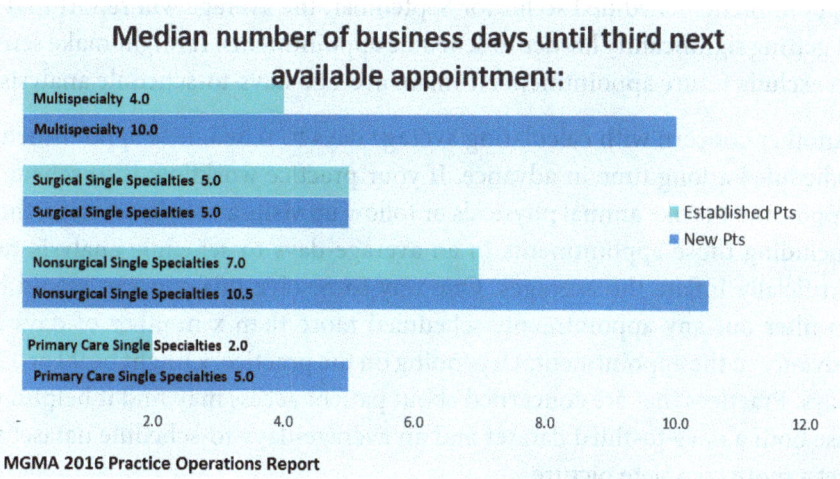

Median number of business days until third next available appointment:

Multispecialty 4.0	
Multispecialty 10.0	
Surgical Single Specialties 5.0	
Surgical Single Specialties 5.0	
Nonsurgical Single Specialties 7.0	
Nonsurgical Single Specialties 10.5	
Primary Care Single Specialties 2.0	
Primary Care Single Specialties 5.0	

Established Pts
New Pts

2.0   4.0   6.0   8.0   10.0   12.0

MGMA 2016 Practice Operations Report

SOURCE: *MGMA 2016 PRACTICE OPERATIONS REPORT: BASED ON 2015 SURVEY DATA*

AVERAGE DAYS TO SCHEDULE APPOINTMENTS

One way to get historical scheduling data is to calculate the average number of days between the date the appointment was created and the actual date of the appointment. Most PM systems store the date a new appointment was created. For example, an appointment created October 7 for a patient to see a provider on October 21 was scheduled 14 days out. Averaging this calculation over time by provider, provider category, location, appointment type, and more can provide considerable insight about patient access to providers over time. You can also track things that the days to third calculation would have a hard time calculating, such as the average days to schedule a new Medicare patient. Another advantage of the average days to schedule is that instead of storing one data point per day like the days to third calculation, the practice has a data point for each patient appointment.

A disadvantage of the average days to schedule calculation relates to future appointments. If today is July 1 and I look at the average-days-to-schedule appointments in September, the only appointments currently scheduled in September are at least 60 days out. Even if there are only two or three appointments scheduled so far for September, the average will report that it is getting significantly harder to schedule appointments. It might make sense to exclude future appointments from an average-days-to-schedule analysis.

Another concern with calculating average days to schedule is appointments scheduled a long time in advance. If your practice workflow is to schedule appointments like annual physicals or follow up visits a year in advance, then including those appointments in an average-days to-schedule analysis can artificially inflate the averages. One way to resolve this concern would be to filter out any appointments scheduled more than x number of days in advance of the appointment. Depending on the practice, x might be 90 or 120 days. Practices that are concerned about patient access may find it helpful to use both a days-to-third dataset and an average-days-to-schedule dataset to get a more complete picture.

Exhibit 6.34 is an example of an average-days-to-schedule analysis. The PivotTable tracks the average days to schedule a new and an established patient appointment over a four-year trend. In this practice, new patients have a much shorter wait to see a provider than established patients do. In 2017, new patient wait times dropped considerably, but it still took over a month to get an established patient appointment with the average provider in this practice.

Exhibit 6.34 Average Days to Schedule Sample – Monthly

Row Labels	New				Established				Grand Total
	2014	2015	2016	2017	2014	2015	2016	2017	
Jan	11.9	19.8	26.6	22.1	40.4	41.5	38.0	42.0	35.0
Feb	9.5	17.6	21.0	19.5	36.4	37.1	34.8	34.6	30.5
Mar	10.2	17.3	20.5	18.6	32.4	36.5	34.2	33.3	29.3
Apr	11.1	17.8	20.4	18.4	34.3	36.7	36.1	35.9	30.6
May	12.4	19.4	18.9	18.5	35.3	36.3	35.7	36.0	30.8
Jun	13.3	21.2	20.0	18.7	36.3	39.1	37.5	35.0	32.1
Jul	12.9	22.1	21.6	20.2	39.1	38.3	36.7	36.4	32.9
Aug	15.1	22.9	22.6	18.8	35.4	36.6	37.1	36.0	32.0
Sep	17.1	24.8	22.9	28.6	36.7	35.9	37.3	49.3	34.5
Oct	17.6	25.5	21.5	50.2	34.9	36.1	36.2	70.6	34.8
Nov	18.4	23.6	22.2	79.5	35.6	37.0	37.5	88.2	34.5
Dec	21.0	25.8	22.5		39.3	38.0	39.0	96.7	34.5
Grand Total	14.2	21.5	21.7	20.2	36.4	37.5	36.6	39.3	32.5

Exhibit 6.35 is a panel from a dashboard that tracks this information on a weekly basis, since patient access is an important issue for this practice. The dashboard compares days to schedule for the current month to last month and last year. The current month column is set to go red if patient access is getting worse. Having this data on a dashboard that can be emailed frequently helps managers focus on the issue. If the data was only on a spreadsheet that managers had to remember to check, the issue would be less likely to receive the same level of focus.

EXHIBIT 6.35 AVERAGE DAYS TO SCHEDULE SAMPLE – WEEKLY

Avg Days to Schedule by Provider Category

Category	New			Established		
	Current	Last Mo	Last Yr	Current	Last Mo	Last Yr
	23.1	22.7	27.9	47.2	44.3	46.9
	4.3	5.6	1.5	31.4	33.5	34.2
	10.8	11.1	7.5	30.0	41.3	31.2
	22.2	17.0	19.8	38.8	34.4	31.3
	9.3	10.5	13.8	33.6	37.1	35.7
	8.3	30.8	8.3	41.2	25.0	42.5

The complete dashboard is shown in Chapter 11.

COMPARING DAYS TO SCHEDULE APPOINTMENTS TO NO-SHOW RATES

Exhibit 6.36 is from a practice administrator who combined no-show data discussed earlier in this chapter with the number of days to schedule a new patient visit. The administrator wanted to see if providers who took longer to get an appointment with had a lower no-show rate. The data is sorted by the highest no-show percentages.

Exhibit 6.36 Days to Schedule vs. No Show Rates

Provider	Days to Schedule	No Show %
Roman, MD	14.20	16.7%
Hale, MD	5.29	15.0%
Valentine, MD	24.21	12.8%
Small, MD	24.71	12.1%
Mercado, MD	3.58	10.3%
Figueroa, MD	23.21	10.4%
Medina, MD	33.55	8.8%
Stuart, MD	16.48	8.2%
Salinas, MD	31.13	8.0%
Morse, MD	15.27	8.0%
Mack, MD	37.03	8.0%
Forbes, MD	48.71	7.9%
Werner, MD	45.74	7.6%
Mejia, MD	28.50	7.6%
Larson, MD	20.48	7.4%
Klein, MD	25.78	7.3%
Harding, MD	18.58	7.1%
Harvey, MD	26.79	7.0%
Cordova, MD	56.66	6.9%
Crawford, MD	24.86	6.8%
Khan, MD	27.55	6.6%
Roth, MD	18.58	6.4%
Mora, MD	22.65	6.2%
Benjamin, MD	24.49	4.9%
Duran, MD	48.95	4.0%
Guerrero, MD	32.17	3.6%
Sweeney, MD	52.74	2.3%

Clearly, the relationship isn't linear, but the administrator was interested to see that two of the providers who were easiest to get an appointment with (Doctors Hale and Mercado) had some of the highest no-show rates. Conversely, providers like Dr. Sweeney and Dr. Duran took seven weeks to get an appointment, but had very low no-show rates. It took over three weeks to get an appointment with Dr. Valentine and Dr. Small, but both have no-show rates over 12%. The practice administrator can start with this data and then search for reasons providers have abnormally high no-show rates. There may be opportunities to double book those providers and get patients in sooner. Drilling down on these rates may help providers reduce their no-show rates and increase patient access.

APPOINTMENTS IN A GLOBAL PERIOD

Patient appointments in a global period after a procedure are not reimbursed by some payers. This is absolutely not an argument to avoid seeing patients who need to be seen during a global period, but the global period was an issue for the following practice. Exhibit 6.37 is from a daily email that summarizes appointments in a global period. This practice wanted to show both appointments occurring in the global period on the email, together with information like the reason, provider, and location for each appointment. The objective of the SSRS email was to ensure the appointments in the global period were based on patient need rather than a scheduling error.

EXHIBIT 6.37 SUMMARY OF GLOBAL APPOINTMENTS SAMPLE

Appointments Potentially Hitting 10 Day Global Period as of 9/1/2017

Acct Num	Later Appt Date	Later Appt Time	Earlier Appt Date	Earlier Appt Time	Later Provider	Earlier Provider	Later Appt Location	Earlier Appt Location	Later Appt Reason	Earlier Appt Reason	Later Appt Memo	Earlier Appt Memo
3182745	8/22/2017	10:30AM	8/15/2017	9:00AM					Spot(s)	Keratosis		PRIVATE PAY 7/27/2017 SR
3183330	8/22/2017	1:30PM	8/18/2017	1:00PM					Mole	Botox	POSSIBLE REMOVAL AROUND HER NOSE AREA- ASYNA INS: MJ	CONSULT WITH TREATMENT/ PRIVATE PAY 8/14/2017 SR
3181087	8/22/2017	1:15PM	8/14/2017	1:45PM					Acne	Acne	MOM WANT TO START ACCUTANE	FU
220305	8/22/2017	2:10PM	8/15/2017	7:30AM					Suture Removal	MOHS	1 week	SCC IS L SUP CENT FOREHEAD/ SCORE:1 / DR
218014	8/22/2017	2:30PM	8/15/2017	7:30AM					Suture Removal	MOHS	1 week	BCC NOD NASAL DORSUM / SCORE 1 / DR
28452	8/22/2017	9:00PM	8/15/2017	7:30AM					Suture Removal	MOHS	De , sr, LN2	SCC IS ARBINO FRM A AK. Left forehead./ SCORE 1 / DR
48273	8/22/2017	3:00PM	8/15/2017	7:30AM					Suture Removal	MOHS	1 week sr, also schedule 2nd site	BCC NOD L SUP MED MALAR CHEEK - SCORE 0 - DF
3077915	8/22/2017	3:15PM	8/15/2017	9:30AM					Spot(s)	Skin Check	UNDER ARMS, RED/ INS VERIFIED- AWARE @ DNS / sk appt pm	INS VERIFIED/ DNS
3116508	8/23/2017	8:00AM	8/17/2017	10:45AM					MOHS	Follow Up	BCC R MEDIAL FOREHEAD /SCORE 0/ SCC R INF CENTRAL MALAR CHEEK /SCORE 1/skin oldie are in situ left central fromtal scalp/dr	6 WEEKS PER PT S REQUEST
3180698	8/25/2017	8:30AM	8/15/2017	2:00PM					MOHS	Follow Up	MALIGNANT SPINDLE CELL L LOWER CUTANEOUS LIP /SCORE2/-DR PT	vs. previously hold and Advanced AK
3026722	8/23/2017	8:30AM	8/21/2017	2:00PM					MOHS	EDxC	BCC L ANTIHELIX /SCORE 1/ REF BY DR	SCC SCC rt. Forearm : held on 08/02/17 -pt aware of
3159918	8/23/2017	11:00AM	8/21/2017	11:15AM					Follow Up	Follow Up	PATCH TEST	PATCH TEST

CATCH AND FIX FUTURE APPOINTMENT ISSUES

Another way to leverage appointment data is to teach the data warehouse rules to watch for in all future appointments and then report any future appointments "breaking" one of the rules. Exhibit 6.38 is a daily email that captures any issues with future appointments so the issues can be resolved before the patient arrives for the appointment. For example, rules include patients who appear to be out of network, patients who have not paid a required deposit, patients who shouldn't be seen by a specific provider or

167

at a given location, and many more. Any time a patient presents for an appointment and there is an issue that could have been resolved in advance, this practice makes a point to add a rule to the data warehouse to prevent that problem occurring in the future.

Note the "Repeated" column on this email. If this is the first time the email is notifying the practice of a potential problem, the column shows "New" and the relevant columns are shaded green. The staff can see at a glance the new appointment problems identified overnight. If the problem isn't new to today's email, the email shows "Repeat" and the date the appointment was scheduled. Appointments do not drop off the email until the issue is resolved or the appointment is past. Dropping items off a report is very important, however. If no mechanism exists for problems to disappear, even if the practice chooses to ignore the problem, the report will eventually become so cluttered that it will be unworkable.

EXHIBIT 6.38 AUTOMATED APPOINTMENT CONFLICT REPORT SAMPLE

Appt Date	Acct Num	Location	Provider	Repeated	Appt Reason	Appt Memo	Schd By
Aetna Medicare HMO Plan							
9/7/2017	3181666			Repeat - Scheduled 08/21/2017	Other	PEELING SKIN ON FINGER / A FEW MOLES ON BACK OF HEAD // INS CONF. BB 08/21/17	
9/7/2017	3183861			New	Skin Check	INS VERIFIED, AWARE REF IS IN PROCESS/ AWARE @ LC. DNH	
Filler Appointment without Deposit							
9/22/2017	207665			Repeat - Scheduled 07/25/2017	Dermal Filler	PER KP. KV 07-25-17	
10/19/2017	3016548			Repeat - Scheduled 08/15/2017	Dermal Filler	botox	
PA with Medicare Patient DIFFERENT Appointment Reason							
9/5/2017	222752			Repeat - Scheduled 08/30/2017	Spot(s)	SPOT ON HEAD/NO INS CHANGES/AWARE@ CT	
9/6/2017	222647			New	Itchy	INJ FOR HIVES// PT STATED SHE USUALLY SEES NURSE FOR SHOT, AND DR. WILL COME IN FOR AFEW MINS. BB 09/01/17	
9/11/2017	3061069			Repeat - Scheduled 08/14/2017	Follow Up	1mo f/u eyelid dermatitis	
10/16/2017	3017321			Repeat - Scheduled 08/25/2017	Skin Check		
Patient in Collections with Appointment							
9/21/2017	60154			Repeat - Scheduled 08/10/2017	Skin Check	SKIN CHECK// INS VERIFIED. BB 08/10/17	

This email is a textbook example of an exception report. The email doesn't show all future appointments. Only appointments with issues needing review by the staff appear on the report. Teaching the data warehouse the rules is far more reliable than having staff, even experienced staff, trying to remember all the rules. Staff members' time is optimized. This email can allow one staff member to review many more providers' appointments than he or she could without the report.

What appointment rules would make the biggest difference in your practice?

UPCOMING APPOINTMENTS MISSING CLINICAL INFORMATION

Another way to leverage appointment data is to combine the appointments with clinical information. Consider the following examples. In Exhibit 6.39, the practice looks for appointments that will require pathology results when the patient is seen. The trick is to identify which appointments need the pathology results and then to determine whether the pathology data is in the patients' electronic charts. One way to identify appointments is by creating an appointment type or a set of appointment types that indicate pathology will be reviewed during the appointment. The SSRS logic can then find appointments needing pathology by looking for appointment types. The next trick is to find the appropriate pathology data in the patients' charts. Simply finding pathology data isn't good enough, since the pathology could relate to a previous appointment. There are a couple of different approaches to solving this problem. One way might be to set date parameters so that a pathology only applies to appointments within a certain number of days. Another way could be to attach an appointment or an appointment date to the pathology information in the EHR so that the pathology data points to the patient appointment. This SSRS email only shows pending pathology reports. If the pathology has been received and is ready for the patient appointment, the appointment automatically drops off the report.

EXHIBIT 6.39 AUTOMATED REPORT FOR PENDING CLINICAL INFORMATION FOR UPCOMING APPOINTMENTS SAMPLE

Pending Path Reports as of 9/1/2017

Collected Date	Provider	Location	Accession	Pt Last Name	ME Acct Num	Next Appt	Corrected Or Revised
8/17/2017			S17-08798		3153630	NONE	
8/21/2017			S17-08890		3183384	NONE	
8/22/2017			S17-08992		3062491	NONE	
8/23/2017			S17-09067		3007973	NONE	
8/24/2017			S17-09130		222811	NONE	
8/24/2017			S17-09133		26477	NONE	
8/24/2017			S17-09128		3065854	NONE	
8/24/2017			S17-09132		3142879	NONE	
8/24/2017			S17-09131		3183603	NONE	
8/24/2017			S17-09126		41207	NONE	

Exhibit 6.40 is a similar report for labs that needs to be received and reviewed before the next patient appointment. This report has a slightly different approach than the pathology example in Exhibit 6.39. This report shows all upcoming appointments that require labs and then highlights appointments to focus on in the "No Labs Received" section. Appointments do not drop off this report until the appointment is past.

EXHIBIT 6.40 AUTOMATED REPORT FOR PENDING CLINICAL INFORMATION FOR UPCOMING APPOINTMENTS SAMPLE – MISSING INFORMATION FOCUSED

Appt Date	Appt Time	Acct Num	Provider	Loc	Appt Reason	Prim Ins	Last Visit	Repeated
Labs Have Been Received for the Following Patients:								
9/5/2017	4:30PM	3177095				SCOTT & WHITE HEALTH PLAN	08/01/2017	Repeat
9/6/2017	8:45AM	3164725				UNITED HEALTHCARE	08/07/2017	Repeat
9/6/2017	10:00AM	3179225				UNITED HEALTHCARE SHARED SERVICES	07/27/2017	Repeat
9/6/2017	3:45PM	3032828				UNITED HEALTHCARE	08/02/2017	Repeat
No Labs Received for these Patients:								
9/5/2017	10:45AM	3083974				UNITED HEALTHCARE	07/28/2017	Repeat
9/5/2017	3:30PM	3178564				BCBS OF TEXAS	08/03/2017	Repeat
9/6/2017	8:00AM	3169201				MERITAIN HEALTH	07/26/2017	Repeat
9/6/2017	9:30AM	3012666				CIGNA	07/31/2017	Repeat
9/6/2017	4:00PM	3179672				BCBS OF TEXAS	07/31/2017	Repeat

For some practices, the exception report approach used in the pathology example is more appropriate. If there are a lot of appointments and few exceptions, an exception report may be the way to go. If the clinical data is very critical to the patient appointment and there are not many appointments, it may be more appropriate to show all appointments, highlighting appointments that need work. The key in Business Intelligence is still customize, customize, customize.

USING APPOINTMENT INFORMATION TO HELP THE FRONT DESK BE MORE EFFICIENT

Clinical staff are not the only department that can be made more efficient with appointment data. Exhibit 6.41 is a daily SSRS email delivered each weekday afternoon to the front desk manager of a practice, and several of her team. The top section is a summary of "Tomorrow's" appointments by location.

(On Friday, the email shows Monday appointments.) The appointments are subtotaled by morning and afternoon so that front desk staff can move between locations during the lunch hour as necessary. The lower section of the report has column charts that show the different types of patient appointments expected "Tomorrow." This practice uses the appointment status to track the different types of patients who present. Those appointment status categories are summarized into four main categories: Updates, Review, New Patient and Benefits Verified. The purpose of the summary is to capture patients who may take longer at patient registration, such a new patient. Patients whose benefits are verified may take very little front desk time. The column charts help identify what the manager calls, "sticky spots," or times during the day when the front desk will be very busy. By seeing these sticky spots in advance, the manager can schedule more staff, ask a patient to come in earlier, or reallocate staff to improve patient flow. The patients' wait time is reduced and the providers in the clinic are not delayed.

EXHIBIT 6.41 FRONT DESK EFFICIENCY: TOMORROW'S APPOINTMENTS REPORT SAMPLE

Tomorrow Appointment Count for 8/25/2017

	Total Appts	Total Updates			New Patients		Portal	
		AM	PM	EVE	AM	PM	AM	PM
	56	8	4				1	
	237	56	31		13	8	3	1
	39	10	6	1	2		1	
	18		1					

Totals	
Appointments	350
Updates	117
New Patients	23
Evening	3
Portal	6

Tomorrow Graph For 8/25/2017

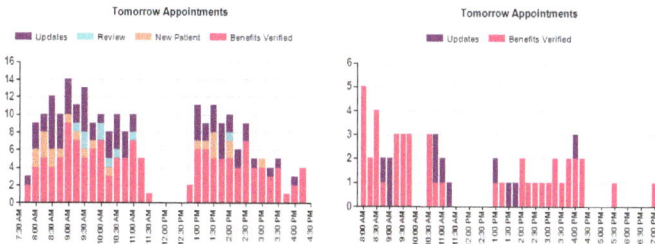

Tomorrow Appointments — Updates, Review, New Patient, Benefits Verified

Tomorrow Appointments — Updates, Benefits Verified

To make this report successful, front desk staff during their downtime used eligibility and benefit information to manually change upcoming appointments' status to reflect the registration status of the patients. The report data become so helpful to the practice that over time the internal IT department developed ways to automate the appointment status change based on data in the PM system. The combination of automating techniques and reports like this have allowed this practice to see 10% more patients yearly without adding front desk staff.

UNSUPERVISED NURSES

This practice uses scheduling data to look for locations where nurses are scheduled to see patients but without a physician also scheduled at the location to supervise those nurse encounters. An example of the SSRS email is shown in Exhibit 6.42. The scheduling information comes straight from the templates in the PM software. Each provider is entered in a separate table in the data warehouse. Part of the provider-specific information tracked in that table is whether the provider *can* supervise nurses, as well as tracking nurses who *need* physician supervision. The SSRS report logic looks for mornings or afternoons where nurses are scheduled but there are no providers scheduled who can supervise those nurses. One of the advantages of using a data warehouse instead of relying solely on PM or EHR data is the ability to track custom information like whether the nurse or other resource actually needs physician supervision.

EXHIBIT 6.42 UNSUPERVISED NURSE REPORT SAMPLE

Unsupervised Nurses in the Next 90 Days

Unsupervised Nurse	Location	Date	AMPM
		9/13/2017	AM

SCHEDULING PROVIDERS

Most PM systems provide a templating system to schedule providers. Some practices build spreadsheets to support the templating process and allocate the practice's providers across multiple locations fairly and efficiently. The example in Exhibit 6.43 was built for a practice whose PM system made it especially difficult to see which providers had been templated in those locations over time. The Excel spreadsheet allows the practice to see an overall view of utilization by location. The spreadsheet also summarizes where clinical staff are scheduled on a separate tab to make it easy for staff to know where they need to be. Most PM systems schedule providers, but scheduling the supporting clinical staff is often overlooked.

EXHIBIT 6.43 SCHEDULING PROVIDERS BY LOCATION SAMPLE

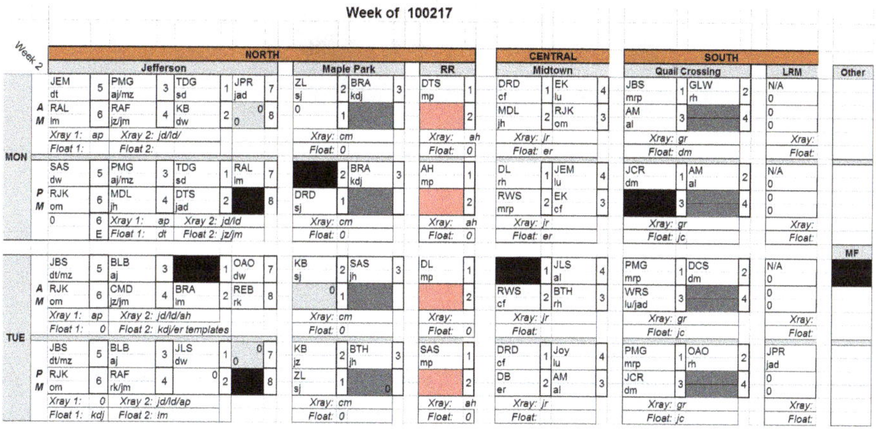

AVAILABLE ADVANCED PRACTITIONERS

This practice generally schedules advanced practitioners to see patients, but the advanced practitioners also have call responsibilities and operating room duties, making scheduling advanced practitioners more complex than other practices. As surgery schedules and call schedules change, the advanced practitioners may occasionally not be scheduled with patients, with providers, or on call. The custom SSRS email in Exhibit 6.44 is a weekly analysis of the upcoming schedule for the next four weeks. This practice's experience is that with enough notice, the advanced practitioners' schedules are much more productive. Before this email was implemented, advanced practitioners would occasionally not be scheduled in the operating room or on call. By the time the practice realized the advanced practitioner was available to see patients, it was too late to fill their schedule. This same approach could be taken with other practice resources in different specialties.

Exhibit 6.44 Advanced Practitioners Scheduling

Midlevels Available in the Next 4 Weeks

Midlevel	Date	AMPM	Provider
	9/5/2017	AM	
	9/28/2017	PM	
	9/29/2017	AM	
	9/29/2017	PM	
	9/15/2017	AM	
	9/19/2017	PM	
	9/5/2017	AM	
	9/5/2017	PM	
	9/19/2017	AM	
	9/19/2017	PM	
	9/26/2017	AM	
	9/26/2017	PM	

The same practice also uses provider schedules to schedule clinical staff. A spreadsheet connected to the data warehouse imports provider schedules. The spreadsheet tracks which providers are in office locations that need clinical staff support and which providers are in surgical locations where the clinic staff are not needed. The spreadsheet quickly highlights providers in office locations who do not have staff assigned. The spreadsheet also tracks providers in surgical locations who do have clinical staff assigned so that the staff can be reassigned to support other providers. An example of the spreadsheet is shown in Exhibit 6.45.

EXHIBIT 6.45 CLINICAL STAFF SCHEDULING

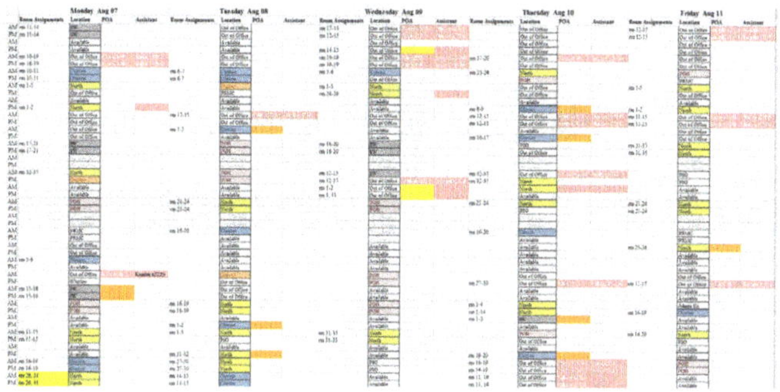

Once that spreadsheet was successful, a second spreadsheet tab summarized the schedule by provider and location for each member of the clinical team. The spreadsheet also helped schedule exam rooms. Over time, good Business Intelligence reports get better as more team members are exposed to them. Often the best ideas to build on existing reports come from end users who use the reports daily.

UPCOMING APPOINTMENTS THAT WILL NOT BE REIMBURSED

This report was designed just in time to make it in this book. The practice had been notified that the local Medicaid plan would only pay for a podiatry visit once every 365 days. The report pulls all future appointments with podiatry providers and compares the appointment date to the date of the patients' last podiatry visit. The daily email to help staff reschedule these appointments is shown in Exhibit 6.46.

EXHIBIT 6.46 UPCOMING APPOINTMENTS WITH NO REIMBURSEMENTS REPORT SAMPLE

Upcoming Medicaid and HIP Podiatry Appointments Less than
1 Year from Last Appointment as of 9/1/2017

Appt Start	Acct Num	Patient Name	Doctor	Last Visit
9/7/2017	10739931			7/31/2017
9/8/2017	10680094			6/9/2017
9/13/2017	10739562			8/11/2017
9/13/2017	10722516			3/23/2017
9/13/2017	10732667			7/27/2017
9/14/2017	10737051			7/27/2017
9/15/2017	10710634			8/2/2017
9/18/2017	821758			8/18/2017
9/19/2017	10144390			6/27/2017
9/21/2017	10679221			7/13/2017
9/21/2017	10710634			8/2/2017
9/21/2017	10738454			7/14/2017
9/22/2017	10717913			8/2/2017

The report isn't fancy, but it does get the practice reimbursed for every visit they can schedule appropriately. The report is another example of something that would be very difficult to get from a canned PM report. What upcoming appointments do your schedulers need to see?

USING SCHEDULES TO MARKET THE PRACTICE

The final example in this chapter comes from an orthopedic practice. The practice wanted a way to tell hospitals and other potential referral sources which orthopedic specialists were at which location tomorrow. The goal was to make it easy for those referral sources to know who was available for a referral tomorrow. This is the only example in this chapter of an email sent outside the practice, but it is an easy way to market the practice and increase patient referrals as long as all necessary precautions to protect patient information are taken.

EXHIBIT 6.47 SCHEDULING REPORT FOR REFERRING PROVIDERS SAMPLE

Sport Doctors In Tomorrow

Location	Doctor	Date	AM PM
		9/5/2017	AM
		9/5/2017	PM
		9/5/2017	AM
		9/5/2017	PM
		9/5/2017	AM
		9/5/2017	PM
		9/5/2017	AM
		9/5/2017	PM
		9/5/2017	AM
		9/5/2017	PM

CHAPTER 7

MEASURING PRODUCTIVITY

Now more than ever, practice managers are being asked to do more with less. Expenses are increasing dramatically, while many specialties are seeing revenue reductions. Many practices are running close to maximum capacity under their current workflows and systems. Simply working harder is likely not the answer. Workflows and systems need to be improved so the practice can work smarter, and that improvement needs to be measured. This chapter focuses on ways to measure and increase productivity across the practice, from providers to the billing office. *Better Data, Better Decisions* included this quote from Thomas S. Monson. "Where performance is measured, performance improves. Where performance is measured and reported, the rate of improvement accelerates." That principle is true in life, but medical practices have another advantage. The ability to measure and compare productivity can motivate providers as much or more than any other factor. When processes to work smarter are measured and shared, a naturally competitive nature often motivates providers to improve.

The examples in this chapter range from measuring physician productivity to the workflow of the billing office staff to the duration of patient appointments. The underlying theme is that each practice found an issue that directly impacted the bottom line in their situation and designed a report or a series of reports to measure that metric over time. The process is often iterative. The lag days report is a good example. Once the practice decided to analyze lag days, the data showed that there was a significant difference based on whether pathology was involved. Drilling down to location identified differences between employed pathologists and outside pathologists. Now the practice has a benchmark to compare both situations over time.

This chapter contains the Front Desk Balances to Collect reports. Productivity driven by these reports can be some of the easiest ways to justify Business Intelligence in a practice. At a minimum, collecting copayments means collecting money from patients sooner than waiting for payers to process claims. Collecting copayments in advance also saves time and effort sending patient statements. In some practices, collecting copayments means a much better chance of collections from patients period. Productivity improvements are a fertile place to look for initial Business Intelligence projects.

MEASURING PROVIDER PRODUCTIVITY USING WORK RVUS

The PivotTable in Exhibit 7.1 is an excerpt from a neurosurgery practice's analysis of work RVUs. Work RVUs in 2018 have dropped considerably. While the overall results are important, using PivotTables provides the ability to understand why the trend is down. The initial analysis by provider helped the practice see that a big part of the decrease was retiring providers, but that was not the entire story. The providers labeled MD A and MD F have decreased as well. By using the PivotTable to continue to filter on procedure code, location, and referring physician, the practice can see how much of the decrease is due to fewer procedures and how much is due to decreased referrals.

EXHIBIT 7.1 MEASURING PROVIDER PRODUCTIVITY WITH wRVUS SAMPLE

Charge Location	(All)
CPT Code	(All)
Department	(All)
Practice	(All)
Primary Financial Class	(All)
Referring Physician	(All)
Zip	(All)
Begin DOS	(All)

Sum of Work RVU	Column Labels			
Row Labels	2016	2017	2018	Grand Total
	21,292	17,804	15,571	54,668
	20,629	17,883	19,793	58,305
	21,608	22,692	23,454	67,754
	20,077	19,617	5,501	45,195
	10,344	11,378	13,519	35,241
	24,781	25,265	26,490	76,537
	18,358	16,787	16,605	51,750
	13,658	15,802	4,197	33,657
	20,184	14,436	4,255	38,875
Grand Total	170,932	161,665	129,386	461,982

The practice administrator uses analyses like this in annual strategy meetings with the partner physicians. Compensation is driven by work RVUs, so physicians are interested in their numbers. It also helps for physicians to see their productivity compared to their peers. Since retiring providers are an important consideration in this practice, the work RVU detail is also factored in decisions about when to bring in another provider.

Since provider revenue is often tied to payer mix, the group looked at changes in payer mix and the impact of those changes in providers' productivity. Sometimes decreases in productivity are outside the providers' control. Schedules and workflows may need to be modified so that providers can work as hard as they want to work.

WHICH PROVIDER TO SEE NEXT

Some practices try to be productive by having advanced practitioners see patients while the patients are working through conservative care requirements imposed by payers. Once patients are approved for surgery, the patient is scheduled to see the surgeon who will perform the surgery. This practice looks at patients seen in a same-day clinic by an advanced practitioner. The SSRS email looks at the next scheduled patient appointment for certain providers. Patients whose last appointment is with an advanced practitioner and whose next appointment is with the surgeon are included in the report. Patients meeting certain criteria for surgery are flagged with the yellow highlight in the first column. Scheduling and clinical staff review those appointments to make sure the appointments are scheduled in accordance with the surgeon's protocols.

EXHIBIT 7.2 SURGERY PROTOCOL SCHEDULING SAMPLE

Yesterday Appointments as of 9/1/2017

Acct Num	Patient Name	Resource	Next Appt Created By	Next Appt Date	Next Appt Resource	Next Appt Category
599991				9/7/2017		Doctor
660824				9/7/2017		Doctor
828990				9/21/2017		Doctor
10729455				9/13/2017		Doctor
10742797				9/13/2017		Doctor
10742827				9/5/2017		Doctor

FRONT DESK BALANCES TO COLLECT

If you are looking for low-hanging Business Intelligence with the potential for a fast return on investment, look no further. Appointment data can be extremely helpful to improve front desk collections. Typically, this involves two emails. The first email lists all the day's appointments at each location and reports the copays and patient balances expected to be collected that day. It's delivered to the front desk staff early each morning. An example is shown in Exhibit 7.3.

EXHIBIT 7.3 TODAY'S APPOINTMENTS AND BALANCES DUE FOR FRONT
DESK SAMPLE

Balances To Collect at Denver Office as of 9/1/2017

Appt Date	Provider	Acct Num	Patient	Appt Type	Copay	Pat Balance
7:30 AM		95009			$0.00	$603.63
7:30 AM		61489			$60.00	$3,840.76
7:30 AM		53631			$50.00	$0.00
7:45 AM		83675			$0.00	$2,495.15
7:45 AM		102146			$40.00	$0.00
8:00 AM		2145			$0.00	$1,329.44
8:00 AM		78009			$0.00	$177.09
8:00 AM		66608			$0.00	$204.20
8:00 AM		1332			$0.00	$49.07
8:30 AM		85549			$50.00	$52.00
8:45 AM		99235			$50.00	$0.00
9:00 AM		102274			$35.00	$0.00
9:00 AM		87121			$90.00	$0.00
9:15 AM		97483			$35.00	$0.00
9:45 AM		101899			$45.00	$0.00
10:00 AM		2145			$0.00	$1,329.44

A dropdown list at the top of the report allows the user to filter by facility. When you subscribe to a report with a parameter like this, SSRS allows you to include the parameter so that the email for the South office front desk team automatically chooses South as the location. The idea behind this report is to show the front desk which patients are coming in today who owe the practice either a copayment or a patient balance.

First, accurate patient insurance information, especially the copayment amount, must be stored in the PM system. The most time-consuming part of the logic is factoring out appointments where a copay isn't required. The logic that determines which patients owe a copayment varies by insurer, specialty, type of care and practice. Most practices focus on the patient's primary insurance to make the copayment determinations. Practices could filter out Medicare patients from owing a copayment, even if those patients may owe coinsurance at the start of the year. Workers compensation or accident patients may be similarly excluded. A practice in the Southwest filters out patients who have a secondary insurance, assuming that the secondary insurance will generally cover the copayment. Another practice records global period information with each procedure code and looks back at prior patient visits to exclude patients who are in a global period from owing a copayment. Some practices use the appointment type to determine which patients owe a copayment. The example above includes an appointment type column. It usually takes some combination of this logic to get a reasonable estimation of the patients owing a copayment. As the report is worked, the front desk will help find additional exceptions to the report so that their percentage collected numbers are accurate.

The goal is to produce a daily list with copayments the front desk should collect. That daily list will become a denominator on tomorrow's report that measures the percentage of copayments collected. If the email incorrectly shows the front desk missed copayments, the front desk will let you know that some patient appointment types need to be filtered out. Be careful not to unduly filter out patient appointments from the denominator since you clearly want the front desk to collect everything the practice is entitled to collect. There is a balance to be struck when setting the copayment denominator. It may be worth setting the front desk copayment collection goal a little lower and including appointments with potential copayments rather than having the front desk collect 100% of a smaller number that excludes potential copayments.

Some practices include a patient balance in the morning email, treating the patient visit as a prime opportunity to collect from the patient. Other practices prefer to let the billing office's system collect patient balances. Part of this decision may be driven by the culture of the practice and the strength of the front desk team. The example in Exhibit 7.3 includes the patient balance at the far right. For this practice, the primary goal is to collect the copayment, but the front desk is encouraged to collect any patient balances as well.

The email in Exhibit 7.3 is an exception report. This email isn't designed to tell the front desk every appointment coming in today. The email only includes patients who either owe a copayment or who have a patient balance.

Usually filtering by location and sorting by appointment time is sufficient for the front desk to collect from patients. A large clinic could also consider adding the provider or resource for the appointment. For example, assume primary care patients check in on the first floor and cardiology patients check in on the third floor. The data warehouse could read the type of provider on the appointment, categorize the appointment, and filter the appointments accordingly. The objective is to make the email as easy as possible for the front desk to use.

A second email is also delivered each morning. This email, Exhibit 7.4, refers to yesterday (or the last day the clinic is open) to evaluate the front desk's performance in collecting copayments and patient balances. The trick with this email is determining who should have collected from the patient. The analysis is grouped by who should have collected the money. The light blue line on the email (the name is masked in the exhibit) shows who should have collected from the patient. Depending on the practice, the staff responsible for collecting from the patient could be the check-in person or the cashier. At one orthopedic practice, the responsibility to collect from the patient varies by location. At some locations, the receptionist is responsible to collect copayments at check in. At other practice locations, the cashier is responsible to collect as the patient checks out. Teach the data warehouse who is responsible to collect the copayment so that the email is correctly informative.

Exhibit 7.4 Outstanding Balance Collections Performance Tracking for Front Desk Staff Sample

Yesterday's Front Desk Collections as of 9/1/2017

Appt Date	Acct	Provider	Appt Type	Primary Ins Group	Copay Collected	Copay To Collect	%	Pt Pmt Collected	Pt Pmt To Collect	%
						$0.00			$178.90	0%
3:30 PM	80954		OV - 15	Aetna		$0.00			$178.90	0%
					$260.00	$330.00	79%	$21.03	$11,863.14	0%
8:00 AM	76171			United Healthcare		$50.00	0%		$0.00	
8:30 AM	94839		CKUP - 30	BCBS	$30.00	$30.00	100%		$0.00	
9:00 AM	84903		OV - 15	United Healthcare		$0.00			$121.92	0%
9:45 AM	97994		OV - 15	Aetna	$15.00	$30.00	50%		$0.00	
10:30 AM	100282			BCBS		$30.00	0%		$0.00	
10:45 AM	81478		OV - 15	Medicare		$0.00			$11,690.19	0%
12:30 PM	95534		OV - 30	HMO	$50.00	$50.00	100%		$0.00	
1:00 PM	34270		OV - 15	PacifiCare SecureHorizons	$50.00	$50.00	100%		$0.00	
1:15 PM	100953			CIGNA	$60.00	$30.00	200%		$30.00	0%
2:00 PM	41694		OV - 15	BCBS	$20.00					
2:00 PM	97399			United Healthcare		$0.00		$21.03	$21.03	100%
3:45 PM	43836		OV - 15	BCBS	$35.00	$60.00	58%		$0.00	
					$755.00	$695.00	109%	$221.10	$2,457.61	9%

Once you know whether to look for the receptionist or the cashier, finding the person in the PM data can be tricky as well. Some systems store the information. Other PM systems store the person who changed the appointment status to "checked in" or "checked out." Still other PM systems show the last person to modify an appointment, which can mean the receptionist or the cashier. This question may take IT help or support from the PM vendor to answer. You might also try experimenting on fake patients to understand how the PM system stores the information you need to make the report accurate.

Based on the amounts expected to be collected yesterday, this report shows the total amounts actually collected as a percentage of the total amounts available to collect. There is also a logic system in place to account for patients who may have multiple appointments on the same day or who were somehow checked in or out multiple times during the day.

Another challenge with this data is identifying patient payments as copayments. Some PM systems make this question easy by tracking copayments as a payment type. Other PM systems need to be configured to create a copayment payment type. Sometimes it is matter of correctly entering payments in the PM system. The front desk workflow may need to change to ensure the copayments are entered in the system as the proper payment type.

If these solutions do not work due to limitations with the PM system or the practice's workflow, then consider a practice in the southeast that matches the date of a payment with the date of a patient appointment. If a patient pays an amount on the same day as a patient appointment, the assumption is that the payment was collected by the front desk. The difficulty with matching the payment date to an appointment date is distinguishing a copayment from payment on a patient balance.

The bottom line is that it can be tricky to determine if a patient owes a copayment, who should collect that copayment, and how much of the copayment was collected. This type of logic is exceedingly difficult to obtain from a canned PM report. Despite these complications, do not let getting the report perfect be the enemy of starting the report at all. Start tracking front desk collections and hold the staff responsible. For many practices, these two email reports are packed with revenue potential. The return on investment for these emails can be weeks, not months or years.

The emails are a daily summary. Copy practice managers on the emails to ensure the front desk knows how important copayments are. PivotTables are a terrific way to analyze trends in front desk collections over time. Use the PivotTable to analyze collections by staff member, location, day of the week, appointment type, and more. Are some staff members better at collecting copayments or patient balances? Those staff members are the trainers. Which locations need more training to collect copayments and which locations need a celebratory lunch after a particularly good month?

THE FOLLOWING BENCHMARKS FROM MGMA'S PRACTICE OPERATIONS REPORT SHOW THE PERCENTAGE OF COPAYMENTS AND PATIENT PAYMENTS COLLECTED AT THE TIME OF SERVICE. MULTISPECIALTY PRACTICES HAVE THE MOST ROOM TO IMPROVE, ESPECIALLY WHEN IT COMES TO COLLECTING PATIENT DUE BALANCES. IDEAS IN THIS SECTION CAN HELP YOUR PRACTICE COLLECT MORE AT THE FRONT DESK.

EXHIBIT 7.5 MEDIAN COPAYMENTS COLLECTED AT TIME OF SERVICE

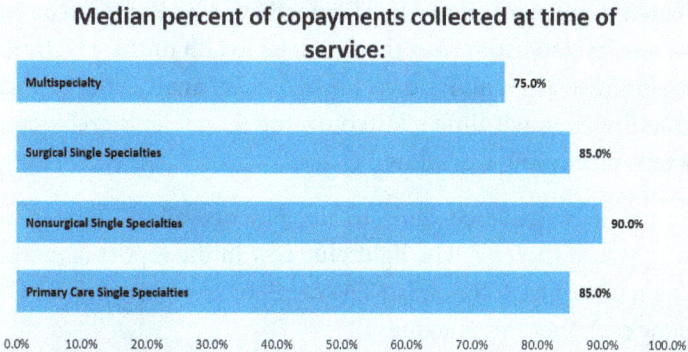

Median percent of copayments collected at time of service:

- Multispecialty: 75.0%
- Surgical Single Specialties: 85.0%
- Nonsurgical Single Specialties: 90.0%
- Primary Care Single Specialties: 85.0%

SOURCE: *MGMA 2016 PRACTICE OPERATIONS REPORT: BASED ON 2015 SURVEY DATA*

EXHIBIT 7.6 MEDIAN OUTSTANDING BALANCES COLLECTED AT TIME OF SERVICE

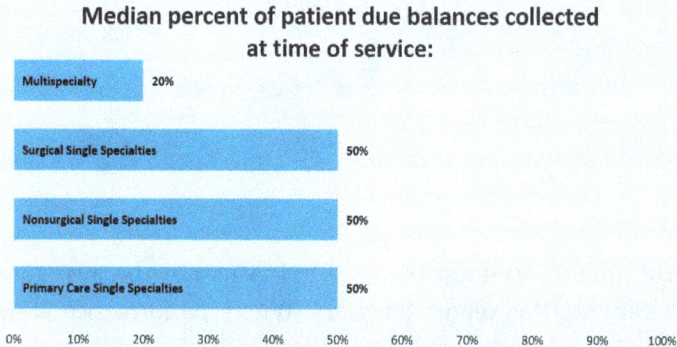

Median percent of patient due balances collected at time of service:

- Multispecialty: 20%
- Surgical Single Specialties: 50%
- Nonsurgical Single Specialties: 50%
- Primary Care Single Specialties: 50%

SOURCE: *MGMA 2016 PRACTICE OPERATIONS REPORT: BASED ON 2015 SURVEY DATA*

189

PHYSICAL THERAPY PRODUCTIVITY

This example comes from a practice that offers physical therapy (PT). The practice administrator came back from a physical therapy conference with a benchmark for PT visits to be 1.5 work RVUs. The intention of the practice was certainly not to bill for services that were not medically necessary, but to make sure that the services that were rendered were captured appropriately. The practice educated the therapists and implemented procedures, but the workflow that made a difference was a reporting mechanism. With reimbursement challenges related to PT, effectively managing and monitoring RVU productivity can assist with the financial health of the practice. It also allows the administrator and PT director to quickly analyze the patients who may not require as much time allotted on the schedule, thereby creating a more efficient scheduling workflow.

This SSRS email is delivered daily to the practice administrator and the director of physical therapy. The light blue row in the report is masked, but it shows the name of each therapist. The detail of any low work RVU visit is shown below each therapist's name.

EXHIBIT 7.7 LOW PROVIDER PRODUCTIVITY WITH LOW wRVUs SAMPLE

Yesterday's Low RVU PT Visits as of 8/26/2016

Enc Number	Patient	Begin DOS	Total Charges	Total Work RVU
1229297		8/18/2016	$116	1.06
1231684		8/25/2016	$80	0.90

It's hard to find an example of low RVU visits now because the practice has been running this report for years. Where performance is measured, performance improves.

LAG DAYS

Productivity reports are not just for providers. This example measures lag days, the number of days between the date of service and the date a claim is billed. Any reduction in lag days increases the speed at which a practice is paid. This example from a gastroenterology group shows how drilling down to root causes can help understand lag days. Some of the lag days calculation is under the providers' control, some of the calculation is under the practice's control, and the practice does not have control over some issues.

The practice has two main drivers of lag days, the time it takes for the provider to document the encounter in the EHR and the time it takes the billing office to file a claim once the documentation is complete. The two columns "Average of Lag Days to EHR" and "Average of Lag Days to Bill" capture these two components. In this practice, the EHR documentation time is significantly longer than the billing office time.

EXHIBIT 7.8 AVERAGE LAG DAYS TO EHR AND BILLING SAMPLE

Row Labels	Average of Lag Days to EHR	Average of Lag Days to Bill	Average of Lag Days
	13.8	0.4	14.2
	13.8	0.3	14.1
	13.6	0.6	14.2
	13.2	0.3	13.5
	13.0	0.5	13.5
	12.7	0.4	13.0
	12.6	0.3	12.9
	12.5	1.4	13.9
Providers	12.1	1.3	13.4
	12.0	1.2	13.2
Are	11.8	0.5	12.3
	11.4	0.5	11.9
	10.8	6.2	16.9
Listed	8.5	6.1	14.6
	7.5	0.9	8.4
Here	7.5	3.8	11.2
	5.8	9.1	14.9
	5.7	8.8	14.5
	5.4	4.8	10.2
	5.0	10.4	15.3
	4.6	7.8	12.3
	4.5	3.7	8.2
	4.3	1.4	5.7
	3.9	5.3	9.2

The practice has two main Lag Days areas of focus: office visits and procedures. Office visits should be documented promptly in the EHR, but procedures take much longer to document because the providers wait for the pathology results before finishing the documentation, and coding staff can better code the diagnosis if they have the final pathology report. In the PivotTable in Exhibit 7.9, place of service has been added below the provider (name masked). The practice administrator uses place of service (11, 21, 22, etc.) as a proxy for office visits vs. procedures. The proxy isn't perfect, as some procedures are done in place of service 11. The PivotTable still shows the dramatic difference between lag days for office procedures compared to non-office procedures.

EXHIBIT 7.9 AVERAGE LAG DAYS TO EHR AND BILLING WITH PLACE OF SERVICE SAMPLE

Row Labels	Average of Lag Days to EHR	Average of Lag Days to Bill	Average of Lag Days
⊟	13.8	0.4	14.2
⊕ 11	8.9	0.7	9.7
⊕ 21	20.6	0.0	20.6
⊕ 22	20.6	0.0	20.6
⊕ 23	20.6	0.0	20.6
⊕ 24	18.4	0.0	18.5
⊟	13.8	0.3	14.1
⊕ 11	8.3	0.7	8.9
⊕ 21	24.6	-1.1	23.6
⊕ 22	20.2	0.0	20.2
⊕ 23	25.7	0.0	25.7
⊕ 24	18.8	0.0	18.9
⊟	13.6	0.6	14.2
⊕ 11	8.0	1.0	9.0
⊕ 21	23.7	0.0	23.7
⊕ 22	21.1	0.0	21.1
⊕ 23	25.0	0.0	25.0
⊕ 24	20.3	0.0	20.3
⊟	13.2	0.3	13.5
⊕ 11	8.8	0.7	9.6
⊕ 21	18.0	0.0	18.0
⊕ 22	18.3	0.0	18.3
⊕ 23	18.7	0.0	18.7
⊕ 24	17.1	0.0	17.0

The average lag days for the billing office is less than one day, which means the billing office is billing most of the claims the same day the claims are documented in the EHR and ready to be billed. Pay attention to the negative 1.1 average days to bill circled in red. Occasionally there will be discrepancies in the data due to billing errors, rebilled claims, or EHR documentation issues. If you see a lot of issues with the data, filter out any lag days less than zero or more than the maximum number of expected lag days. In this practice, you might filter out lag days calculated over 45 or 60 days. Each practice must decide how to best to filter outliers without accidentally filtering out valid data.

Some locations are supported by in-house pathology. Other locations rely on outside pathology so the wait time for results is outside of the practice's control. In Exhibit 7.10 the location names (masked) have been added below the place of service. For the first provider, the average lag days for place of service 11 is 8.9, but that average is made up of three separate locations with averages of 18.3, 1.9, and 17.8 respectively. The 1.9 average is office visits. The 18.3 and 17.8 locations are locations where procedures are performed. The longer lag days locations in Exhibit 7.10 are locations where the practice does not control the pathology. With this level of detail, the practice can focus on providers whose documentation for evaluation and management visits is slow. The practice can ensure that the billing office is filing claims in a timely manner. The practice can compare pathology times for employed pathologists to that of outside pathologists. Each of these calculations can be trended over time. Where performance is measured and reported, the rate of improvement accelerates.

EXHIBIT 7.10 AVERAGE LAG DAYS TO EHR AND BILLING WITH PLACE OF SERVICE AND LOCATION SAMPLE

Row Labels	Average of Lag Days to EHR	Average of Lag Days to Bill	Average of Lag Days
	13.8	0.4	14.2
11	8.9	0.7	9.7
	18.3	0.0	18.3
	1.9	1.3	3.1
	17.8	0.0	17.8
21	20.6	0.0	20.6
	20.6	0.0	20.6
22	20.6	0.0	20.6
	18.3	0.0	18.3
	18.2	0.1	18.2
	21.1	0.0	21.1
	31.1	0.0	31.2
	0.0	0.0	0.0
23	20.6	0.0	20.6
	20.6	0.0	20.6
24	18.4	0.0	18.5
	7.0	0.0	7.0
	18.4	0.0	18.5

Here is MGMA's benchmark lag time data from the 2016 *Practice Operations Report*. Surgical single specialties have the longest lag time. How do your providers and locations compare to these benchmarks? What ideas from this section will help your lag days decrease?

Exhibit 7.11 Median Charge Posting Lag Time - in Days

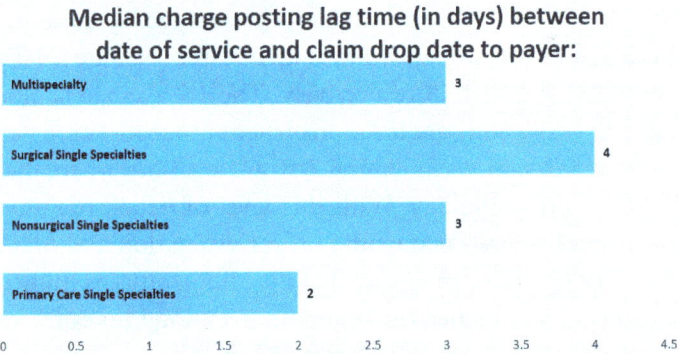

Median charge posting lag time (in days) between date of service and claim drop date to payer:

Specialty	Value
Multispecialty	3
Surgical Single Specialties	4
Nonsurgical Single Specialties	3
Primary Care Single Specialties	2

Source: *MGMA 2016 Practice Operations Report: Based on 2015 Survey Data*

DATA ENTRY

Exhibits 7.12 and 7.13 are examples of how one practice tracks data entry activities in the billing office. Exhibit 7.12 tracks the number of charges entered by the login of the staff entering the charges. The heading to the SSRS dashboard indicates that quality codes are excluded from the count. The SSRS report separates and subtotals charges by staff member in the first column. The practice also separates charges entered by the place of service (OFF stands for office and NOF stands for non-office charges). Generally non-office procedures are more time consuming to enter. The manager of this department can easily see workloads and trends by staff member and can reassign staff as necessary.

EXHIBIT 7.12 CHARGES ENTERED BY CLINICAL STAFF LOGIN TRACKING SAMPLE

Count Charges Entered as of 9/1/2017
by Line Item (Quality Codes Excluded)

Created By	Off Or Nof	Jan	Feb	Mar	Apr	May	Jun	Jul	Aug	Sep	Total
	NOF	4	1	17	12	22	50	21	18		145
	OFF	1,798	5,218	5,060	4,230	4,334	4,962	3,020	4,102	316	33,040
	Total	1,802	5,219	5,077	4,242	4,356	5,012	3,041	4,120	316	33,185
	NOF	7	4	12	1	22	34	27	8		115
	OFF	2,374	3,582	4,362	3,407	4,045	4,665	3,113	3,567	119	29,234
	Total	2,381	3,586	4,374	3,408	4,067	4,699	3,140	3,575	119	29,349
	NOF	688	1,400	1,727	1,381	1,773	1,570	1,434	1,780		11,753
	OFF			1							1
	Total	688	1,400	1,728	1,381	1,773	1,570	1,434	1,780		11,754
	NOF	584	808								1,392
	OFF	5									5
	Total	589	808								1,397
	NOF	908	1,277	1,782	1,053	1,338	1,649	1,020	1,779		10,806
	OFF	1	3	4	4		1		2		15
	Total	909	1,280	1,786	1,057	1,338	1,650	1,020	1,781		10,821
	NOF	446	377	665	316	480	347	208	428		3,267
	OFF	16	27	39	191	311	532	720	619		2,455
	Total	462	404	704	507	791	879	928	1,047		5,722
	NOF		2	3	5	11	9	3			33
	OFF	698	3,941	5,411	5,470	6,807	6,432	4,791	4,755	191	38,496
	Total	698	3,943	5,414	5,475	6,818	6,441	4,794	4,755	191	38,529
	NOF	681	1,162	1,453	1,212	1,313	1,310	1,023	1,618	230	10,002
	OFF	14	12	1	20	100	9	975	1,031	14	2,176
	Total	695	1,174	1,454	1,232	1,413	1,319	1,998	2,649	244	12,178
	NOF		1		1		5	1			8
	OFF		1	3	1,450	3,818	4,739	244			10,255
	Total		2	3	1,451	3,818	4,744	245			10,263

Exhibit 7.13 does the same analysis for payments entered. Most payments in this practice are entered by uploading electronic remittances into the PM system, but patient payments are generally entered manually. This SSRS dashboard (which is also emailed at the first of each month) is a rolling 12-month report as opposed to the calendar year charges report. The underlying dataset drives the date range of the report. SSRS can easily report on either date range. Both reports are customized to the needs of the managers overseeing the department and are designed to measure the workload of the charge entry and payment entry departments.

Exhibit 7.13 Payment Entered by Staff Login Tracking Sample

Count Payments Entered Last 12 Months as of 9/1/2017

Staff	Sep 2016	Oct 2016	Nov 2016	Dec 2016	Jan 2017	Feb 2017	Mar 2017	Apr 2017	May 2017	Jun 2017	Jul 2017	Aug 2017	Total
	6,090	5,790	5,244	4,637	4,857	4,993	5,758	4,762	6,112	5,864	5,501	5,767	65,375
	5,283	7,130	4,335	5,526	4,832	4,183	6,006	5,296	5,199	5,497	3,954	4,171	61,412
	548	749	692	415	608	432	1,199	484	1,077	655	592	719	8,170
	8,747	6,792	6,329	3,688	5,046	4,870	6,089	3,220	5,759	4,787	3,922	3,955	63,204
Total	20,668	20,461	16,600	14,266	15,343	14,478	19,052	13,762	18,147	16,803	13,969	14,612	198,161

MGMA's *Practice Operations Report* provides helpful benchmark information here. The first chart is encounters processed per day, and the second chart is claims processed per day. Multispecialty practices do better on these measures, followed by primary care and single specialty practices. A daily, weekly, and monthly email detailing encounters and claims processed per day by staff member, compared to these benchmarks, has the potential to dramatically increase billing office productivity in your practice.

Exhibit 7.14 Median Encounters Processed Per Day By CODING Staff

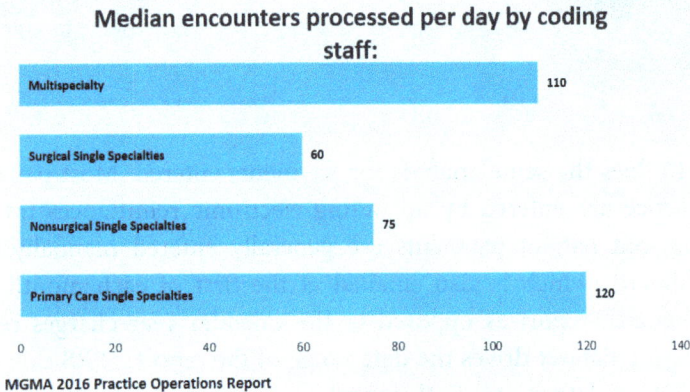

Median encounters processed per day by coding staff:

- Multispecialty — 110
- Surgical Single Specialties — 60
- Nonsurgical Single Specialties — 75
- Primary Care Single Specialties — 120

MGMA 2016 Practice Operations Report

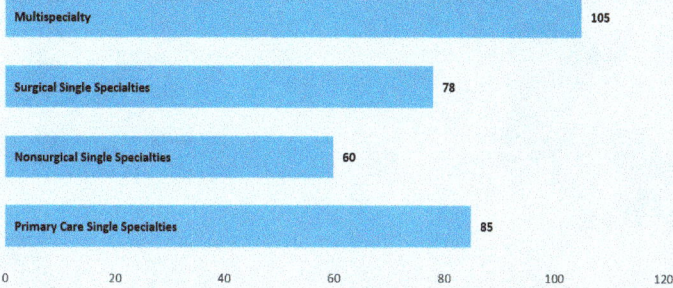

EXHIBIT 7.15 MEDIAN CLAIMS PROCESSED PER DAY BY CODING STAFF

Median claims processed per day by coding staff:

Multispecialty — 105
Surgical Single Specialties — 78
Nonsurgical Single Specialties — 60
Primary Care Single Specialties — 85

SOURCE: *MGMA 2016 PRACTICE OPERATIONS REPORT: BASED ON 2015 SURVEY DATA*

COLLECTION ACTIVITIES

Exhibit 7.16 takes workflow changes to gather the data this practice administrator wanted to see. The practice wanted to know if it was cost-effective for billing department staff to make outbound collections calls and how many calls were being made. The PM software does not track collection calls, so the first step was to ask the staff making the calls to change their workflow. Each time they made a call, the staff put a dummy transaction code in the patient's encounter. The dummy code doesn't appear on insurance claims or patient statements, but it does allow SQL Server to find every time that code is entered. The PM system tracks who entered the code, so the SSRS report can show who made the call and can count those calls by month. The PM system also stores the date the code was entered, so the SQL Server logic can also look for patient payments made up to 20 days after the call. The combined data is shown in Exhibit 7.16.

You can see that SSRS allows the collections and the number of calls made to be shown in the same cell. Collections are shown with a dollar amount and the number of outbound calls is shown in parentheses. The staff names are masked in the first column.

197

EXHIBIT 7.16 PATIENT PAYMENTS AFTER COLLECTIONS CALLS TRACKING SAMPLE

Patient Payments After Collection Call as of 9/1/2017

Staff	Turned	Apr 2017	May 2017	Jun 2017	Jul 2017	Aug 2017
Call to Patient re:						
	Not Turned	$0.00 (0)	$0.00 (0)	$45.00 (1)	$0.00 (0)	$0.00 (0)
	Not Turned	$1,098.51 (5)	$1,133.56 (5)	$341.00 (3)	$559.04 (10)	$117.00 (1)
	Turned	$100.00 (1)	$50.00 (1)	$0.00 (0)	$313.87 (2)	$0.00 (0)
	Not Turned	$184.68 (2)	$5,818.59 (16)	$7,096.63 (19)	$3,804.15 (10)	$311.99 (3)
	Turned	$0.00 (0)	$4,951.16 (2)	$156.51 (5)	$195.00 (3)	$0.00 (0)
	Not Turned	$2,888.01 (13)	$1,033.75 (5)	$5,092.17 (11)	$901.80 (3)	$250.60 (3)
	Turned	$165.00 (2)	$181.00 (3)	$165.00 (3)	$77.00 (1)	$134.03 (1)
	Not Turned	$1,104.05 (8)	$336.15 (6)	$2,579.58 (11)	$2,730.08 (8)	$3,116.70 (10)
	Turned	$62.26 (2)	$0.00 (0)	$1,950.00 (4)	$30.00 (2)	$169.00 (2)
	Not Turned	$832.02 (9)	$2,349.00 (5)	$7,112.77 (7)	$5,025.47 (15)	$7,158.01 (16)
	Turned	$0.00 (0)	$71.01 (2)	$0.00 (0)	$485.62 (2)	$829.27 (10)
	Subtotal	$6,434.53 (43)	$15,924.22 (45)	$24,538.66 (64)	$14,122.03 (56)	$12,086.60 (46)

Once this report had been running for a few months, the next question was whether patients who had been turned to collection would be more likely or less likely to respond to a call from the billing department. The "Turned" column tracks patients who have been turned to collection. Now the manager can see how many calls have been made to patients in each category and can decide whether it is beneficial to call patients who have been sent to collection in the past.

CLINICAL SCHEDULING

One of the duties of clinical staff in this medical practice is to ensure that certain patients always have a next visit scheduled or a recall reminder set up to make a future appointment. A list of follow up protocols is created per provider with the pertinent details and then a report is created to look for any patients who are not scheduled within the set parameters. This practice uses this daily SSRS email to track that objective.

Managers can easily compare the follow-up objective by provider using this daily email. Since the clinical staff getting a copy of the email know that managers are watching this objective, the rate of performance on this objective has increased.

EXHIBIT 7.17 PATIENT FOLLOW-UP CALL LOG SAMPLE

Follow Up After Yesterday's Appointments as of 9/1/2017

Appt	Location	Acct Num	Pat Last Name	Future Appt/Recall Date
Next Visit Scheduled				
1:00 PM		3118405		10/05/2017
1:15 PM		3142818		10/10/2017
2:30 PM		3113712		09/12/2017
4:00 PM		3175743		09/07/2017
Active Recall				
1:30 PM		3182925		01/01/2018 RTC
2:00 PM		3157584		07/01/2018 RTC
2:15 PM		3183578		10/01/2017 RTC
2:45 PM		3095574		07/01/2018 RTC
3:00 PM		3182916		10/01/2017 RTC
4:00 PM		3162926		01/01/2018 RTC
No Future Appt or Recall				
1:00 PM		3184297		
1:30 PM		3153920		
1:45 PM		3183557		
2:30 PM		3183629		
3:00 PM		3182823		
3:15 PM		3183611		
3:30 PM		3183315		

DURATION

This orthopedic practice makes a serious, concerted effort to measure the duration of their office visits. The practice tracks the time the patient arrives, the time the patient spent in registration, and the time until the patient was ready to see a provider. The practice also tracks the time a patient was roomed and the time the patient left the practice. To get this level of detail, the IT group needed timestamps, date and time information stored in the PM and EHR at each milestone as the patient flows through the practice. Some of the timestamps were available in the existing software, but the IT group created additional timestamps to refine and build on the process. The underlying objective is to measure the duration of a patient appointment and then optimize that duration. From a patient's perspective, the time with the provider is the reason for the visit. Anything that can be done to reduce the duration of the rest of the appointment is a big patient satisfier. Reducing the appointment duration also makes the practice more efficient. Of course, reducing time patients spend in the lobby also makes patients happy.

Exhibit 7.18 is an example of the duration calculation in a PivotTable. The average wait time is only about a minute longer at Location 2, but the average duration of the entire patient appointment is almost 10 minutes longer. Friday appointments are longer at Locations 1 and 2, but Tuesdays are longest at Location 3. The PivotTable allows the clinical team to look at duration by doctor or the front desk team to analyze wait time by appointment type. Prior year data is available, and the practice can also trend duration by month. A recent addition to the PivotTable logic is whether the patient went to casting during the visit. The logic flags casting procedure codes during the visit to track the impact of casting on overall patient duration. The PivotTable measures reductions in wait time for patients who register with the portal and the average wait time for new patients compared to established patients.

EXHIBIT 7.18 AVERAGE WAIT TIME CALCULATIONS SAMPLE

Appt Type	(All)	
Appt Start	(All)	
Years	2017	.T
Doctor	(All)	
Week Number	(All)	
Casting During Visit	(All)	
Appt Time	(All)	

Row Labels	Average of Wait Time	Average of Duration
− Location 1	8.77	47.65
Monday	9.07	47.09
Tuesday	9.04	45.81
Wednesday	8.41	46.97
Thursday	8.29	48.63
Friday	9.15	50.92
− Location 2	8.81	55.59
Monday	9.00	57.66
Tuesday	8.67	54.43
Wednesday	9.40	53.70
Thursday	7.96	56.92
Friday	9.07	55.14
− Location 3	7.60	50.09
Monday	6.60	51.86
Tuesday	8.47	53.41
Wednesday	7.79	49.64
Thursday	7.60	47.65
Friday	7.65	46.28
Grand Total	8.57	51.96

Exhibit 7.19 is a separate, more detailed duration analysis focused on the time difference between when a patient is marked as ready by the front desk and when the patient is roomed. Using timestamps within the PM and EHR system to get this sort of data to make your practice better is almost the perfect case of custom Business Intelligence reporting. Integrating a "patient ready" timestamp in the PM and a roomed timestamp in the EHR produces very powerful data that can be used to make a practice better in the eyes of patients, practitioners, and shareholders. In this example, location 2 is the location most likely to get patients in a room within five minutes, but that percentage has been decreasing in 2017. Location 3 is meeting the goal half as often as Location 1 and one third as often as Location 2.

EXHIBIT 7.19 TIME BETWEEN PATIENT CHECK-IN AND ROOMING CALCULATIONS SAMPLE

PATIENTS ROOMED WITHIN 5 MINUTES OF READY

Weekday Name	(All)		
Doctor	(All)		
Appt Type	(All)		
Years	2017		

Count of Patient Name	Column Labels		
	⊟ Location 1	⊟ Location 2	⊟ Location 3
Row Labels	Y	Y	Y
Jan	10.51%	15.69%	4.91%
Feb	10.73%	15.44%	6.27%
Mar	9.70%	15.87%	5.20%
Apr	10.23%	13.94%	4.99%
May	9.41%	14.46%	5.33%
Jun	9.30%	14.27%	6.79%
Jul	8.67%	12.22%	6.22%
Aug	8.98%	12.57%	6.36%
Grand Total	**9.68%**	**14.31%**	**5.75%**

DURATION FOR WALK-IN CLINICS

These physicians started offering a walk-in clinic staffed by advanced practitioners. A key metric for the walk-in clinic was the number of patients seen by the advanced practitioner within 30 minutes. Waits longer than 30 minutes are categorized as a "Long Wait." Exhibit 7.20 is the PivotTable that analyzes patients at the walk-in clinic. The patient count is included so the percentage of long wait patients can be tracked. So far, almost 75% of patients wait less than 30 minutes, with an average wait of 12.2 minutes. For patients who wait longer than 30 minutes, the average wait is 52.4 minutes. Wednesdays and Thursdays are equally busy, but there are far fewer long waits on Wednesday.

EXHIBIT 7.20 WALK-IN CLINIC WAIT TIMES CALCULATIONS SAMPLE

Years	(All)
Appt Date	(All)
Doctor	(All)
Facility	(All)

	Column Labels					
	Less than 30 Minutes		Long Wait		Total Avg Duration	Total Patient Count
Row Labels	Avg Duration	Patient Count	Avg Duration	Patient Count		
Monday	12.7	478	53.2	203	24.7	681
Tuesday	13.2	285	53.6	130	25.9	415
Wednesday	11.2	383	50.1	78	17.8	461
Thursday	12.1	315	52.7	168	26.2	483
Friday	11.9	404	50.6	116	20.5	520
Grand Total	12.2	1,865	52.4	695	23.1	2,560

Armed with this analysis, management can decide how best to improve the patient experience and how to market the walk-in clinic. Management can also track the number of surgeries that result from patients whose first visit was to the walk-in clinic as shown in Exhibit 7.21. The "Avg Days to Surgery" column measures the average number of days from the patient's first visit at the walk-in clinic to the patient's surgery.

EXHIBIT 7.21 SURGERY PATIENT TRACKING SAMPLE

Surgeon	Patient Count	Surgery Revenues	Avg Days to Surgery
	16	$16,067	61.3
	6	$11,947	77.8
	14	$8,874	68.3
	2	$8,151	183.0
	16	$8,043	117.8
	13	$7,202	112.2
	5	$6,602	116.6
	6	$5,805	53.2
	4	$5,388	63.8
	13	$4,355	50.3
	8	$3,729	52.3
	1	$3,384	76.0

Productivity is measured two ways for the walk-in clinic. Patient wait times measures patient satisfaction, while measuring surgeries resulting from the walk-in clinic drives revenue.

ON-TIME BOARD

Exhibit 7.22 is an example of how a practice took their appointment lobby wait times and created an awesome patient satisfaction tool. The practice administrator stated it this way. "Our practice has a long history of trying to keep patients apprised of delays in the clinic flow. Like many practices, you would see the 'if you have waited more than 20 minutes, see our receptionist' message. We attempted to display this using chalk boards and magnets, but this required communication between the front desk and clinical teams, and often failed at the busiest times. Using our PM and EHR data we created automated display boards that update every 60 seconds, located in each of our main clinic locations. The on-time board in the patient lobby lists the providers in that location that day and if they are on time. If the provider is behind, the on-time board shows an estimate of how far behind the provider is. The process is automated on a television behind each receptionist, visible to guests in the lobby." Exhibit 7.22 is a sample on-time board.

EXHIBIT 7.22 ON TIME BOARD SAMPLE

ONE	ORTHO NORTHEAST	
WELCOME TO THE ONE SOUTHWEST MEDICAL OFFICE		
Today Is: Tuesday, November 22, 2016		
Andersen MD. Lane R		OnTime
Bailey MD, William R		OnTime
Casey MD, Ben G		OnTime
Adham MD, Mehdi		20 Min. Late

The on-time board reads the daily schedule to know which providers are scheduled in each clinic. As patients arrive and are registered, the on-time board logic starts the clock. As patients are roomed, the on-time board recognizes the patient is no longer waiting. The longest-waiting patient by provider drives the determination of whether the provider is on time and the calculation of how far behind a provider is. The on-time board logic also drives a related television screen display in the back office so that providers, nurses, and the rooming team know how many patients are waiting in the lobby and whether the provider is showing as behind in the front lobby. The immediate feedback to the back office has reduced patient wait time and the overall appointment duration while increasing patient satisfaction. These physicians' long-standing commitment to transparency and patient care has served the practice well.

RESOURCE UTILIZATION

When designing this analysis, the following practice described their objective as "to show the effectiveness of a resource's time, our practice uses a time-based calculation comparing the available capacity as defined by the resource template against the time filled to determine the unfilled time. This helps identify when a particular resource is over or under-utilized for a period of time, uncovering trends that can be further analyzed for clues on root causes and corrective actions." These physicians have several different categories of providers and offer ancillary services. The top left part of the SSRS management dashboard shown in Chapter 11 is the chart in Exhibit 7.23. Resource utilization for providers is a relatively straight-forward calculation for most physicians, the total number of minutes appointment slots are booked divided by the total minutes appointment slots are available each day. Ancillary services are a more complex calculation. Some ancillary services are calculated using a fixed capacity. Once any portion of that capacity is "sold" or used by a patient, the remaining capacity cannot be used by another patient, so any usage of the service results in 100% capacity for that day. Other ancillary services have a fixed capacity per day but different slots can be sold to different patients. Still other ancillary services may have different hours or availability by location. The group that created this dashboard spent considerable time working with department heads to segregate and analyze ancillary services to maximize the physicians' investment in those services.

EXHIBIT 7.23 SSRS MANAGEMENT DASHBOARD: RESOURCE UTILIZATION

Resource Utilization

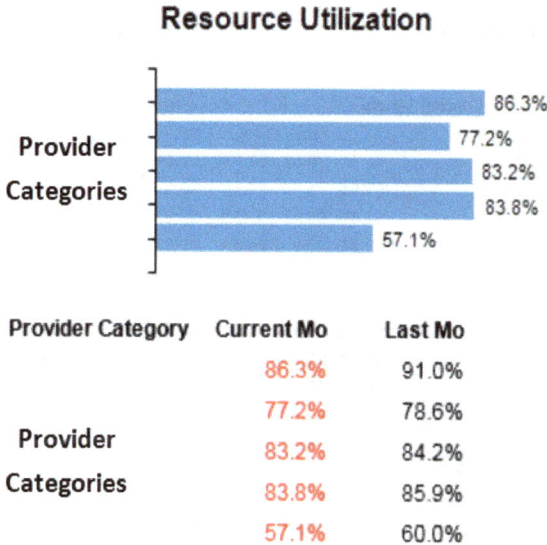

Provider Category	Current Mo	Last Mo
	86.3%	91.0%
	77.2%	78.6%
Provider	83.2%	84.2%
Categories	83.8%	85.9%
	57.1%	60.0%

Exhibit 7.24 is a PivotTable the management team used to validate the initial dashboard and to analyze trends in resource utilization going forward. Some of the physicians' utilization is over 100% (highlighted in green). Physician capacity varies by type of physician and by the philosophy of the practice. If a physician overbooks a schedule, resource utilization can rise over 100%. How to deal with overbooking when calculating utilization is a practice preference. A medical practice in Texas has some physicians who routinely hit 110% of capacity. Other practices will say that if a physician typically schedules that many patients, the benchmark should be 100%, not 110%. Vacation time is factored out of the denominator for resource utilization, so it may be helpful to compare physician capacity to other providers' denominators over time. Is a physician who books 23 of 24 20-minute appointments as productive as a physician who books 45 of 48 10-minute appointments that same day? How do call, rounds, medical director responsibilities and other duties factor into utilization? Each physician group may answer these questions differently based on the culture, the compensation and other characteristics unique to

that situation. The key is agreeing on a calculation and then measuring the utilization of the most important financial resources in the business.

EXHIBIT 7.24 RESOURCE UTILIZATION TRENDS TRACKING SAMPLE

Sum of Utilization%	Column Labels							
Row Labels	Jun	Jul	Aug	Sep	Oct	Nov	Dec	Grand Total
Provider 1		84.0%	76.5%	94.9%	67.6%	79.0%	86.0%	70.2%	79.0%
Provider 2		67.6%	71.6%	87.2%	89.3%	92.0%	93.0%	90.3%	81.6%
Provider 3		94.4%	96.4%	97.5%	97.9%	93.0%	94.5%	92.0%	95.3%
Provider 4		89.4%	85.9%	93.0%	89.8%	80.4%	86.7%	79.4%	86.8%
Provider 5		94.3%	97.3%	98.3%	101.6%	96.5%	91.4%	100.5%	96.8%
Provider 6		86.7%	84.6%	87.2%	85.7%	91.6%	90.3%	88.4%	87.4%
Provider 7		90.3%	83.8%	87.7%	92.6%	89.3%	93.3%	89.4%	89.2%
Provider 8		89.2%	95.5%	92.2%	89.7%	77.5%	87.7%	92.3%	89.9%
Provider 9		66.5%	85.3%	87.8%	90.1%	82.1%	86.1%	89.4%	83.0%
Provider 10		93.1%	92.1%	88.2%	87.4%	84.6%	85.2%	88.9%	89.0%
Provider 11		75.0%	96.4%	86.5%	97.5%	100.0%	83.3%	97.5%	91.3%
Provider 12		84.8%	87.7%	93.0%	95.5%	82.5%	69.6%	84.6%	83.0%
Provider 13		84.9%	82.0%	87.5%	87.6%	84.9%	88.4%	84.2%	85.5%
Provider 14		66.3%	59.5%	86.6%	88.0%	59.3%	66.8%	70.7%	70.8%
Provider 15		87.8%	88.1%	90.5%	89.1%	91.6%	85.8%	95.2%	89.3%
Provider 16		82.7%	87.9%	91.3%	93.8%	93.0%	92.1%	82.2%	88.4%
Grand Total		83.8%	86.4%	90.4%	90.4%	86.3%	86.8%	87.7%	87.3%

Remember the adage: "Where performance is measured, performance improves. Where performance is measured and reported, the rate of improvement accelerates." Whether measuring productivity of physicians or staff, make the metrics readily available and put the data to work. SSRS is a fabulous way to automate reporting so that performance continues to accelerate across the practice.

CHAPTER 8

DON'T TELL THE BOSS HOW EASY THIS IS: AUTOMATING RECURRING REPORTS

S ometimes one of the first Business Intelligence projects a medical practice starts with is automating an existing report. In this situation, the practice isn't usually getting new information. Instead, they are saving significant time by avoiding downloading, cleaning, and combining data to build reports day after day, month after month.

One of the dashboards in Chapter 11 saved the practice 2-3 days each month of dumping data to Excel, cleaning up the data, and recreating the analysis. Dumping and cleaning data has at least three potential downsides. First, since the process is manual, dumping and cleaning data introduces the opportunity for errors to creep into calculations. Second, dumping and cleaning takes time that the management team could be using to act on data instead of simply creating the analysis. Third, because dumping and cleaning takes so much time, physicians or administrators begin to believe that reports lag behind their usefulness.

Some canned reports in PM systems help with some of this burden, but canned reports often report more information than the busy manager wants to know. Canned reports often don't translate into Excel from the vendor's format. Canned reports can also require managers to run multiple reports and combine data to see the patterns and correlations they need. The dumping and cleaning problem begins all over again. The following examples, therefore, are focused on a specific issue displayed exactly the way the manager preferred to see it.

Another project common to many groups is pulling data out of PM or EMR systems that isn't currently available to be dumped to a spreadsheet and cleaned. Many of these projects involve so much protected health information that they aren't exhibited in this chapter. For example, a family practice group in the Pacific Northwest provides physical exams for patients to pass Department of Transportation requirements for commercial driver's licenses. The state required reports documenting the visits. In this case, the documentation was in the EHR, but was not readily available to meet the compliance requirements. The automated report eliminates retyping the information and provides just what the state requires in the proper format.

In another scenario, a physician group in Texas focuses their custom Business Intelligence projects on exception reporting. These email reports only show patient records with missing information, like missing dictation, missing labs, or missing a quality measure. Some emails come daily, while especially important emails may come several times a day. These emails helped the practice meet meaningful use requirements in the past and will help meet future quality metrics as well. The key for this practice is to only send SSRS emails when there is missing information. Send the emails to the people who can act on the missing information in time to fix the problem (before a claim goes out, before the patient arrives for their appointment, etc.)

This chapter is about not telling the boss how easy it is to have reports available in minutes instead of hours, but this example is just the opposite. Timely exception reports make the supervisor's job much easier. For critical issues, the staff may get an email several times a day. The manager only gets an email if any issues from yesterday remain unresolved. The boss knows that the staff have the information they need to do their job and that there will be a notification if something slips through the cracks.

In a different example, a group practice wanted to outsource old receivables to a collections agency, but couldn't get the patients' email addresses on the report. The canned report also failed to tell the collections agency which phone numbers corresponded to home, cell, and work numbers so that the collection agency could contact the patients accordingly. The solution to this problem was to create a report with information just the way the collection agency needed it in a spreadsheet that refreshed with current data every time the spreadsheet opened. The staff simply opened the spreadsheet, saved the data as a csv file, and sent the information securely to the agency. SSIS (discussed in Chapter 3) can automate these processes further by saving the data as a csv file in a Secure File Transfer Protocol (SFTP) location for a collection agency to automatically transfer.

To summarize, physicians and administrators pay medical practice executives for their expertise in running a business, not for running reports. It is expensive and frustrating when reports take hours to run and still need to be cleaned, modified or merged with other reports before the data is valuable. It is even more exasperating when that process must be repeated day after day, month after month. The more the report process can be automated, the more reliable the process is, the more time managers can spend acting on reports, and the more often those reports can be run. Faster, focused, friendly reports are the objectives here.

CHANGES IN CHARGES AND PAYMENTS

Exhibit 8.1 is a good example of a report that used to take a manager a long time to manually generate. A director of revenue services wanted to see potential problems before a much larger problem developed. The premise of this SSRS email is a straight-forward exception report showing the top providers whose charges or payments decreased last month relative to a 12-month moving average. The SSRS report sorts the providers two ways, by dollar decrease and percentage decrease. At a glance, she can see exactly which providers are a concern. She knows many of the reasons for the decreases (a provider was on vacation, took a medical leave, etc.) but with this report she can quickly identify variances she did not expect. Since SSRS delivers the email automatically early each month, she gets an automatic reminder to watch this metric.

EXHIBIT 8.1 PROVIDERS WITH DECREASING CHARGES TRACKING SAMPLE

Doctors with Decreasing Charges Last Month

Provider	Last Month Charges	12 Mo Avg Charges	$ Change	Provider	Last Month Charges	12 Mo Avg Charges	% Change
	$202,818	$352,227	($149,409)		$202,818	$352,227	-42.4%
	$403,200	$522,614	($119,414)		$106,239	$165,598	-35.8%
	$298,503	$365,731	($67,228)		$137,975	$197,537	-30.2%
	$137,975	$197,537	($59,562)		$403,200	$522,614	-22.8%
	$346,240	$405,653	($59,413)		$298,503	$365,731	-18.4%
	$106,239	$165,598	($59,359)		$239,698	$282,467	-15.1%
	$577,216	$635,706	($58,490)		$346,240	$405,653	-14.6%
	$360,602	$414,899	($54,297)		$360,602	$414,899	-13.1%
	$385,851	$439,440	($53,589)		$385,851	$439,440	-12.2%
	$239,698	$282,467	($42,769)		$321,099	$356,869	-10.0%
	$321,099	$356,869	($35,770)		$577,216	$635,706	-9.2%
	$338,917	$344,770	($5,853)		$338,917	$344,770	-1.7%
	$162,951	$163,551	($600)		$162,951	$163,551	-0.4%

Doctors with Decreasing Payments Last Month

Provider	Last Month Payments	12 Mo Avg Payments	$ Change	Provider	Last Month Payments	12 Mo Avg Payments	% Change
	$113,919	$151,894	($37,975)		$113,919	$151,894	-25.0%
	$64,652	$92,935	($28,283)		$64,652	$92,935	-30.4%
	$90,445	$116,432	($25,987)		$90,445	$116,432	-22.3%
	$107,407	$133,063	($25,656)		$107,407	$133,063	-19.3%
	$82,149	$106,796	($24,647)		$82,149	$106,796	-23.1%
	$22,635	$42,811	($20,176)		$22,635	$42,811	-47.1%
	$81,939	$100,174	($18,235)		$81,939	$100,174	-18.2%
	$45,055	$62,003	($16,948)		$45,055	$62,003	-27.3%
	$94,353	$109,561	($15,208)		$94,353	$109,561	-13.9%
	$115,737	$128,085	($12,348)		$115,737	$128,085	-9.6%
	$94,776	$105,377	($10,601)		$94,776	$105,377	-10.1%
	$43,793	$52,611	($8,818)		$43,793	$52,611	-16.8%
	$146,902	$154,858	($7,956)		$146,902	$154,858	-5.1%
	$134,748	$142,257	($7,509)		$134,748	$142,257	-5.3%
	$113,096	$119,771	($6,675)		$113,096	$119,771	-5.6%
	$92,047	$96,537	($4,490)		$92,047	$96,537	-4.7%
	$117,565	$121,964	($4,400)		$117,565	$121,964	-3.6%

Both Charges and Payments are caclulated based on Date of Entry. 12 month averages include actual number of months with charges or payments if less than 12

PAYER MIX CHANGES

A similar monthly email evaluates changes in the practice payer mix over time. The business office categorizes insurance plans into insurance groups to make it easy to trend overall changes by carrier. As the payer mix by insurance group changes, Exhibit 8.2 shows the five largest changes (positive or negative). Depending on the payer and the contract, increases may be good or bad. Changes in payer mix have a direct impact on reimbursement and the bottom line. This monthly SSRS email helps the revenue cycle manager get a broad sense of what the bottom line will look like in the future.

EXHIBIT 8.2 TOP 5 LARGEST CHANGES IN PAYER MIX SAMPLE

Top 5 Payer Mix Changes (Rolling 6 Month Average)

Insurance Group	Prior Year	Current Year	Change
	1.3%	3.0%	1.7%
	4.6%	6.0%	1.4%
	15.9%	14.5%	-1.4%
	3.1%	1.9%	-1.3%
	11.3%	12.4%	1.2%

TRENDING ACCOUNTS RECEIVABLE BALANCES

Monitoring accounts receivable balances is critical to the financial health of almost any practice. Trending accounts receivable is difficult because receivables fluidly change as charges are entered and payments and adjustments are posted.

One way to trend accounts receivable is to simply recalculate accounts receivable as of a date in time by adding all charges and subtracting all payments and adjustments up to that date. In a large practice with years of history, this calculation can take quite a while. Recalculation has worked for some practices, but recalculation misses some data. For example, it is difficult to recalculate whether a primary or a secondary insurance was responsible for a claim on a given date, especially if the primary insurance only pays part of the procedure codes on the claim or if some of the codes are underpaid and appealed.

To work around those issues, store accounts receivable balances and key metrics in the data warehouse each week. Exhibit 8.3 is an example of a stored accounts receivable report. The report is focused on only balances due from patients and stores several key metrics to trend over time. The thought process behind this SSRS email is to give the patient billing manager a sense of how the department is doing over time. This is a new report. The practice expects to store more metrics as they get more experience with the data.

EXHIBIT 8.3 ACCOUNTS RECEIVABLE BALANCES REPORT SAMPLE

Patient A/R History as of 9/1/2017

Category	This Week		Last Week		Last Month	
Balance Over 12 Months	205	$50,676	236	$69,810	231	$68,824
No Statement in 2 Months	942	$248,068	1,007	$354,406	970	$343,951
Balance Over $2,000	159	$889,551	164	$924,274	166	$937,779
Total Patient A/R	6,941	$2,197,851	7,209	$2,348,533	7,068	$2,337,778

TRENDING PATIENT CREDIT BALANCES

Exhibit 8.4 is a similar approach to trending receivables. The data is presented in a chart, with the objective of giving the manager a sense for how the department is doing. The credit balances are categorized into four main buckets and then trended by day. This approach helps flag sudden changes that may result from a data entry error or longer-term trends that need to be addressed. The SSRS email is delivered weekly to the patient billing manager and her supervisor so both managers can see progress or potential problems.

EXHIBIT 8.4 TRENDING ACCOUNTS RECEIVABLE REPORT SAMPLE

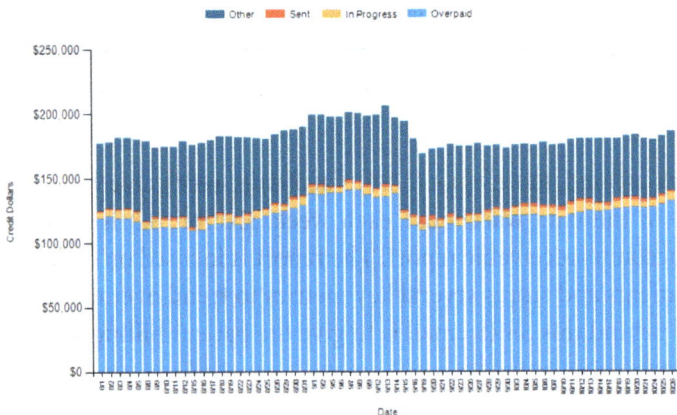

Patient Credit Balances as of

PRE-AUTHORIZATION

These days, pre-authorization departments are busier everywhere. An orthopedic practice became concerned about the growing demands and constant drama within the department. A almost consistent flow of last-minute emergency efforts to pre-authorize a case frustrated patients, providers, managers, and staff. It was past time to make the process easier! Their two-part solution involved a spreadsheet tool to help the pre-authorization team know which surgical case to work on next, and the SSRS email shown in Exhibit 8.5.

The daily email to the pre-authorization department (and management) charts the number of cases on the y-axis and the days remaining until the surgical appointment on the x-axis. The chart on the left is the next 30 days. The chart on the right is days 31-60. The staff changed their process by adding an asterisk in the pre-authorization number field when they request pre-authorization. If nothing had been entered in the pre-authorization, the pre-authorization had not been started. If an asterisk had been added, pre-authorization would have commenced, while any other entry save an asterisk indicated the pre-authorization was complete.

EXHIBIT 8.5 OUTSTANDING PRE-AUTHORIZATIONS AND DAYS UNTIL SURGERY

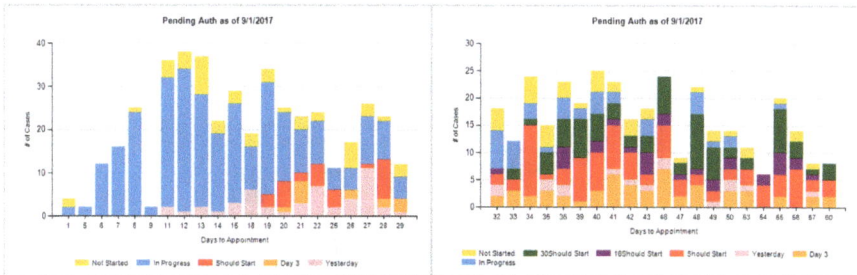

With this information, the chart in Exhibit 8.5 categorizes each case. Light blue represents pre-authorizations that are in progress. Yellow represents pre-authorizations that have not been started and that the procedure to

authorize has been on the schedule for less than two days. On the left chart, almost all pre-authorizations in the next 30 days have been started. The colors on the right chart display other colors that indicate how long a case has been on the schedule and not yet started. The color black indicates that a scheduled case cannot yet be started because that insurer doesn't allow cases that far out to be pre-authorized.

With the spreadsheet tool and this daily email, drama in the pre-authorization department has been significantly reduced. There will always be a case added on to the schedule with very little notice for prior authorization, but because the rest of the cases are under control, the pre-authorization team can respond to those cases without disrupting the rest of the cases that need to be addressed. The right tool and daily insight from SSRS helped make pre-authorization much less painful.

The pre-authorization tools were so effective in illustrating surgery authorizations that this practice built a similar tool to manage pre-authorizations for office-based procedures. In the office email, the color scheme represents each office location, rather than how long the appointment has been on the schedule, but the principle is the same. Both tools give staff the visibility of potential problems and the perspective to manage the potential problems effectively. Exhibit 8.6 is an example of the office-based pre-authorization daily email.

EXHIBIT 8.6 OFFICE PRE-AUTHORIZATION TRACKING SAMPLE

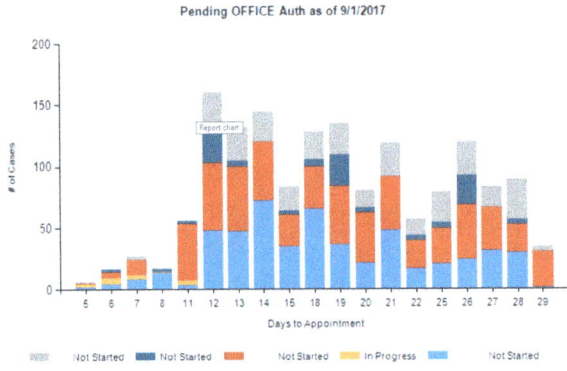

USING SSRS TO SOLVE TEMPORARY ISSUES

Exhibit 8.7 was a simple solution to a problem for a practice where Medicare claims were failing to crossover to Medicaid. While the issue was being worked out, this basic email captured claims that may not have crossed over to Medicaid. The report is filtered to only include claims that may have an issue. The staff just needs to follow up on these claims to make sure that Medicaid received the information.

EXHIBIT 8.7 SOLUTION FOR TEMPORARY PROBLEM – MEDICAID CROSSOVER SAMPLE

Medicaid Crossover Issues as of 9/1/2017

Ticket Number
3126651
3129671
3133812
3133916
3133950

TRACKING POTENTIAL DATA ENTRY PROBLEMS

Exhibit 8.8 is an SSRS email designed to track problems this business office has with a data entry issue. The PM system allows the rendering provider on a charge to be different from the provider on the encounter. The billing office's policy is for both providers to be the same on all claims. Capturing billing issues prior to claim submission prevents denials as well as time in the billing department having to correct claims, improving a practice's revenue cycle.

This daily email catches these errors so that the providers can be reconciled and fixed before there is an issue with claim. The Medicaid Crossover email only included the ticket number, since that was the only piece of information the staff needed. This email contains lots of additional information to help the staff resolve the problem by looking at the email.

Mismatch Chg Enc Providers as of

Patient	Chg Create Date	Chg Last Modified	Service Item	Chg Status	Enc Status	Charge Rendering Physician	Encounter Rendering Physician
	11:22	11:22	99213	Billed	Billed		
	11:10	11:10	99204	Billed	Billed		
	11:9	11:9	99213	Billed	Billed		
	10:5	10:10	99214	Billed	Billed		
	9:15	9:15		Billed	Billed		
	9:13	9:13		Billed	Billed		
	9:6	9:6		Billed	Billed		
	8:30	9:15	99214	History	History		

Some issues include data entry errors that can be resolved by training. For those types of issues, include the login of the staff member making the error on the email. You might even summarize the errors by staff member so that it is easy to see who is making the errors and provide training to keep the error from happening again.

TRACKING SPECIFIC PATIENTS

This Business Intelligence example in Exhibit 8.9 comes from a group of physicians who treat a lot of Workers Compensation patients. The market is competitive for those patients, so a specific team tracks the Workers Compensation patients. The team frequently communicates with the case manager to ensure the care is received timely so the patients return to work quickly. To make that process easier, this daily email tracks all Workers Compensation appointments scheduled yesterday. (Monday's report shows Friday appointments.)

This quick notification tool allows the staff to track each Workers Compensation patient through the system and update the case manager as necessary. The extra service to keep the case manager happy helps the practice attract more Workers Compensation patients.

Exhibit 8.9 Tracking Workers Patients Sample

New Work Comp Appts Scheduled Yesterday as of 9/2/2017

Appt Start	Patient Name	Acct Num	Provider	Appt Type
9/12/2017 9:30 AM		723554		Work Comp New Patient
9/12/2017 10:45 AM		723554		Work Comp New Patient
9/11/2017 2:45 PM		10742836		Work Comp New Patient
9/5/2017 9:30 AM		10742856		Work Comp New Patient
9/7/2017 10:15 AM		10742858		Work Comp New Patient

STAFF TOOLS THAT MAKE IT EASY TO DO THE RIGHT THING

Notice the heading to the Excel Table in Exhibit 8.10. The underlying dataset filters all accounts receivable to only display secondary claims where there has been no insurance payment for claims filed more than 30 days ago. The dataset does all the filtering for the billing office. Then Excel sorts the data to show the largest balances first. As soon as the billing office team opens the spreadsheet, they know exactly what claims need to be worked. This beats sorting through a canned report with an alphabetized list of patients that includes many claims that do not need to be followed up on. Rather, this tool focuses on the most important claims first.

Exhibit 8.10 Accounts Receivable Management Tool Sample

UNPAID SECONDARY CLAIMS WITH NO INSURANCE PAYMENT AFTER LAST FILE DATE
FOR CLAIMS FILED MORE THAN 30 DAYS AGO

Ticket #	Account #	Patient	Balance	Current Insurance	Current Ins Level	Last Filed Date
3164845	726586		$46.20	Medicare Trad** 4854 MCR	2	7/14/2017
3131189	10751896		$27.53	Combined Ins COMM 16546	2	7/27/2017
3177212	10739842		$125.25	Cigna Medicare Supplement 16446	2	8/1/2017
3171567	715180		$20.00	Cigna Medicare Supplement 16446	2	7/24/2017
3171568	715180		$17.93	Cigna Medicare Supplement 16446	2	7/24/2017
3171569	715180		$17.93	Cigna Medicare Supplement 16446	2	7/24/2017
3131092	770275		$85.87	Cigna Medicare Supplement 16446	2	8/1/2017
3174364	758328		$50.62	Cigna Medicare Supplement 16446	2	7/27/2017
3131307	10709464		$31.30	Manhattan Life Ins Co 16419 COMM	2	8/1/2017
3131309	10735001		$54.59	Aetna Continental Ins Co16262	2	8/1/2017
3125523	9502430		$50.22	Aetna Continental Ins Co16262	2	7/21/2017
3130045	10604230		$13.95	Medico Ins Co 16293 COMM	2	7/27/2017
3130961	849807		$11.86	Medico Ins Co 16293 COMM	2	8/1/2017
3170622	656447		$34.17	Forethought Life Ins Co 15954 COMM	2	7/21/2017
3169003	9773890		$82.62	First Health Life and Health Ins 15536 COMM	2	7/20/2017
3130917	643217		$20.57	Aetna United Security Life and Health 15558	2	8/1/2017
3174390	10664708		$267.52	UHC 15467	2	7/27/2017
3130842	767514		$20.66	UMR UHC** 15476	2	8/1/2017
3165900	10666857		$19.22	Anthem 15393	2	7/21/2017
3129564	10641200		$568.00	Anthem 15393	2	7/18/2017
3130990	10697523		$13.95	Anthem 15393	2	7/31/2017
3128104	10703420		$6.86	Anthem 15393	2	7/18/2017

Apparently, college students need "trigger warnings" when a book or discussion might offend them. Consider this your "technical discussion warning," especially for a chapter talking about how easy reports can be. The remainder of this chapter addresses a technical issue with how refreshing data automatically can impact certain reports. The potential solutions are technical, but it is a topic either you or your IT team may want to consider.

Spreadsheet tools like Exhibit 8.10 can be set to refresh with current data every time the spreadsheet opens. It is very helpful to always have current data in the spreadsheet, but the downside of the refresh is that any notes or data entered into the spreadsheet will be scrambled or overwritten as new claims refresh. There are several ways to address the problem of keeping track of data—such as which claims are worked—in a spreadsheet that is set to refresh.

Assume that a billing office team member named Joy worked the first 10 unpaid secondary claims today. Even if Joy contacted the payers and confirmed that all 10 tickets will be paid, the tickets will not be paid by the time the spreadsheet refreshes tomorrow, so the tickets will still appear on the spreadsheet. How does Joy keep track of which claims she worked so that she doesn't call the same payers and try to work the same claims tomorrow?

One solution is to enter the extra data into the PM system so that when the data refreshes, the refresh includes the data Joy needs to filter worked claims on the spreadsheet. In the receivables example, if Joy enters a note or a code in the PM system, the dataset can filter out claims that have a note within the past 15 days, 30 days, or whatever interval you prefer. Alternatively, the report can include the note as part of the refreshed data in the spreadsheet, including the date the note was made. Making notes in the PM system allows the dataset to mine the notes. Making notes in Excel may not.

If there is no easy place to enter notes into the PM system, another solution is to make the notes on a separate tab in Excel and then use VLOOKUP to automatically pull the data onto the main tab after the spreadsheet refreshes. The example in Exhibit 8.11 is from a group that stores demographic information in two different systems, the PM system and a pathology system. The pathology system isn't based in SQL Server, so an SSIS routine (introduced in Chapter 3) imports the data from an old database format into SQL Server. Once the data is in SQL Server, it is much easier to manipulate in Excel.

This spreadsheet is a tool to make sure the demographics match between the two systems. Occasionally there is a reason the PM system will never match the pathology database. Those patients would never be removed from this spreadsheet and would clutter the list in the future. There was no easy way to tell either the PM system or the pathology system to ignore those patients. Exhibit 8.11 is the solution the practice devised.

Exhibit 8.11 Comparing Demographics Tools Sample

COMPARE PM DEMOGRAPHICS TO PATHOLOGY DEMOGRAPHICS

							From Pathology Software								
	Accession	Status	Date Collected	Overall Test	Error Column	Ignore Error	Acct Num	Last Name	First Name	Sex	DOB	Provider	Location	Test First Name	Test Last Name
1020	S16-10579	Signed	10/12/2016	FALSE	Test First Name	FALSE	3171359			F				FALSE	FALSE
1162	S16-10730	Signed	10/17/2016	FALSE	Test First Name	FALSE	3151508			F				FALSE	FALSE
1593	S16-11165	Signed	10/26/2016	FALSE	Test First Name	FALSE	3114019			F				FALSE	FALSE

All the columns except column G refresh every time the spreadsheet refreshes. Column G pulls from a separate spreadsheet tab based on a VLOOKUP formula. The VLOOKUP formula returns true if the pathology accession number is found on the list of patients to ignore. The Excel Table filters out any patients where Ignore Error is set to true, thus removing the patients from the future list of demographics that do not match. The downside is that the staff must enter (or copy/paste) a unique reference number each time they want to remove the patient from the spreadsheet. The spreadsheet tabs are shown in Exhibit 8.12.

Exhibit 8.12 Spreadsheet Tabs

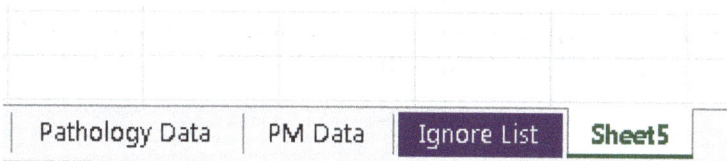

The Ignore List tab is highlighted to make it easier for the staff to find. A sample of the Ignore List tab is shown in Exhibit 8.13.

EXHIBIT 8.13 IGNORE LIST TAB SAMPLE

Put Accession Numbers you'd like to ignore matching errors in the table below

Accession Number
S12-02068
S12-01923
S12-01899
S12-01392
S12-02223
S12-02183
S12-02324
S12-02109
S12-02078
S12-02076
S12-01989
S12-01817

This solution is more appropriate for smaller practices or smaller datasets. You would not want to have hundreds of thousands of lines of lookup every time the spreadsheet refreshed. For a smaller issue, this solution has worked for this practice for years. For reference, in four years, the ignore list is about 900 patients. For more information about using VLOOKUP, please see the VLOOKUP Excel Mastery page at mooresolutionsinc.com/em-vlookup/.

A third solution is to control or limit the automatic data refresh on the spreadsheet. To see outside data sources connected to an Excel spreadsheet, click Connections (circled in red) from the Data tab on the Ribbon, as shown in Exhibit 8.14. Choose the connection you want to review from the list of connections (many spreadsheets only have one connection) and click the Properties button (also circled in red).

EXHIBIT 8.14 CONTROLLING OR LIMITING THE AUTOMATIC DATA REFRESH TOOL: PART 1

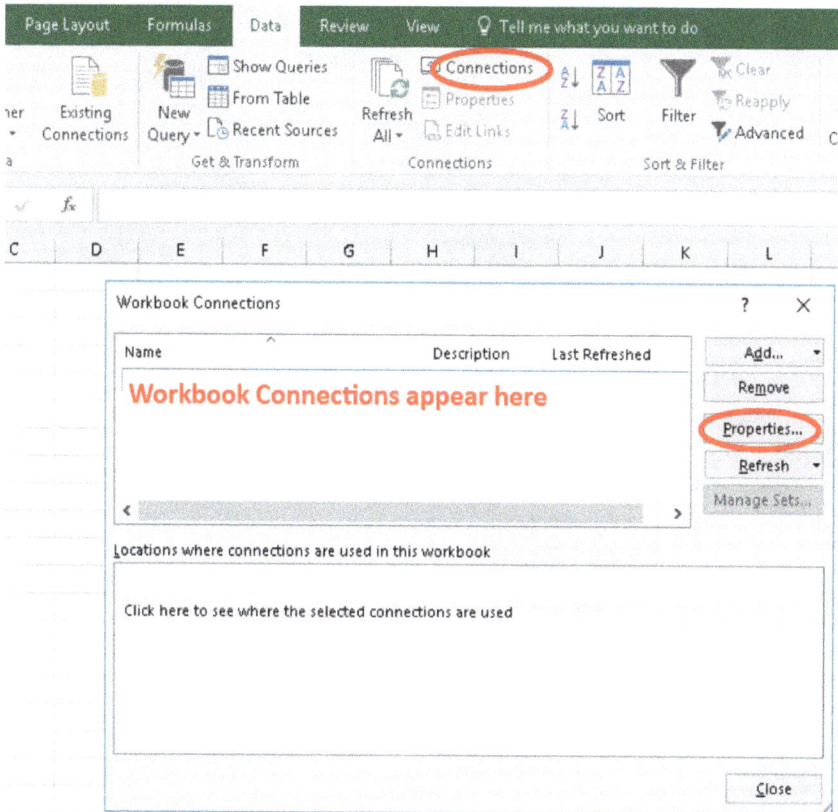

You should see the screen shown in Exhibit 8.15. The key is the box circled in red. If Refresh data when opening the file is checked, Excel will refresh the data every time the spreadsheet is opened, potentially overwriting any manual changes made outside the refreshed data. Uncheck this box and the spreadsheet will no longer refresh when the data as the spreadsheet is opened, but Excel will retain the information on how to connect to the outside data.

EXHIBIT 8.15 CONTROLLING OR LIMITING THE AUTOMATIC DATA
REFRESH TOOL: PART 2

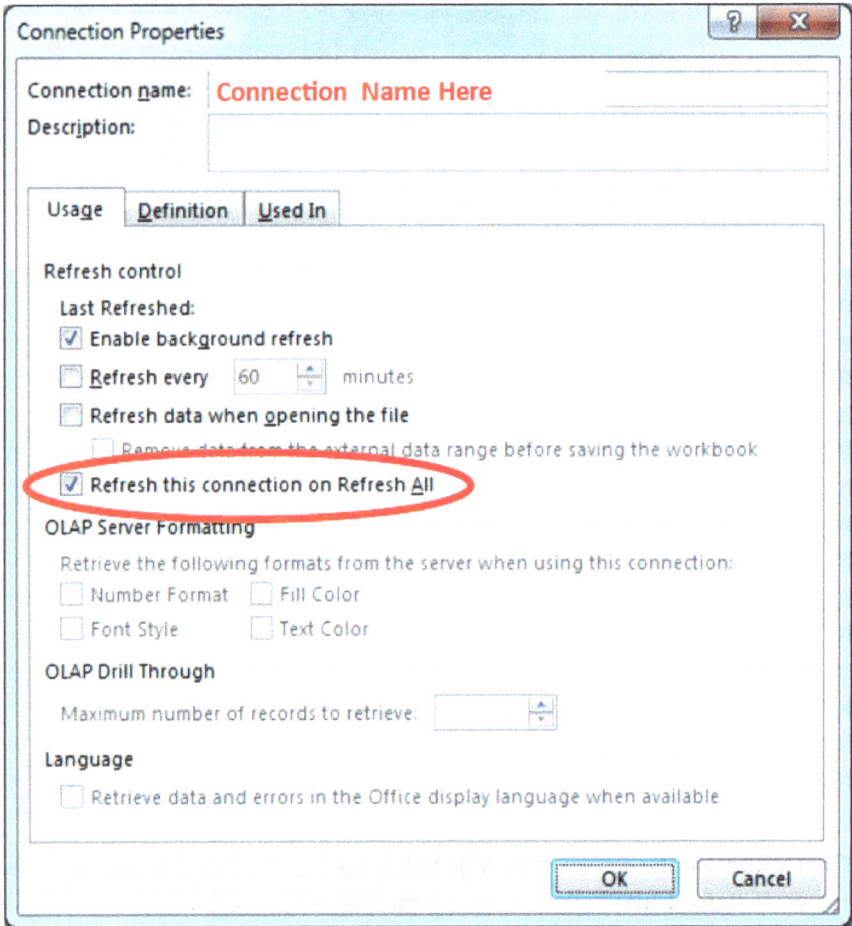

When you want to refresh the data, simply click Refresh or Refresh All from the data tab, as shown in Exhibit 8.16. The trick is to remember to refresh the data when you need new data, since the spreadsheet doesn't automatically refresh.

EXHIBIT 8.16 CONTROLLING OR LIMITING THE AUTOMATIC DATA REFRESH TOOLBAR

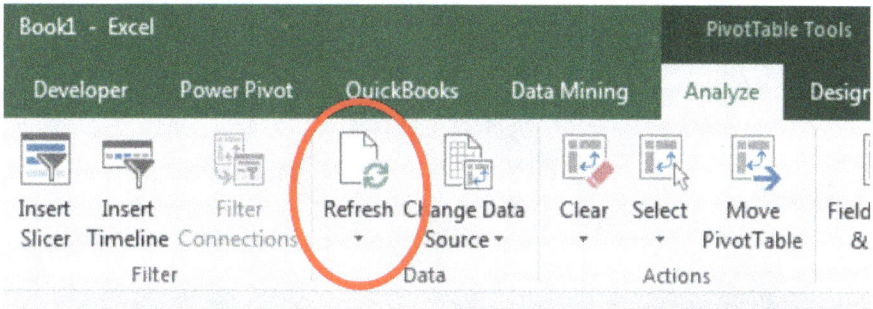

Another solution is to use Save As to save a spreadsheet with a different name, and then use the Remove button in Exhibit 8.14 above to delete the connection from the revised spreadsheet. The revised spreadsheet will no longer refresh. Be sure to use Save As so that the original spreadsheet can still connect to the data. The initial connection to the data often requires IT help, so do not break the original spreadsheet connection to your data in SQL Server.

Mix and match these solutions to get the results you need for a specific tool or application. The issue is spreadsheets that need to refresh but have data in Excel that will be overwritten during the refresh. Receivables is the classic example. Once you have worked a claim, you want the claim to be removed from your list for a number of days. Remember that Excel spreadsheets connected to outside data sources like SQL Server can lose data entered separately in Excel. Use one of these strategies to prevent problems.

CHAPTER 9

BUSINESS INTELLIGENCE WITH CLINICAL AND EHR DATA

A group of surgeons thought they wanted to build a comprehensive database to track a wide variety of clinical data around several different types of surgical procedures. When the surgeons saw how much additional effort was required to track all the information, they became discouraged and progress slowed. The practice found more success by starting again with a shorter list of procedures and a smaller list of required data, focusing specifically on clinical data already available in the PM system.

It might seem counter-intuitive to look for clinical data in the PM system, but PM data is generally the lower-hanging fruit when it comes to Business Intelligence. PM data is more standardized across practices due to decades of data exchanged between practices and payers. Organizations like the American Medical Association (AMA), CMS, Council for Affordable Quality Healthcare (CAQH) and the World Health Organization have specifically designed the meaning of CPT codes and ICD-10 codes. This standardization process defines the reporting and meaning of the data as it pertains to work in medical practices.

In contrast, EHR data is often significantly more specialty and practice specific. One group of cardiologists may create a workflow or metric in their documentation that specifically meets the needs of their organization, while another group of cardiologists tracks different measures and outcomes. Although there is significant effort in the industry to standardize outcomes measures, there is a long way to go before this is as well defined as the exchange of claims and payment data files. And even though CMS has attempted to certify EHR systems and define how providers should use these systems, there is still considerable variability in how customizable a system is, how (and when) the data collection occurs and in the ease of storing discrete data. Discrete data is much easier to mine than free-text data that might be found in a traditional dictation environment.

Even though EHR data has shortcomings, this chapter offers a variety of ideas to get started using Business Intelligence tools with clinical data. Some of the examples combine PM data like appointments or charges with clinical data to identify patients who need to be seen. The most extensive example comes from a practice that significantly optimized their x-ray department to predict which patients would need an x-ray. There are also examples where EHR data is used to ensure that protocols are followed from prescribing narcotics to lab tests for new patients. The end of the clinical examples circles back to a financial issue as a practice uses clinical data to search for missing charges.

FOLLOWING UP ON NO SHOWS AND APPOINTMENT CANCELLATIONS

Exhibit 9.1 is an email combination of the appointments ideas in Chapter 6 and the EHR ideas in this chapter. Some no shows and appointment cancellations are more important to follow up on than other appointments. For example, a dermatology practice might follow up on missed melanoma appointments more persistently than missed acne appointments. Exhibit 9.1 is an example of an SSRS email that tracks patients with specific appointment types who missed an appointment.

EXHIBIT 9.1 NO SHOWS AND CANCELS WITHOUT FUTURE APPOINTMENT SAMPLE

MOHS No Shows and Cancels Without Future Appt as of 9/2/2017

Appt	Acct Num	Provider
No show		
8/1/2017 7:30 AM	3062967	
Cancel		
6/7/2017 8:00 AM	2334476	
6/12/2017 9:00 AM	10227	
6/20/2017 9:00 AM	3099925	
6/20/2017 9:00 AM	3178823	
6/22/2017 9:00 AM	2346318	
6/26/2017 8:00 AM	3061869	
7/17/2017 7:30 AM	3023675	
7/19/2017 1:00 PM	3170159	
7/25/2017 7:30 AM	2345716	
7/25/2017 7:30 AM	3179505	

There are a couple of issues to consider with a report like this. The first is how to identify more serious appointments. In the dermatology example, how can a practice distinguish between melanoma patients and acne patients? Which missed appointments need to be followed up on, and is the follow up from a nurse or from the scheduling staff? One way to distinguish appointments is by an appointment type or appointment reason field. Build a workflow so that all melanoma patients are assigned a specific appointment type or reason so that melanoma appointments can be found and acted on. Another method might be to look back at the patients' diagnosis codes or procedure codes billed over a prior time period.

A second issue is how to get missed appointments off a report like this. Once the staff has followed up on the missed appointment, there needs to be a mechanism to remove the patient from the list so the patient doesn't receive repeat calls for the same missed appointment. One way to remove patients is to find an unused field in the appointment area of the PM system and put something in the field so that logic can be written to exclude the appointment from the report. The field could even be filled with the name of the person following up on the appointment (much like in Chapter 8's prior authorization example) or the date the follow up occurred so that mining the data to look for appointments to exclude also gives information about who followed up or when the follow up happened.

The unused field should be in the appointment section of the PM, not the patient section. The objective isn't to exclude the patient from any future follow up calls. The objective is to exclude that specific missed appointment from future calls.

Another approach is to only show patients once on an SSRS email. Once the missed appointment has been reported, it will not appear on another email. Whenever staff are on vacation or get behind, the emails will be saved in a folder until the patients are contacted. For more ideas about how to remove items from lists, see the last section of Chapter 8.

PATIENTS WHO NEED AN X-RAY

Exhibit 9.2 is a different clinical example.

The Problem – How Many X-ray Rooms Does the Clinic Need?

The story is that an orthopedic clinic was remodeling their main location and had to decide if they needed to build four x-ray rooms, or if they could manage with three. There are major costs in adding a fourth x-ray room, including purchasing the equipment, shielding the room, and staffing the room on an ongoing basis. The clinical team met with the IT staff to find a way to use three x-ray rooms more efficiently so that the fourth room would not be needed. The patient throughput needed to be fast enough so that providers were not kept waiting for patients to receive an x-ray. The other consideration was not to hold up exam rooms while patients were waiting for the x-ray team. As with most practices, both providers' time and exam rooms are scarce resources to be optimized.

The Solution – Show Which Patients Need an X-Ray

The solution was to give the x-ray team better insight into which patients would need an x-ray during their visit. If the x-ray team could predict patient volume by location, the manager could staff the locations accordingly, even moving staff between locations during the lunch hour if necessary. Furthermore, if the x-ray team knew enough information about the patient and the x-ray that would be needed, many patients could receive an x-ray before being assigned an exam room. And rather than the provider waiting to see the patient, ordering an x-ray, escorting the patient to the x-ray room to receive the x-ray, and waiting to see the patient again, the patient could have an x-ray before seeing the provider. The patient saves time, the provider saves time, and the exam room is made available to help more patients.

Hurdle # 1 – Did the Provider Order a Future X-Ray with Sufficient Details

The trick was helping the x-ray staff determine which patients needed to have an x-ray. That insight included which body part need to be to x-rayed, which views the provider wanted to see, and whether a cast should be on or off during the x-ray. Capturing all this information required a major workflow change and IT help. The IT staff changed the patient form in the

EHR to capture body part, views, casting, and other information necessary to prepare the x-ray staff to properly x-ray the patient before the patient saw the provider. Once IT had the new form built, the providers had to get in the habit of ordering an x-ray for the next patient visit, including all the required details.

Hurdle #2 – Has the Patient Already Received the Ordered X-Ray?

The next hurdle was applying logic in the data warehouse to find patients who have an upcoming appointment and who have an outstanding order for an x-ray. If the patient has already been seen after the date of the last x-ray order, the patient appointment needs to be excluded from the list, since the ordered x-ray has already been filled. Careful, complex logic was written to determine if a patient had already been seen. Seen could mean the patient saw the provider who ordered the x-ray, but seen could also mean that the patient met with an advanced practitioner who commonly works with the provider. Seen could also mean the patient saw the provider who supervises the advanced practitioner who ordered the x-ray. Seen could also mean the patient met with another provider in the same subspecialty. Those patient appointments need to be filtered off the x-ray list so that a patient doesn't receive an unnecessary x-ray. On the other hand, if a patient is being seen for a wrist injury, a visit with a provider specializing in hips shouldn't be considered as being seen for the purposes of a wrist x-ray order.

Hurdle #3 – How Confident is the Assessment that the Patient Needs an X-Ray?

Given the complexity of the workflow and the logic, the clinic's system could not be certain that a patient did or did not need an x-ray. This hurdle was ultimately resolved by assigning a color code to each appointment. A green appointment is one that has met all criteria for a patient with an outstanding x-ray order requiring an x-ray (with a provider ordering the x-ray who matches the provider scheduled to see the patient that day). A yellow appointment meant that the ordering provider did not match the appointment provider, but the x-ray might still be required (the x-ray staff manually reviews these patients' charts to see if the x-ray should be done). A red appointment means that the appointment most likely doesn't require an x-ray during that day's visit. The colors appear as a column on Exhibit 9.2 so that staff can filter to make sure the green appointments have an x-ray and the yellow appointments are more carefully vetted.

The Result

The IT support, workflow changes, and report logic took time to develop and test. The x-ray team took time to assure themselves that the report was accurate and that the x-rays requested should be performed. Over time, the process was a major success. Today the location only requires three x-ray rooms because they are used much more efficiently. The overall duration of a patient appointment is down, saving the patients time and the practice money.

When the project was initially considered, data showed that only about one-third of patient visits that ultimately required an x-ray could be accurately forecast in advance. The other two-thirds were patients who presented with a new injury, patients who initially visited the emergency room, or patients with other issues. So far, the efficiencies gained by providing the information in Exhibit 9.2 are enough for the practice to use three x-ray rooms successfully.

The Lessons

One of the lessons from this project is to not let the perfect be the enemy of the good. Rather than try to overcomplicate an already complex process, focus on factors the practice can control (changing the EHR form and the providers' workflow, for example) to get enough information for the project to be successful. The green/yellow/red confidence color educated and thus reassured the staff over whether an x-ray was required without needing perfect certainty to move the project forward. As the project advanced, opportunities to perfect the process manifested and the x-ray team continued to improve.

The second lesson is that for the practice to solve the problem, it did not need to successfully predict every x-ray. Optimizing the one-third of patients whose x-ray could be reasonably known in advance was enough for the project to be successful. The solution lay in defining the problem as increasing x-ray efficiency sufficiently enough to avoid a fourth x-ray room instead of defining the problem as predicting every x-ray.

EXHIBIT 9.2 PATIENTS WHO MAY NEED AN X-RAY AT THEIR NE4XT VISIT SAMPLE

PATIENTS WHO MAY NEED AN XRAY AT THEIR NEXT VISIT

Appt Date	Appt Time	Patient Name	Account Number	Resource	Body Part Needing Xray	Xray Order Date	Follow Up Provider	Follow Up Plan	Appt Type	Color
9/1/2017	6:45 AM		797415		Lumbar*AP, Lateral**LUMI	8/23/2017			X-Ray 15	GREEN
9/1/2017	7:45 AM		811219		(51") Long Leg*AP*50**Ste	8/3/2017			X-Ray 15	GREEN
9/1/2017	8:00 AM		755003		TSA*Axillery, Grashey*RT**	8/2/2017			X-Ray 15	GREEN
9/1/2017	8:15 AM		9153650		TKA*standing AP, Lateral, N	8/15/2017			X-Ray 15	GREEN
9/1/2017	8:30 AM		796787		THA*AP, AP pelvis, X Table I	8/8/2017			X-Ray 15	GREEN
9/1/2017	8:30 AM		10704700		TKA*standing AP, Lateral, N	8/8/2017			Post Op 15	GREEN
9/1/2017	8:45 AM		9653140		THA*AP, AP pelvis, X Table I	7/24/2017			X-Ray 15	GREEN
9/1/2017	9:45 AM		851924		Lumbar*AP, Lateral***Alar	7/21/2017			X-Ray 15	GREEN
9/1/2017	10:00 AM		10176230		Shoulder*Axillary, Grashey*	7/20/2017			X-Ray 15	GREEN
9/1/2017	11:00 AM		808430		Lumbar*AP, Lateral**LUMI	7/21/2017			X-Ray 15	GREEN
9/1/2017	11:00 AM		9428360		Lumbar*AP, Lateral**ARTH	7/24/2017			X-Ray 15	GREEN
9/1/2017	12:00 PM		10362990		Cervical*Lateral***Alan W	3/13/2017			X-Ray 15	GREEN
9/1/2017	12:15 PM		634061		Lumbar*AP, Lateral***Alar	7/10/2017			X-Ray 15	GREEN
9/1/2017	1:00 PM		10734843		THA*AP, AP pelvis, X Table I	7/17/2017			X-Ray 15	GREEN
9/1/2017	1:00 PM		9611250		TKA*standing AP, Lateral, N	6/26/2017			X-Ray 15	GREEN
9/1/2017	4:15 PM		10176670		Wrist*Lateral, PA*LT*LEFT	7/28/2017			X-Ray 15	GREEN
9/5/2017	7:45 AM		684814		Cervical*AP, extension, flex	6/8/2017			Recheck 15	GREEN
9/5/2017	7:45 AM		750322		Lumbar*AP, extension, flex	7/11/2017			Recheck 15	GREEN
9/5/2017	7:45 AM		740753		Shoulder*AP, Y/Outlet, A/C	8/9/2017			Recheck 15	GREEN
9/5/2017	8:00 AM		9308160		Cervical*Lateral**John I.	6/8/2017			Recheck 15	GREEN
9/5/2017	8:00 AM		987830		Elbow*AP, Lateral*RT**Ala	8/9/2017			Recheck 15	GREEN
9/5/2017	8:00 AM		9721780		Shoulder*AP, Y/Outlet*LT*	8/8/2017			Work Comp Recheck	GREEN
9/5/2017	8:00 AM		10666310		Knee*standing AP, Lateral,	8/22/2017			Recheck 15	GREEN
9/5/2017	8:15 AM		667058		TKA*standing AP, Lateral, N	7/20/2017			Recheck 15	GREEN
9/5/2017	8:15 AM		10739849		Scoliosis*AP, Lateral***Mi	7/21/2017			Recheck 15	GREEN
9/5/2017	8:15 AM		10739603		Foot*AP, Lateral, oblique*F	8/8/2017			Recheck 15	GREEN
9/5/2017	8:15 AM		782453		Shoulder*AP, Y/Outlet, A/C	8/9/2017			Auth Required 15	GREEN

Exhibit 9.2 shows the data the x-ray staff reviews each morning. The data is presented as a Table in a spreadsheet so that the staff can filter by provider, facility, appointment type, and more. Columns help the staff recognize information about the x-ray to be performed, including body part and views. It helps to show the provider information, since the x-ray technicians are familiar with each provider's x-ray preferences.

Once the practice got the spreadsheet version of this report tested and successfully working, their next step was to integrate the x-ray data with known patient scheduling information. The practice tracks patients who have checked in and have not been roomed. Now the x-ray staff can see patients who have checked in and who need an x-ray. Those patients can be called from the waiting room and have the x-ray performed. Sharing with the x-ray team the patient check-in status has made the x-ray department even more efficient because they can see how many patients are coming in with pre-ordered x-rays and how many x-rays are in the queue to be performed. The practice that made this project work uses GE's Centricity® PM/EHR and won a national award from GE for their efforts.

NARCOTICS PRESCRIBED WITHOUT AN APPOINTMENT

This spreadsheet was requested by the nurse in charge of clinical operations at a practice that has pain providers. Exhibit 9.3 mines the electronic prescription data, pulls all prescriptions written for narcotics and then compares the date of the prescription to appointment data in the PM system. Narcotics with a prescription date without a matching appointment date are stored in the dataset that feeds this spreadsheet.

EXHIBIT 9.3 NARCOTIC PRESCRIPTION TRACKING SAMPLE

NARCOTICS PRESCRIBED WITHOUT AN APPOINTMENT ON DATE PRESCRIBED

Prescrip Date	Patient	Provider	Created By	Signed By	Description	Product Name	Dose Form	Strength	Generic Name	Quantity	Refills
9/1/2017					TYLENOL/CODEINE #3 300-30 MG	TYLENOL WITH CO	TABS	300-30 MG	ACETAMINOPHEN-C	30 Tablet	
9/1/2017					NORCO 5-325 MG TABS	NORCO	TABS	5-325 MG	HYDROCODONE-ACI	30 Tablet	0
9/1/2017					NORCO 5-325 MG TABS	NORCO	TABS	5-325 MG	HYDROCODONE-ACI	30 Tablet	0
9/1/2017					NORCO 5-325 MG TABS	NORCO	TABS	5-325 MG	HYDROCODONE-ACI	30	0
9/1/2017					NORCO 10-325 MG TABS	NORCO	TABS	10-325 MG	HYDROCODONE-ACI	120	0
9/1/2017					MS CONTIN 30 MG T812	MS CONTIN	CR-TABS	30 MG	MORPHINE SULFATI	90	0
9/1/2017					NORCO 7.5-325 MG TABS	NORCO	TABS	7.5-325 MG	HYDROCODONE-ACI	180	0
9/1/2017					PERCOCET 10-325 MG TABS	PERCOCET	TABS	10-325 MG	OXYCODONE-ACETA	120 Tablet	0
9/1/2017					PERCOCET 10-325 MG TABS	PERCOCET	TABS	10-325 MG	OXYCODONE-ACETA	150 Tablet	0
9/1/2017					MS CONTIN 15 MG CR-TABS	MS CONTIN	CR-TABS	15 MG	MORPHINE SULFATE	90	0
9/1/2017					NORCO 10-325 MG TABS	NORCO	TABS	10-325 MG	HYDROCODONE-ACI	150	0
9/1/2017					NORCO 5-325 MG TABS	NORCO	TABS	5-325 MG	HYDROCODONE-ACI	30	0
9/1/2017					NORCO 10-325 MG TABS	NORCO	TABS	10-325 MG	HYDROCODONE-ACI	120	0
9/1/2017					PERCOCET 7.5-325 MG TABS	PERCOCET	TABS	7.5-325 MG	OXYCODONE-ACETA	120	0
9/1/2017					PERCOCET 7.5-325 MG TABS	PERCOCET	TABS	7.5-325 MG	OXYCODONE-ACETA	120 Tablet	0
9/1/2017					PERCOCET 7.5-325 MG TABS	PERCOCET	TABS	7.5-325 MG	OXYCODONE-ACETA	120 Tablet	0
9/1/2017					NORCO 5-325 MG TABS	NORCO	TABS	5-325 MG	HYDROCODONE-ACI	90 Tablet	0
9/1/2017					NORCO 5-325 MG TABS	NORCO	TABS	5-325 MG	HYDROCODONE-ACI	90	0
9/1/2017					NORCO 5-325 MG TABS	NORCO	TABS	5-325 MG	HYDROCODONE-ACI	60 Tablet	0
9/1/2017					NORCO 5-325 MG TABS	NORCO	TABS	5-325 MG	HYDROCODONE-ACI	60 Tablet	0
9/1/2017					DILAUDID 4 MG TABS	DILAUDID	TABS	4 MG	HYDROMORPHONE	180	0
9/1/2017					MS CONTIN 100 MG CR-TABS	MS CONTIN	CR-TABS	100 MG	MORPHINE SULFATI	60 Tablet	0
9/1/2017					NORCO 5-325 MG TABS	NORCO	TABS	5-325 MG	HYDROCODONE-ACI	50	0
9/1/2017					PERCOCET 5-325 MG TABS	PERCOCET	TABS	5-325 MG	OXYCODONE-ACETA	90 Tablet	0
9/1/2017					PERCOCET 7.5-325 MG TABS	PERCOCET	TABS	7.5-325 MG	OXYCODONE-ACETA	40 Tablet	0

The spreadsheet shows the prescription date, the patient, the patient's pain provider, and who created and signed the electronic prescriptions. There is data about the type of narcotics, dosage, strength, quantity and refills. The spreadsheet has more data than can fit in Exhibit 9.3. (For example, there is information about where the prescription was filled.) The practice can also track the last time the patient was in the clinic for an appointment. The nurse can review this detailed Excel Table for patterns. She can also summarize the dataset in a PivotTable to find patterns by patient, provider and by who is signing off on narcotics prescriptions without an appointment.

Narcotics prescribed without an appointment draws from appointment data and electronic prescribing data. Some of the most effective custom Business

Intelligence reports combine data from various systems across diverse practice areas. Reports crossing different software systems and practice areas are also some of the hardest reports to replicate using traditional canned reporting methods.

Narcotics compliance has become much more time consuming for this practice. Exhibit 10.4 in chapter 10 is in the compliance chapter, and is a good example of how the practice combines appointment data with clinical data to keep the pain providers compliant with several different regulations and policies.

UPCOMING APPOINTMENTS NEEDING CLINICAL DATA

All too many practices spend staff time reviewing past visit information to prepare for upcoming appointments. This is often referred to as "chart prep." An example of a solution created to replace some chart prep prior to appointments is an SSRS email in Exhibit 9.4 that was requested by a physician group that uses pathology. The objective is to ensure that patients with a follow up appointment that expect pathology results have those results in time for the appointment. This is a common chart prep function for many medical practices.

Two different processes go into creating this report. First, a document management system's database is mined to track the status of scanned pathology reports. (Other practices might look for data in their EHR that has been electronically integrated.) Each pathology case is matched to the related patient appointment and checked to determine if the pathology results are complete. Second, this data is matched to upcoming appointments. The key is to identify appointments that require pathology results. This practice uses the appointment type field to indicate those appointments. The dataset finds patient appointments in the next five days that need pathology, filtering out appointments that have matching, complete pathology. Because staff should only follow up on charts without the required pathology report, the SSRS email becomes an exception report. The email is delivered daily to the clinical staff, saving significant time.

EXHIBIT 9.4 PENDING PATHOLOGY REPORTS FOR UPCOMING APPOINTMENTS SAMPLE

Pending Path Reports with Appt in Next 5 Days as of 9/2/2017

Collected Date	Accession	Next Appt	Provider	Location	PM Last Name	ME Acct Num	Corrected Or Revised
8/28/2017	S17-09266	9/8/2017				3169840	
8/29/2017	S17-09280	9/8/2017				3020193	
8/29/2017	S17-09272	9/5/2017				3018651	
8/29/2017	S17-09281	9/7/2017				5979	
8/30/2017	S17-09365	9/5/2017				3149730	
8/30/2017	S17-09340	9/7/2017				3182569	
8/31/2017	S17-09434	9/7/2017				3183905	

One reason to include Exhibit 9.4 in this chapter is that the clinical data isn't in the EHR. The challenge of clinical data outside the EHR, but required for an upcoming appointment, isn't limited to this pathology example. What data does your practice have from an outside source that isn't integrated in the EHR? How much time does your staff spend opening every electronic chart to make sure data has been received from labs, imaging, or outside consultants? Short of an expensive HL7 interface, what customized Business Intelligence solution would save your practice time and money?

FOLLOWING CLINICAL PROTOCOLS

Exhibit 9.5 is an email from a practice that has a treatment protocol for new and established patient visits. The SSRS report specifically focuses on tests performed by a set of providers to make sure that providers are following the agreed upon protocol. There is a daily version of this email which is then summarized by a weekly and a monthly version of the email as well.

EXHIBIT 9.5 FOLLOWING CLINICAL PROTOCOLS TRACKING SAMPLE

Wed 1/18/2017 7:00 AM

R reports@

Yesterday Lab Dashboard ran at 1/18/2017 7:00:08 AM

To
Cc

If there are problems with how this message is displayed, click here to view it in a web browser.

1/17/2017 Testing Dashboard

Rendering Physician	New Pt	New Pt Tests	Est Pt	Est Pt Tests
	2	0	5	1
	2	2	11	5
	8	6	28	6
	2	2	12	0

As reimbursement models change to focus more on performance and results, and less on volumes and procedures, following protocols will becoming increasingly important. Whether those protocols are created internally or imposed externally by a payer, the ability to track conformance with clinical rules will differentiate practices in the future.

EXHIBIT 9.5 INCLUDES SOME OF THE LINES FROM THE ORIGINAL EMAIL IN THIS REPORT, AFTER MASKING THE EMAIL ADDRESSES. MOST SSRS REPORTS ARE EMBEDDED IN THE BODY OF THE EMAIL, AS THIS REPORT IS. FOR MORE COMPLEX OR LARGER REPORTS, ATTACH THE REPORT AS A PDF FILE TO AN SSRS EMAIL. SSRS MAKES IT EASY TO SWITCH FORMATS. IF USERS WANT A MORE CONSISTENT EXPERIENCE FROM A PHONE SCREEN THROUGH A TABLET-SIZED SCREEN TO A COMPUTER MONITOR, PDF FILES ARE THE WAY TO GO. THE ADVANTAGE OF EMBEDDED EMAILS LIKE THIS EXAMPLE IS THAT THE BOTTOM LINE INFORMATION IS EASY TO SEE AS SOON AS THE EMAIL IS OPENED WITHOUT HAVING TO OPEN A SEPARATE PDF FILE.

TRACKING SPECIFIC DISEASES

As alternative payment methods continue to grow, savvy physicians are tracking patients by disease. Patients can be tracked by outcome, side effects, or by compliance with a practice protocol. Exhibit 9.6 is an example to track melanoma patients. As melanoma patients are first identified in the practice, this SSRS dashboard helps the clinical staff ensure that the patient is included in the protocol for melanoma patients and that each patient receives the appropriate follow-up care.

EXHIBIT 9.6 TRACKING SPECIFIC DISEASES AND FOLLOW-UP CARE SAMPLE

Malignant Melanoma as of 9/2/2017

Accession #	Dx Cat	Date Reported	ME Acct Num	PM Last Name	Primary Ins	Provider	Location	Pathologist	PCP Notify
Medicare									
S17-08392	MM6	8/17/2017	3071478		MEDICARE PART B				
S17-08465	MM1	8/16/2017	3181390		MEDICARE PART B				
S17-08251	MM1	8/9/2017	3017321		MEDICARE PART B				
S17-07672	MM1	7/29/2017	3014279		MEDICARE PART B				
S17-07517	MM1	7/26/2017	3066346		MEDICARE PART B				
S17-06866	MM3	7/10/2017	57069		MEDICARE PART B				CGMM
S17-06720	MM1	6/29/2017	42488		MEDICARE PART B				
S17-06494	MM1	6/24/2017	3073702		MEDICARE PART B				
S17-06031	MM3	6/14/2017	3004268		MEDICARE PART B				
S17-04726	MM1	5/11/2017	1214		MEDICARE PART B				
S17-03119	MM3	3/30/2017	2335766		MEDICARE PART B				CGMM
S17-03029	MM1	3/29/2017	3057137		MEDICARE PART B				
S17-02900	MM3	3/26/2017	3176355		MEDICARE PART B				
S17-02249	MM3	3/3/2017	3176056		MEDICARE PART B				CGMM
S17-01945	MM1	2/22/2017	2345099		MEDICARE PART B				
S17-01945	MM1	2/22/2017	2345099		MEDICARE PART B				
S17-01610	MM1	2/15/2017	3174402		MEDICARE PART B				
S17-01597	MM3	2/15/2017	3057137		MEDICARE PART B				
S17-01508	MM3	2/12/2017	2345099		MEDICARE PART B				
S17-01249	MM3	2/3/2017	3175254		MEDICARE PART B				

This dashboard essentially monitors and enrolls patients in an internal disease tracking system. It is the first step to track a specific diagnosis internally. As the practice continues to treat these patients, they will include and track many more details. Some of the detail may be available in an EHR system, but for many diseases and treatments a significant amount of the data is stored outside the physician practice. Start building an internal disease tracking system now by reviewing EHR forms, requiring essential data to be completed, and replacing free-text data with standardized choices so that the data can be mined later.

EXTERNAL REGISTRIES

External disease tracking systems or registries are a challenge of a different magnitude. First, registries typically require specific minimum information to participate. That minimum information may be imposed by a payer, including CMS, or by the registry. Gathering that minimum data can require a change in workflow to capture specific data in the first place. For example, to submit data to a clinical registry a surgical group in the Southeast had to manually record data in the practice's EHR system that formerly was only available in hospital records.

Second, standardizing information can be a fluid, time-consuming process. A large group in the Midwest thought they had carefully defined and tracked case outcomes only to find the registry changed outcome definitions the following year. The practice built forms, created workflows, trained physicians on those forms and workflows, only to see the rules change. Because the registry responds to CMS rules, submitting data can be a moving target. The large group in the Midwest often doesn't have final registry submission rules for the current year until April or May of that year.

Third, submitting data in the form the registry requires is challenging. Some registries will accept csv files, which can be created by downloading practice data to Excel and then saving as a csv file. Other registries require formats such as Extensible Markup Language (XML) that generally requires customized reporting well beyond Excel's capabilities. Registries can be very specific about how data is formatted. Basic formatting issues include the way dates are formatted or how a patient's gender is defined (M/F, Male/Female, 1/0, etc.) More challenging requirements include mapping diseases to a specific list of diseases maintained by the registry.

A small practice in the Midwest encountered all three problems when attempting to submit quality data to an external registry. Their PM did not track all the information required to submit data to the registry. Gathering the required information from hospital records was time consuming, and since the PM system did not have a place to store the data, the staff entered the data into spreadsheets that had to be merged with the PM data. Once the data was successfully merged, it had to be converted to XML to submit to the registry. Submitting data to a registry is a process that takes time.

The lessons learned for external registry submission include:

- Start early. Registry submission can have time-consuming land mines that take work to resolve.
- Meet the minimums. Understand the minimum data required to submit data to a registry and compare that minimum data to what is available in your PM/EHR systems.
- Watch definitions. Ensure that your providers' understanding of outcomes, diseases, and quality measures is consistent with what the registry requires.
- Build a quality system. Establish workflows and data entry standards, including key terms definitions. Monitor providers and data entry staff compliance. Train, and then train again.
- Test submission processes. Ensure that the practice can successfully submit data to the registry in the format the registry requires.
- Keep watching. Registries are relatively new. Requirements change frequently. Meeting this year's requirements is no guarantee that the rules have not changed for next year.

MINING CLINICAL DATA TO IMPROVE PATIENT CARE

Exhibit 9.7 is an (fictitious) example created for an MGMA Annual Conference presentation a few years ago. The example is based on a report created for a multi-specialty practice in Texas, though no real data was used. Two datasets combine to create the report. First, the practice found all active patients who met the demographic profile (female patients between ages 50 to 74). For this practice, an active patient is a patient who was seen in the past 18 months.

EXHIBIT 9.7 COMBINED DATA SET FOR DEMOGRAPHIC PROFILE SAMPLE

WOMEN AGE 50-74 SEEN IN THE PAST 36 MONTHS WITHOUT A REFERRAL FOR MAMMOGRAM IN THE PAST 12 MONTHS

Patient	DOB	Address	City	State	Zip
Mingo, Stefania	12/29/1963	425 Main Street	Las Vegas	NV	89104
Bohrer, Joni	11/3/1947	742 Main Street	Las Vegas	NV	89102
Wertman, Willena	11/2/1961	1075 Main Street	Las Vegas	NV	89102
Vega, Caron	7/29/1946	43 Main Street	Las Vegas	NV	89106
Gaxiola, Gabriella	2/12/1942	1182 Main Street	Las Vegas	NV	89103
Lackey, Tamera	1/18/1957	1263 Main Street	Las Vegas	NV	89101
Hunn, Emelda	7/6/1946	145 Main Street	Las Vegas	NV	89103
Treadway, Mozell	11/7/1945	181 Main Street	Las Vegas	NV	89105
Prude, Bettyann	4/16/1943	795 Main Street	Las Vegas	NV	89106
Rhymes, Lannie	2/5/1954	1351 Main Street	Las Vegas	NV	89103
Pedro, Coral	1/18/1945	617 Main Street	Las Vegas	NV	89102
Matlock, Marlyn	11/28/1962	848 Main Street	Las Vegas	NV	89105
Perkinson, Jenniffer	6/21/1948	1020 Main Street	Las Vegas	NV	89104
Irizarry, Angela	4/18/1955	1260 Main Street	Las Vegas	NV	89106
Truss, Taylor	6/30/1957	298 Main Street	Las Vegas	NV	89105
Rolfe, Vesta	6/29/1944	607 Main Street	Las Vegas	NV	89102
Dowler, Rosalee	2/10/1951	676 Main Street	Las Vegas	NV	89102

Once the list of patients was generated, the next step was to determine who had been referred for a mammogram. Some practices are much more consistent about tracking incoming referrals compared to outgoing referrals. Incoming referrals are clearly a source of revenue, but if physicians and management knew how much business was referred to outside providers, that volume may justify providing the service internally. Tracking outbound referrals is also becoming more important in patient care. Part of the challenge with outside referrals is knowing whether the referred service or treatment happened. In this case, the patient was referred for a mammogram, but did she receive it? That data will become increasingly relevant as alternative payment models increase.

USING CLINICAL DATA TO FIND MISSING CHARGES

Charge capture from many EHR systems is often automated, but it literally pays to make sure. This orthopedic practice employs anesthesiologists. The logic behind the dataset in Exhibit 9.8 looks for cases billed by surgeons in locations where the billing office should also bill for anesthesia. If the dataset finds a surgical case in those locations without finding corresponding anesthesia charges for the same patient on the same date of service, the case shows up on this spreadsheet.

After this section of the book was written, but before the book went to press, the practice identified another concern commonly reported from this same type of data. Now the report also looks at charges with a QK modifier (indicating an anesthesiologist supervised a case with a Certified Registered Nurse Anesthetist (CRNA)) without a charge with a QX modifier (billed by the CRNA) for the same patient on the same date of service. Good Business Intelligence is never finished. There is always a way to capture data to save the practice more money.

EXHIBIT 9.8 USING CLINICAL DATA TO FIND MISSING CHARGES SAMPLE

POTENTIAL MISSING ANESTHESIA CHARGES

Patient	Patient ID	Ticket Number	Date Of Service From	Facility	Provider
Patient 1	10741651	3198599	8/17/2017	Mercy Hospital	Provider A
Patient 2	720488	3195699	8/18/2017	St. Mark's	Provider B
Patient 3	711327	3198918	8/10/2017	St. Mark's	Provider C
Patient 4	9876500	3200635	8/24/2017	St. Mark's	Provider B

The point of including this example is not for the limited number of orthopedic or surgical practices that employ anesthesiologists. This example could apply to practices that want to monitor for assistant surgeon's claims, ER patients treated, patients who have fractures without casts applied, and so forth. What unique logic to your practice could find unbilled charges? Are there injections prescribed in the EHR but not billed in the PM system? Are there post-op visits without a surgery being billed? Is there some way to reconcile surgical appointments or pre-authorizations to actual charges? This logic becomes more important the greater the number of lag days required to bill surgery. Any time a billing office discovers charges that should have been billed but were not, carefully investigate what when wrong. Search for timely filing denials that indicate charges were not billed until it was too late. Identify logic that could be implemented to automatically report any time that failure, however rare, happens again.

Financial reporting from PM systems is still the optimal ideal for many practices starting Business Intelligence. The future of payer contracting and the future of patient-centered medicine will draw more and more from clinical data. For most software packages, the canned PM reporting, however weak, is much better than the canned reports for clinical data. The ability to mine and act on clinical data will only become more of a competitive advantage in the coming years.

CHAPTER 10

COPING WITH COMPLIANCE

Please resist the temptation to skip a chapter with the word "compliance" in the title. Compliance is too often about filling out paperwork instead of helping patients. Hopefully that perspective motivates you to make compliance as efficient as possible so time can be better spent adding value to a medical practice. There are financial examples of compliance in this chapter (Medicare credit balances) as well as clinical examples (narcotics patients). You will also see compliance examples in terms of CMS compliance programs and clinical registry reports. The government changes program names, but the amount of work required to comply and get paid continues to increase.

This chapter will also include examples from a physical therapy group that uses reports to ensure billing complies with payer requirements.

MEDICARE CREDIT BALANCES

You do not have to spend much time in medical billing to understand how complex the process can be. Even the most conscientious practices will end up with overpayments due to coordination of benefits, coding issues, and human error. Exhibit 10.1 is one practice's approach to tracking and resolving credit balances, specifically focused on Medicare patients. This practice uses the spreadsheet to quickly identify and research credit balances so that unresolved balances are repaid in a timely manner.

EXHIBIT 10.1 MEDICARE CREDIT BALANCES TRACKING SAMPLE

MEDICARE CREDIT BALANCES

Ticket Number	Visit Date	Patient Name	Ins Balance	Current Insurance Group	Provider
3191297	8/18/2017		$ (9.83)		
3177139	7/20/2017		$ (9.48)		
3172721	7/19/2017		$ (2.77)		
3172729	7/18/2017		$ (3.20)		
3173004	7/16/2017		$ (37.17)		
3173002	7/15/2017		$ (31.59)		
3173001	7/14/2017		$ (95.46)		
3159287	7/5/2017		$ (1.65)		
3161670	6/29/2017		$ (3.20)		
3159536	6/29/2017		$ (20.98)		
3158055	6/28/2017		$ (9.83)		
3157579	6/27/2017		$ (5.58)		
3154058	6/27/2017		$ (53.20)		
3156307	6/27/2017		$ (10.00)		
3155432	6/23/2017		$ (65.62)		
3155751	6/23/2017		$ (49.28)		
3159604	6/21/2017		$ (4.75)		
3153445	6/21/2017		$ (147.74)		
3170261	6/20/2017		$ (28.28)		
3152357	6/20/2017		$ (624.82)		
3151970	6/19/2017		$ (3.84)		

The objective of the spreadsheet is to find the credit balances so that the billing team can spend their time addressing the credit balances to determine if refunds are due. If there are issues that caused the refunds, this tool provides the ability to sort and trend credit balances. This spreadsheet has the same exception report approach with credit balances as other reports throughout the book; only show the report user what he or she needs to see. Rather than spend time looking for the balances that may need to be refunded, use Business Intelligence to make the research easier and use the staff time more effectively.

TRACKING COMPLIANCE IN QUALITY REPORTING

Compliance with government quality reporting programs is only getting more complicated. The government changes the rules for how and what is measured annually. The carrots are more appealing and the sticks are more daunting. Even when providers and staff are educated on what this year's requirements are, processes and work flows can fall through the cracks. Measures that used to be easy to meet are now not being met because a form was too much trouble to give to a patient or a box was not checked. A button on an EHR form that used to indicate compliance was changed in an upgrade or the clinical team did not correctly follow a prescribed workflow. Challenges like this happen to the best practices.

The practice that created Exhibit 10.2 has 70 providers trying to qualify for government quality incentives. The billing office uses the PivotTable to carefully track compliance by provider and by measure. The measures are color coded based on whether the provider is meeting the standard. The PivotTable allows filtering by dates of service and provider. The PivotTable columns track the numerator, denominator, and the exclusions. Whether your practice reports via claims or via a registry, it is critical to know which providers are meeting the measure throughout the year to avoid a crisis at year end. The PivotTable structure makes it easy to double-click any value and get the underlying detail. If a provider is missing compliance codes, the PivotTable can tell you exactly which claims, which patients, and which locations are in trouble so corrective action can be taken.

EXHIBIT 10.2 COMPLIANCE BY PROVIDER AND MEASURE TRACKING SAMPLE

Domain/Measure & Measure Description	Sum of Numerator	Sum of Denominator	Sum of Exclusion	Sum of Completeness	Sum of Performance %
DOS	(All)				
Provider	(All)				
⊟ Effective Clinical Care	248	446		91.9%	60.5%
⊟ 1 - Diabetes: Hemoglobin A1c Poor Control	109	285		89.1%	42.9%
(blank)	0	31		0.0%	0.0%
3046F-8P - A1c level was not performed	78	78		100.0%	100.0%
3044F - A1c level < 7.0%	0	96		100.0%	0.0%
3046F - A1c level > 9.0%	31	31		100.0%	100.0%
3045F - A1c level 7.0 to 9.0%	0	49		100.0%	0.0%
⊟ 145 - Radiology Exposure Time	139	161		96.9%	89.1%
G9500 - Radiation exposure indices, or exposure time & number of images documented	139	139		100.0%	100.0%
G9501 - Radiation exposure indices, or exposure time & number of images NOT documented	0	17		100.0%	0.0%
(blank)	0	5		0.0%	0.0%
⊟ Patient Safety	2,899	3,318	3908	99.1%	89.1%
⊟ 154 - Fall Risk Assessment	1,581	1,992	3908	99.1%	81.7%
1101F - No falls or 1 fall with no injury	0	0	3908	100.0%	0.0%
3288F and 1100F - Fall risk documented, 2 or more falls or fall with injury	1,581	1,581	0	100.0%	100.0%
3288F-8P and 1100F - Fall risk assessment not completed	0	355	0	100.0%	0.0%
(blank)	0	56		0.0%	0.0%
⊟ 21 - Peri-Operative Care: Selection of Prophylactic Antibiotic - 1st or 2nd Generation Cephalos	708	715		99.0%	100.0%

MISSING QUALITY CODES

Exhibit 10.3 is an email that is sent throughout the day to notify the billing office team about claims missing Medicare quality codes. This practice is submitting codes via claims rather than through a registry, so it is critical to get the codes added before claims are submitted, but practices using a registry would also benefit from knowing which claims are missing codes before the claims go to the registry.

EXHIBIT 10.3 MISSING QUALITY CODES TRACKING SAMPLE

Missing Quality Codes Entered Yesterday as of 9/2/2017

Ticket Number	Patient Id	Patient	Measure	Coder
2969535	9787430		No MIPS Codes	
2970715	10645862		No MIPS Codes	
2972741	757284		No MIPS Codes	
2977661	10704107		No MIPS Codes	
3012481	621741		No MIPS Codes	
3075874	9369560		No MIPS Codes	
3075977	9803160		No MIPS Codes	
3098603	10732447		No MIPS Codes	
3164601	748915		No MIPS Codes	
3191811	9768140		No MIPS Codes	
3200223	10730165		No MIPS Codes	
3200316	682311		No MIPS Codes	
3201797	775824		No MIPS Codes	

The report has custom BI logic to recognize claims that should have a quality code. This email is also an exception report. The only claims that appear on the email are claims missing a code. The exception approach keeps the email short and very relevant to the billing staff. Even if a particular claim went out without getting fixed, this report is one that a manager might want to see, to at least notify providers of failures to meet quality expectations. The rightmost column on the email tracks the coder who billed the claim. The exception report makes it easy to know which coders need additional training on each measure.

This process is evolving to become more of a claim scrubbing system. If we can look for missing quality codes, what else can we look for before a claim goes out the door? Many practices use claim scrubbers to catch these kinds of issues. Is your claim scrubber flexible enough to catch all the issues you need to find before releasing a claim?

SIMPLIFY COMPLIANCE FOR PAIN MANAGEMENT PROVIDERS

Exhibit 10.4 is a custom SSRS dashboard designed for busy pain management providers. The dashboard's objective is to help the clinical team comply with the state's requirements for narcotics patients. At the top of the dashboard are SSRS parameters that allow the user to enter a beginning date, an ending date, and the appointment resource to analyze. With these inputs, the dashboard generates upcoming appointments for a pain management provider. The Business Intelligence behind the report determines whether the patient is treated as a narcotic patient, as indicated in the third column. The physicians in the practice have different requests for data that defines which patients should be included in the dashboard, and the custom Business Intelligence logic incorporates those physician preferences. The Narcotic Patient column also identifies new patients who cannot yet be classified as a narcotic patient.

The last six columns search the EHR data for compliance with practice protocols for pain and narcotic patients. The Last Narcotic Contract Date tracks signed patient management contracts with the provider. (INSPECT is a controlled substance report required in the state of Indiana.) Business Intelligence logic in SSRS highlights (in red) patients whose documents have expired and need to be signed again. The document expiration date also varies by provider. The SSRS logic highlights columns based on the provider-specific logic. The same logic applies to urine drug screens, again customizable by provider preference. The EKG Date column only applies to methadone patients. SSRS checks to see if the patient is on methadone and then reports the date of the last EKG in the EHR.

EXHIBIT 10.4 NARCOTICS TRACKING SAMPLE

Beg Date 9/11/2017　　　　End Date 9/15/2017

Appt Resource

|◁ < 1 of 1 > ▷| ↻ ⊕ 100% ▾ 🖫▾ 🖨   Find | Next

Appointments for   Between 9/11/2017 and 9/15/2017 as of 9/2/2017

Patient	Patient ID	Narcotic Pt	Appt Start	Location	Last Narcotic Contract Date	Last INSPECT Date	Last Point of Care UDS Date	Last UDS Confirm Date	Last Non Compliant UDS Date	Last EKG Date
	10740722		9/13/2017 2:30 PM							Not methadone
	787322		9/13/2017 2:45 PM			7/18/2017				Not methadone
	1072004l		9/13/2017 3:00 PM			8/18/2017		2/23/2017		Not methadone
	786262		9/13/2017 3:15 PM			8/9/2017				Not methadone
	9615110	Narcotic Pt	9/13/2017 3:30 PM		Narcotic Pt	6/14/2017				Not methadone
	687255		9/13/2017 3:45 PM			8/1/2017	5/25/2016	5/25/2016	5/31/2016	Not methadone
	806611	Narcotic Pt	9/14/2017 8:30 AM		Narcotic Pt	1/28/2017	7/20/2011	1/30/2017		Not methadone
	9943570		9/14/2017 8:45 AM			8/18/2017		5/11/2017		Not methadone
	10735250		9/14/2017 9:30 AM			8/31/2017		4/26/2017		Not methadone

The objective of the compliance dashboard is to ensure the providers have all the necessary documents and that tests are completed and current before the patient arrives. This dashboard can save a significant amount of time eliminating chart prep activity since clinical staff do not have to open each electronic chart to get the information they need to prepare for the appointment. Nurses simply scan the dashboard for missing data (blanks) and outdated data (highlighted in red) to make sure they are ready for upcoming appointments. More importantly, the dashboard can prevent human error. Once again, the approach is an exception report.

TESTING DATA BEFORE SUBMITTING TO A REGISTRY

The spreadsheet in Exhibit 10.5 is an example of data about to submitted to the Anesthesia Quality Institute (AQI), a Qualified Clinical Data Registry (QCDR). AQI requires the data to be submitted in an XML format. XML is an extensible markup language that is efficient for submitting data but a difficult format to review data before submission. This spreadsheet reviews the data before converting to XML for submission.

EXHIBIT 10.5 TESTING DATA FOR REGISTRY SUBMISSION SAMPLE

AQI DATA

CaseId	Start From Time	Start Thru Time	Date of Service	CRNA ID	MD ID	Supervising ID	CRNA Staff Type	MD Staff Type	SUPER Staff Type
44659977_20170220_732	732	1114	2/20/2017	460		669	Certified Registered Nurse Anesthetist		Anesthesiologist
44660348_20170308_828	828	859	3/8/2017	442		669			Anesthesiologist
44660645_20170330_830	830	855	3/30/2017	529	668		Certified Registered Nurse Anesthetist	Anesthesiologist	
44660868_20170425_834	834	858	4/25/2017		637			Anesthesiologist	
44660975_20170216_134	1342	1500	2/16/2017	454	626		Certified Registered Nurse Anesthetist	Anesthesiologist	
44661098_20170324_114	1147	1224	3/24/2017	463	652		Certified Registered Nurse Anesthetist	Anesthesiologist	
44661098_20170412_115	1159	1239	4/12/2017	464	532		Certified Registered Nurse Anesthetist	Anesthesiologist	
44661130_20170413_122	1229	1344	4/13/2017	530	660		Certified Registered Nurse Anesthetist	Anesthesiologist	
44661544_20170306_732	732	954	3/6/2017	483		004	Certified Registered Nurse Anesthetist		Anesthesiologist
44662195_20170328_721	721	1345	3/28/2017	527	609		Certified Registered Nurse Anesthetist	Anesthesiologist	
44662534_20170220_140	1408	1435	2/20/2017	482		004	Certified Registered Nurse Anesthetist		Anesthesiologist
44662997_20170308_161	1617	1832	3/8/2017	631				Anesthesiologist	
44663193_20170405_908	908	1107	4/5/2017	444	649		Certified Registered Nurse Anesthetist	Anesthesiologist	
44664449_20170307_720	720	846	3/7/2017	442		671	Certified Registered Nurse Anesthetist		Anesthesiologist
44665149_20170421_134	1342	1355	4/21/2017	499		004	Certified Registered Nurse Anesthetist		Anesthesiologist
44665297_20170210_758	758	810	2/10/2017	350		641	Certified Registered Nurse Anesthetist		Anesthesiologist
44665529_20170212_183	1830	2045	2/12/2017	407	639		Certified Registered Nurse Anesthetist	Anesthesiologist	
44665867_20170214_102	1023	1359	2/14/2017	377	649		Certified Registered Nurse Anesthetist	Anesthesiologist	
44666303_20170407_160	1603	1712	4/7/2017	525		667	Certified Registered Nurse Anesthetist		Anesthesiologist

THE EXCEL TABLE FORMAT HAS A DROP-DOWN COLUMN IN EACH COLUMN TO MAKE IT EASY TO SORT AND FILTER THE DATA IN THE COLUMN. TO CREATE A TABLE IN EXCEL, DO THE FOLLOWING:

SELECT THE DATA YOU WANT TO FORMAT, EITHER BY SELECTING THE ENTIRE RANGE OF DATA OR BY SIMPLY SELECTING A CELL THAT IS PART OF YOUR DATA.

CHOOSE FORMAT AS A TABLE FROM THE HOME TAB, AS SHOWN IN EXHIBIT 10.6.

EXHIBIT 10.6 CREATING A TABLE: PART 1

Excel will bring up a screen of style choices for the Table, as shown in Exhibit 10.7.

Exhibit 10.7 Creating a Table: Part 2

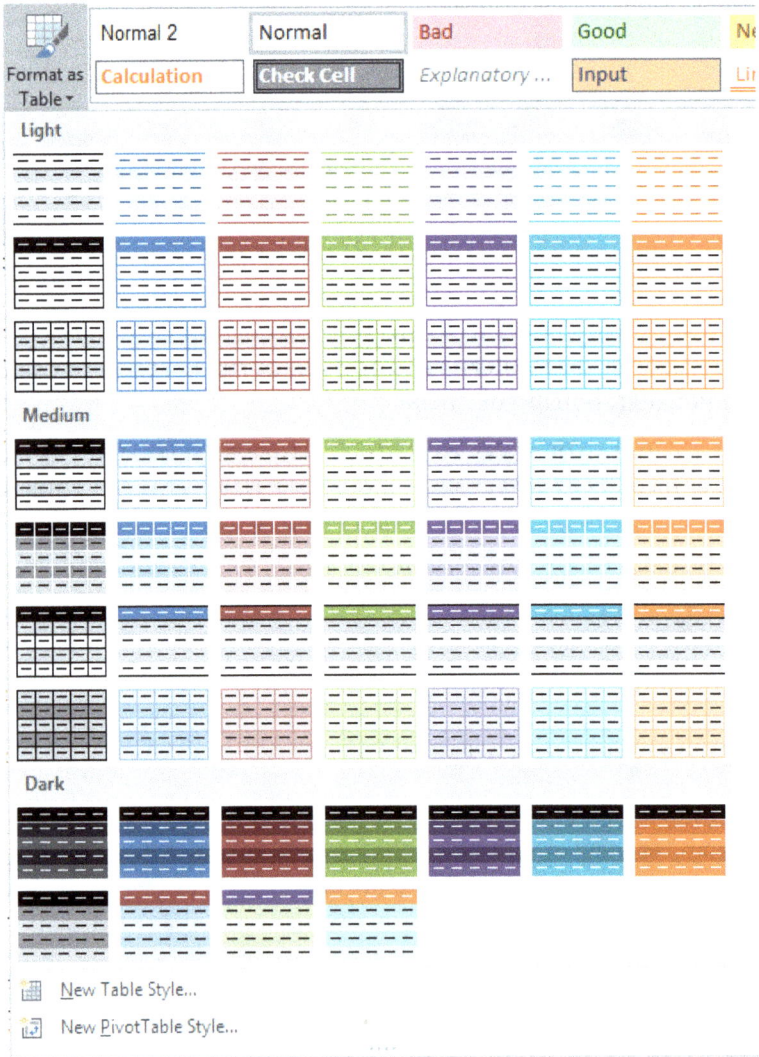

CHOOSE A STYLE THAT WORKS FOR YOUR SPREADSHEET. STYLES IN THE MEDIUM CATEGORY WORK WELL.

THE NEXT WINDOW CONFIRMS THAT THE RANGE OF CELLS TO BE INCLUDED IN THE TABLE IS CORRECT, AS SHOWN IN EXHIBIT 10.8

EXHIBIT 10.8 CREATING A TABLE: PART 3

Claim	Balance	Date	Due From	PSTP	Patient	Aging	Location	Doctor
12013	697.21	4/13/2018	Medicare	Primary	Hunt, Paul	0-30 Days	Main	Dr. Lincoln
12025	381.97	4/2/2018	CIGNA	Primary	Yates, Mike	0-30 Days	South	Dr. Jefferson
12038	525.42	9/20/2017	AETNA	Primary	Norris, Ellis	Over 120 Days	South	Dr. Jefferson
12046	1762.81	4/13/2018	Patient	Patient	Scott, Lee	0-30 Days	Lincoln	Dr. Lincoln
12053	1557.4	3/29/2018	Patient	Patient	Cox, Cory	0-30 Days	Lincoln	Dr. Roosevelt
12054	1125.69	4/9/2018	Patient	Patient	Gray, Nora	0-30 Days	Main	Dr. Washington
12066	264.98	4/13/2018	Medicare	Pri		0-30 Days	Main	Dr. Lincoln
12077	491.03	11/30/2017	Patient	Pat		Over 120 Days	Columbus	Dr. Roosevelt
12087	828.99	3/25/2018	Patient	Pat		0-30 Days	St. Anne	Dr. Kennedy
12091	818.34	1/24/2018	Patient	Pat		61-90 Days	Lincoln	Dr. Lincoln
12097	1848.7	3/30/2018	Medicare	Pri		0-30 Days	South	Dr. Roosevelt
12100	405.29	12/20/2017	Medicare	Pri		91-120 Days	South	Dr. Roosevelt
12102	1681.91	3/21/2018	Patient	Patient	Robbins, Nadine	0-30 Days	Lincoln	Dr. Roosevelt
12114	1302.11	2/20/2018	Patient	Patient	Hines, Rufus	31-60 Days	Lincoln	Dr. Sacagewea
12119	1578.43	1/8/2018	Patient	Patient	Castillo, Cary	91-120 Days	Lincoln	Dr. Roosevelt
12123	745.42	3/1/2018	Patient	Patient	Ramsey, Sheryl	31-60 Days	Columbus	Dr. Sacagewea
12127	962.62	3/29/2018	Blue Cross	Primary	Duncan, Reginald	0-30 Days	South	Dr. Lincoln
12131	253.6	3/15/2018	CIGNA	Primary	Myers, Sheryl	31-60 Days	Columbus	Dr. Kennedy
12138	9.75	4/1/2018	Patient	Patient	Brady, Robin	0-30 Days	Columbus	Dr. Lincoln
12144	1296.7	3/24/2018	CIGNA	Primary	Joseph, Sheryl	0-30 Days	Lincoln	Dr. Kennedy

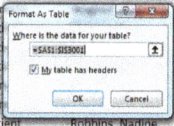

Format As Table dialog box overlaid: "Where is the data for your table? =$A$1:$I$300 / My table has headers / OK Cancel"

MODIFY THE CELL RANGE IF NECESSARY, AND CLICK OK.

EXCEL THEN CREATES A TABLE, AS SHOWN IN EXHIBIT 10.9

EXHIBIT 10.9 CREATING A TABLE: PART 4

Claim	Balance	Date	Due From	PSTP	Patient	Aging	Location	Doctor
12013	697.21	4/13/2018	Medicare	Primary	Hunt, Paul	0-30 Days	Main	Dr. Lincoln
12025	381.97	4/2/2018	CIGNA	Primary	Yates, Mike	0-30 Days	South	Dr. Jefferson
12038	525.42	9/20/2017	AETNA	Primary	Norris, Ellis	Over 120 Days	South	Dr. Jefferson
12046	1762.81	4/13/2018	Patient	Patient	Scott, Lee	0-30 Days	Lincoln	Dr. Lincoln
12053	1557.4	3/29/2018	Patient	Patient	Cox, Cory	0-30 Days	Lincoln	Dr. Roosevelt
12054	1125.69	4/9/2018	Patient	Patient	Gray, Nora	0-30 Days	Main	Dr. Washington
12066	264.98	4/13/2018	Medicare	Primary	Wagner, Kristine	0-30 Days	Main	Dr. Lincoln
12077	491.03	11/30/2017	Patient	Patient	Nichols, Troy	Over 120 Days	Columbus	Dr. Roosevelt
12087	828.99	3/25/2018	Patient	Patient	Curtis, Lucia	0-30 Days	St. Anne	Dr. Kennedy
12091	818.34	1/24/2018	Patient	Patient	Harper, Monica	61-90 Days	Lincoln	Dr. Lincoln
12097	1848.7	3/30/2018	Medicare	Primary	Klein, Jonathan	0-30 Days	South	Dr. Roosevelt
12100	405.29	12/20/2017	Medicare	Primary	Barber, Shawna	91-120 Days	South	Dr. Roosevelt
12102	1681.91	3/21/2018	Patient	Patient	Robbins, Nadine	0-30 Days	Lincoln	Dr. Roosevelt
12114	1302.11	2/20/2018	Patient	Patient	Hines, Rufus	31-60 Days	Lincoln	Dr. Sacagewea
12119	1578.43	1/8/2018	Patient	Patient	Castillo, Cary	91-120 Days	Lincoln	Dr. Roosevelt
12123	745.42	3/1/2018	Patient	Patient	Ramsey, Sheryl	31-60 Days	Columbus	Dr. Sacagewea
12127	962.62	3/29/2018	Blue Cross	Primary	Duncan, Reginald	0-30 Days	South	Dr. Lincoln
12131	253.6	3/15/2018	CIGNA	Primary	Myers, Dora	31-60 Days	Columbus	Dr. Kennedy
12138	9.75	4/1/2018	Patient	Patient	Brady, Robin	0-30 Days	Columbus	Dr. Lincoln
12144	1296.7	3/24/2018	CIGNA	Primary	Joseph, Sheryl	0-30 Days	Lincoln	Dr. Kennedy

Excel automatically shades every other row and creates a drop-down box in each column. The drop-down box makes sorting and filtering the Table data very simple. A sample drop-down box for the Date field is shown in Exhibit 10.10.

Exhibit 10.10 Creating a Table: Part 5

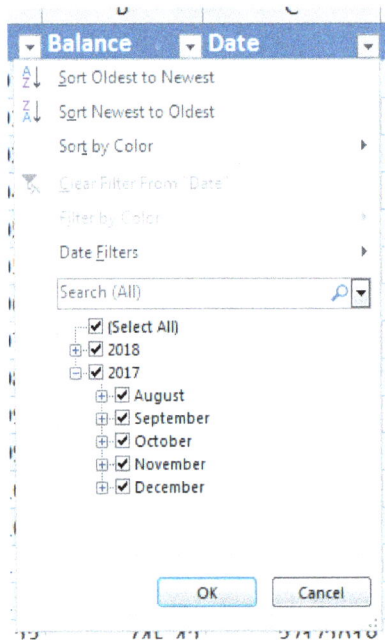

This practice generally submits data as an XML file to AQI monthly after carefully reviewing this spreadsheet. Having a straightforward way to analyze the quality data's completeness and accuracy makes compliance easier for this practice. The practice also uses the data in the Excel Table for their own internal quality measures and analysis.

To make compliance measures easier for the providers to follow, this practice has designed a simple one-page form for the provider to fill out. The form asks for clinical terms that the providers understand. Logic inside the program converts the clinical terms into the appropriate measures. For example, the form may ask questions like whether an inhalation agent was used (during a given procedure), whether there were three or more risk factors for nausea and vomiting, and whether two anti-emetics were used to combat this. The logic converts the answers to those questions to the appropriate quality codes for a measure. It is easy for providers to answer the questions about inhalation agents. Asking providers straight-forward clinical questions rather than requiring them to fill in quality codes that change yearly leads to more accurate data. The program logic must be updated annually, but it is faster and simpler to change the program logic than it is to re-educate all the providers.

COMPLIANCE WITH BILLING REQUIREMENTS

Exhibits 10.11 and 10.12 were designed in conjunction with a practice that provides physical therapy (PT). PT has specific requirements regarding how often a progress note must be documented in the patients' charts. Discharged patients also require a specific note in the patients' charts. The logic behind these reports captures the billing intervals and identifies patients that need billing notes or who have stopped attending appointments and need to be discharged (even if the patient quit without being discharged) to make sure that the documentation is appropriate.

EXHIBIT 10.11 COMPLIANCE: FOLLOW-UP APPOINTMENT TRACKING SAMPLE

Future Appts Needing Progress Note as of 9/2/2017

Scheduled Therapist	Appt Date	Appt Type	Initial Treating Therapist
	9/5/2017	PT Followup	
	9/5/2017	PT Followup	
	9/7/2017	PT Followup	
	9/6/2017	PT Followup	
	9/6/2017	PT Followup	
	9/8/2017	PT Followup	
	9/5/2017	PT Followup	
	9/5/2017	PT Followup	
	9/7/2017	PT Followup	
	9/7/2017	PT Followup	
	9/5/2017	PT Followup	
	9/8/2017	PT Followup	
	9/11/2017	PT Followup	
	9/14/2017	PT Followup	

EXHIBIT 10.12 COMPLIANCE: DISCHARGE NOTES TRACKING SAMPLE

Need Progress or Discharge Note as of 9/2/2017

Patient	Last Appt Date	Appt Type	Initial Treating Therapist
	8/3/2017	PT Followup	
	8/3/2017	PT Followup	
	8/23/2017	PT Followup	
	9/1/2017	PT Progress	
	8/3/2017	PT Followup	
	8/30/2017	PT Followup	
	8/3/2017	PT Followup	
	9/1/2017	PT Followup	
	8/28/2017	PT Followup	

Though the examples are specific to PT, there are plenty of other applications for Business Intelligence in billing compliance. For example, this exhibit from *Better Data Better Decisions* tracks evaluation and management codes by provider. The chart makes it easy to compare providers against peers or similar subspecialty averages to look for anomalies.

EXHIBIT 10.13 NEW PATIENT CODING LEVELS

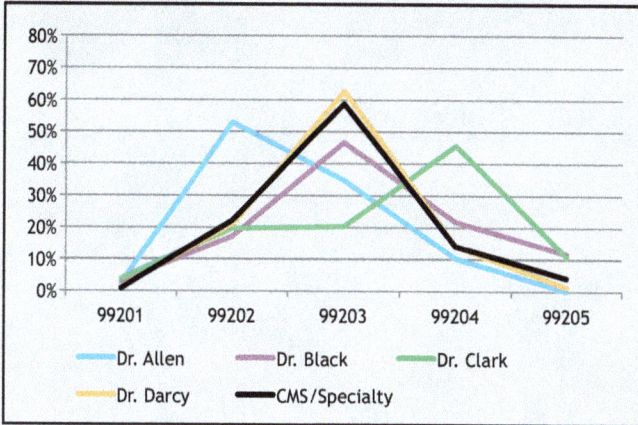

Another billing compliance report might track a specific issue raised on a previous internal or external audit. For example, a radiation oncology group that wanted to ensure that the providers reviewed and approved each image before the next patient treatment. The report helps confirm that the practice is billing in accordance with radiation therapy guidelines. As you would expect, the compliance report identifies exceptions so training physicians and staff is more efficient. The additional training can be tailored based on the providers' exceptions.

Compliance is very important and it is often extremely time-consuming. The Business Intelligence objective is to make compliance work accurate, fast and simple. The less time the staff spends identifying problems, the more time the staff has available to fix problems. Similarly, if a report can confirm that a previous compliance issue is now under control, staff do not need to spend time checking to see that the issue is still fixed.

CHAPTER 11

DASHBOARDS

If you could have one page of information automatically emailed to you every day, what would be on that page? What key information would make the biggest difference in your practice? If you could have one page of information emailed to your physicians weekly or monthly, what would be on that page? What would a one-page email to your billing department, your clinical staff, or your front desk contain?

Start small. Maybe that one-page email isn't full yet. If it could only be one piece of information emailed to you daily, what would make the biggest difference in your practice? Would it be future appointments, current revenues, or physician productivity? How do you choose your candidate for that one piece of information? Is the candidate on the list because you cannot get that information at all or because it takes hours and days to get that information? Do you choose your candidate because it will influence physician behavior, or will the candidate have the most impact on the practice's bottom line?

When a practice starts with Business Intelligence, one of the first things they ask for is a dashboard. Dashboards are terrific, and custom dashboards are even better, but a dashboard that simply says *things are still broken like they were last month* is not the place to start. A practice may instead focus on giving team members tools to better do their jobs so that once a custom dashboard is implemented the numbers improve from month to month. For example, if accounts receivable balances are taking longer and longer to collect, the prettiest, fanciest dashboard in the world won't hasten accounts receivable's efforts along any better. The practice may be better served by building a spreadsheet, an email, or some combination of tools to identify claims over 30 days, claims that need to be appealed, and/or patient balances that could be collected at an upcoming appointment. The balance between tools for staff and custom dashboards for managers differs by practice, but recognizing the balance and making sure the staff have tools to succeed is part of the consideration for any dashboard.

There are plenty of custom dashboard examples in this chapter. And each dashboard is unique. Your practice may benefit from a measure or a component from another practice's dashboard, but each practice has unique concerns and opportunities that these dashboards are designed to address. Several of these examples are designed by numbers-driven certified public accountants, but others are designed by savvy practice managers who know what their providers need to see.

DASHBOARD SUMMARY OF A PRACTICE

The first example is Exhibit 11.1, the summary page of a complex, very customized dashboard. First, notice the heading at the top of the dashboard. The heading reflects the SSRS parameters the user chose to filter the dashboard. This dashboard by default always reports based on last month's date so there are no date filters, but users can filter by location, provider, procedure classes, plan classes (primary insurance), departments, and places of service. With six independent filters, the dashboard offers very specific, granular data to deeply understand the practice from multiple perspectives. The practice has chosen seven key metrics to measure: charges, receipts, work RVUs, receipts per work RVU, new patients, cases, and case mix.

Cases represents the number of surgical cases during the period. Surgical cases can be hard to calculate from a canned PM report. PM reports display charges by procedure code. Since there is often more than one procedure code billed on a case, it can be hard not to double count the same procedure for the same patient. This dashboard uses SQL Server code to count unique patients with procedure codes in a specific range of CPT codes as a case. The beauty of a custom dashboard is the ability to define and completely tailor measures that matter most to your practice.

As an example of customizing metrics that matter to a practice, consider the Case Mix calculation at the bottom of Exhibit 11.1. Case mix is the amount of work RVUs per case. The practice administrator states they use case mix as, "a quasi-indicator of patient severity, though not severity adjusted, of course. It is calculated like the way a hospital would calculate case mix. When a granular analysis is needed to determine collections trends we look first at collections, next at payer mix, and third I will review case mix to determine if the trend is driven by 'sicker' patients. Beyond that, if still not explained, we would then begin to look at denial data. Case mix could also be used to indicate a change in coding. If a physician feels that he is doing a similar basket of cases this year compared to last year and his case mix has increased or declined, that would be an indication that we have somehow changed our coding." The practice administrator created a custom metric and then uses that metric to benchmark performance and explain variances.

The dashboard measures five different time periods: current month, current six months, last six months (the six-month period prior to the current six-month period), year-to-date, and prior year-to-date. With all that detail, the dashboard also measures the change and variance for the current six-month period and current year-to-date compared to prior periods. The page-one summary is a concise yet detailed overview of metrics the chief executive officer uses to manage the group.

EXHIBIT 11.1 DASHBOARDS: SUMMARY SAMPLE

Locations: ALL Providers: ALL
Procedure Classes: ALL Plan Classes: ALL
Departments: ALL POS: ALL

Collection and Production Summary									
	Current Mo	Current 6	Last 6	Chg	Var	YTD	PYTD	Chg	Var
Total Charges	$16,266,607	$83,758,230	$87,190,317	($3,432,087)	-3.9%	$112,319,081	$100,751,061	$11,568,021	11.5%
Total Receipts	$2,687,303	$16,226,323	$17,024,210	($797,887)	-4.7%	$22,208,964	$22,287,566	($78,602)	-0.4%
Work RVUs	21,484	115,824	117,766	(1,942)	-1.6%	154,426	157,056	(2,630)	-1.7%
Receipts/wRVU	$125.08	$140.10	$144.56	($4.46)	-3.1%	$143.82	$141.91	$1.91	1.3%
New Patients	957	5,529	5,246	283	5.4%	7,293	7,612	(319)	-4.2%
Cases	1,427	7,780	7,680	100	1.3%	10,274	9,786	488	5.0%
Case Mix	15.1	14.9	15.3	(0.4)	-2.9%	15.0	16.0	(1.0)	-6.3%

> SSRS can format the numbers red or green, like conditional formatting in Excel. Conditional formatting in Excel is easier since you can format one cell and copy the conditional formatting to other cells. You must conditionally format each cell in SSRS. SSRS does allow more powerful conditional formatting formulas than are available in Excel.

KEY INDICATORS

Immediately below the summary are 13 additional metrics that are measured on the last full month ("This mo" on the dashboard) and the average of the past six months. The trending red and green arrows are some of the many indicators available in SSRS. Several of the measure descriptions are abbreviated for space in this section of the dashboard. "OTC collections" are over-the-counter collections, or collections at the front desk. "Days to Scd NP" is the number of days required to schedule a new patient appointment. "Days to Scd Surg" are the number of days required to schedule a surgery. The percentage of new patients compared to the total number of new and established patient visits is labeled as "% of New Patients."

Exhibit 11.2 Dashboards: Key Indicators Sample

Key Indicators							
	This mo	6 mo Avg	Trend		This mo	6 mo Avg	Trend
AR Balance	$14,653,071			# NP office visits	957	922	⬆
Days in AR	31.3			# EP office visits	1,745	1,506	⬆
% AR over 120 Days	$1,877,095 (13%)			# Post-op visits	1,225	1,165	
Avg days to bill	6.7	12.1	⬆	Total office visits	3,927	3,592	⬆
Gross Collect %	16.5%	19.4%	⬇	# NP hospital visits	73	49	⬆
OTC collections	$125,002	$168,453	⬇	# Round/Admits	960	709	⬆
Days to Scd NP	10.9	10.3	⬆	% New Patients	25.8%	26.6%	⬇
Days to Scd Surg	29.4	29.3	⬆	# Surgery Cases	1,427	1,297	⬆

Accounts-receivable-related measures do not have a six-month average, so they cannot be trended. In this PM system, calculating accounts receivable as of prior time periods is difficult. Historical accounts receivable can be a challenge in many PM systems. Some practices store accounts receivable data in the data warehouse monthly to make trending accounts receivable easier. If trending accounts receivable is important to your practice, consider storing data at the end of each month in a data warehouse. If you do store accounts receivable data, store the responsible party for the outstanding claims when you store the accounts receivable data. Without this detail, it is very difficult to know whether primary or secondary insurance or the patient is responsible for a claim at a given point in time. Storing the responsible party instead of trying to calculate the responsible party is much simpler.

PROCEDURE TRENDS

A key metric for many practices is to trend data by procedures. The practice that developed this dashboard makes a concerted effort to classify each procedure code into an overall procedure category so that the categories can be trended over time similar to the summary in Exhibit 11.3. Organizing procedures into categories can be challenging because some procedures might include many CPT codes. Over time, CPT codes are redefined, often changing the definition of what a single procedure really means.

Defining a procedure is something that may or may not be done when the PM system is installed and configured. Even if the procedures are categorized at the time a practice installs a new PM system, new CPT codes and procedures may not be included in the categories. If the procedure categories are not available on a canned report used by practice, there is no reason to take the time to maintain the procedure categories. If the procedure categories were available on a canned report, uncategorized procedures would serve as a reminder to maintain the categories. Once good reporting is available, classifications matter.

Whenever possible, maintain classifications like procedure category in the PM or EHR system rather than in the data warehouse. The PM or EHR system has a menu and functionality to maintain the categories that the end user can access. Some PM and EHR systems limit access to those menus, but generally someone at the practice can modify categories. If the categories are stored in the data warehouse, a practice either needs to create a mechanism to maintain categories in the data warehouse or work with IT or an outside consultant every time a procedure is added or a category changes. Build a workflow that reminds you to change the category every time procedures change.

Exhibit 11.3 Dashboards: Procedure Trends Sample

	Procedure Trends ($$ and wRvu)							
Procedure	Current 6	Last 6	Chg	Var	YTD	PYTD	Chg	Var
Receipts	$1,687,634	$1,537,122	$150,512	9.8%	$2,205,298	$2,562,792	($357,493)	-13.9%
wRVUs	11,805	11,168	637	5.7%	15,264	15,490	(226)	-1.5%
Receipts	$304,877	$314,268	($9,392)	-3.0%	$406,971	$447,655	($40,684)	-9.1%
wRVUs	2,931	3,309	(378)	-11.4%	4,074	4,690	(617)	-13.1%
Receipts	$830,950	$843,005	($12,055)	-1.4%	$1,161,082	$1,082,155	$78,927	7.3%
wRVUs	11,297	11,794	(497)	-4.2%	15,192	13,736	1,456	10.6%
Receipts	$652,581	$842,953	($190,372)	-22.6%	$877,673	$780,693	$96,980	12.4%
wRVUs	0	0	0	0.0%	0	0	0	0.0%
Receipts	$1,562,945	$1,560,555	$2,389	0.2%	$2,076,523	$2,099,978	($23,455)	-1.1%
wRVUs	22,163	21,614	549	2.5%	29,321	29,624	(303)	-1.0%
Receipts	$162,964	$210,427	($47,463)	-22.6%	$228,299	$313,110	($84,811)	-27.1%
wRVUs	1,870	2,467	(597)	-24.2%	2,653	3,334	(681)	-20.4%
Receipts	$1,045,476	$1,103,095	($57,619)	-5.2%	$1,440,220	$1,325,345	$114,876	8.7%
wRVUs	11,294	11,544	(249)	-2.2%	15,037	14,648	389	2.7%
Receipts	$1,728,437	$1,543,921	$184,516	12.0%	$2,286,838	$1,935,299	$351,539	18.2%
wRVUs	15,390	15,448	(58)	-0.4%	20,380	21,069	(689)	-3.3%
Receipts	$784,168	$920,502	($136,335)	-14.8%	$1,159,461	$1,051,760	$107,701	10.2%
wRVUs	9,270	10,739	(1,469)	-13.7%	12,711	12,953	(242)	-1.9%
Receipts	$396,250	$359,542	$36,708	10.2%	$503,176	$437,975	$65,201	14.9%
wRVUs	2,258	2,105	153	7.3%	2,991	2,681	310	11.6%

The dashboard includes tables like Exhibit 11.3 that trend data by payer and department instead of by procedure code. All the tables respond to changes in the filters set at the top of the dashboard, so it is easy to trend procedures for one payer or location or to trend payer data by provider or place of service.

CLEARLY, THIS DASHBOARD HAS A LOT OF DATA AND A LOT OF CALCULATIONS. SSRS ALLOWS DASHBOARDS TO BE CACHED. WHEN SSRS CACHES A DASHBOARD, ALL THE CALCULATIONS AND DATA ARE SAVED AT CERTAIN TIMES EACH DAY SO THAT THE DASHBOARD RUNS BASED ON THE STORED DATA INSTEAD OF CALCULATING EVERYTHING AT RUNTIME. TO MAKE SURE THE DASHBOARDS DO NOT SLOW DOWN THE DAY-TO-DAY OPERATIONS IN A PRACTICE, PRACTICES TYPICALLY PULL DATA OVERNIGHT SO THAT REPORTING DOESN'T IMPACT SERVER PERFORMANCE. IN THIS PRACTICE, THE DASHBOARD IS CACHED IMMEDIATELY AFTER FINISHING THE OVERNIGHT DATA PULL SO THAT DASHBOARDS DURING THE DAY RUN MUCH FASTER THAN THEY WOULD WITHOUT CACHING. THE PRACTICE KNOWS THE DATA WILL NOT REFRESH FOR 24 HOURS, SO CACHING THE DATA IS AN EFFECTIVE WAY TO GET FASTER DASHBOARDS WITHOUT COMPRISING THE QUALITY OF THE DATA IN THE DASHBOARDS.

PAYER MIX

Exhibit 11.4 is a simple bar chart comparing payer mix by payer groups. Payer groups are maintained like procedure categories discussed in the last section. For example, the payer group Medicare might contain traditional Medicare, Railroad Medicare, or Medicare Advantage plans. It is helpful to understand changes in payer mix over time. The practice's largest payer is almost four percentage points larger year-to-date compared to the prior year. If this is a better payer for the practice, that could be wonderful news. If this payer has higher deductibles to collect and more denials to appeal, the increase may not be such good news. The filters in the dashboard can help management understand whether this change in payer mix is especially relevant for a certain location, procedure group, or department in the practice.

EXHIBIT 11.4 DASHBOARDS: PAYER GROUP MIX SAMPLE

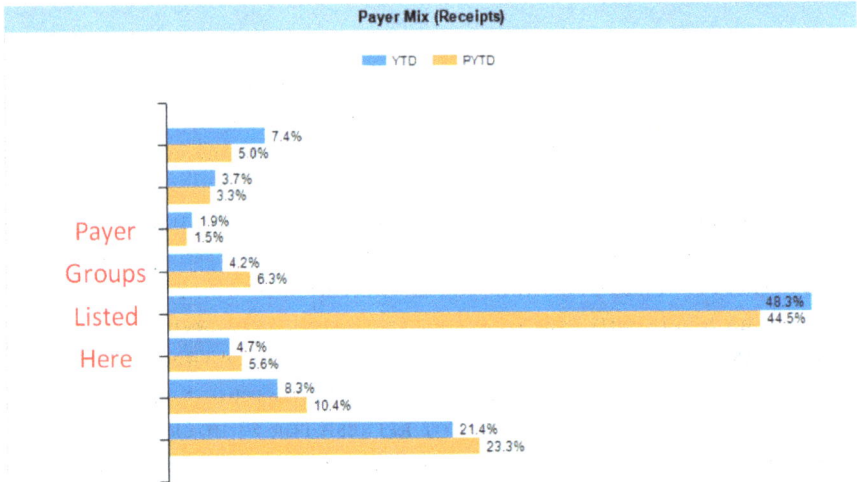

Payer Mix (Receipts)

■ YTD   ■ PYTD

Payer Groups Listed Here:
- 7.4% / 5.0%
- 3.7% / 3.3%
- 1.9% / 1.5%
- 4.2% / 6.3%
- 48.3% / 44.5%
- 4.7% / 5.6%
- 8.3% / 10.4%
- 21.4% / 23.3%

The dashboard also includes monthly trending charts by receipts, work RVUs, receipts per work RVU, total surgery cases, and new patient visits. As the practice manager notices a trend, the dashboard makes it easy to drill down to determine which areas of the practices will be most affected by the change.

The dashboard also includes a chart analyzing payer mix by work RVU. Comparing payer mix by receipts to payer mix work RVUs can be very instructive. A payer who represents more work (as measured by work RVUs) but is a lower percentage of receipts is not a good payer relative to the other payers in the practice. If that payer's business is growing, the practice has reason to be concerned about working harder for less.

RECEIPTS PER WORK RVU

That idea of working harder for less is captured in the practice's receipts per work RVU measure. The chief executive officer uses the metric to compare procedures and payers across providers. A relatively new addition to the dashboard is a series of charts like Exhibit 11.5 that trend receipts per work RVU over time. The dashboard includes several similar charts that analyze groups of five procedure categories.

EXHIBIT 11.5 DASHBOARDS: RECEIPTS PER wRVU TREND CHART SAMPLE

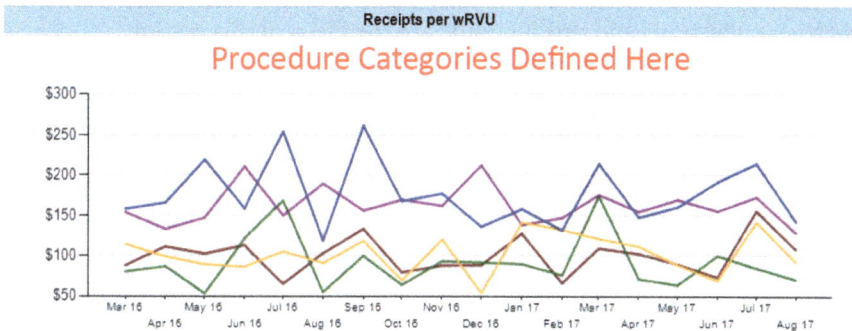

Since receipts per work RVU is such an important metric for this practice, the dashboard also includes similar charts trending receipts and work RVUs separately for each procedure category. Charting receipts and work RVUs separately makes it easier to explain differences in the measure over time. In this case, the practice does not match the month receipts were collected to the month that the work RVUs were rendered.

Other practices match charges and receipts in the same month and trend that data. Consider an example of a service rendered in April. The practice may receive a copayment in April, a primary insurance payment in May, and a secondary insurance payment in June. It will likely take several months to record most of the revenues against April charges. This lag in payments received against charges introduces a delay before the trend matching charges and receipts is available for the month. Though matching charges against receipts does have a lag, the advantage is that the receipts are measured against the charges that generated the receipts.

PHYSICIAN TRENDS

The last section of this dashboard analyzes receipts and work RVUs by individual provider. Again, the filters at the top of the dashboard can isolate this information for a specific payer or group of payers, a procedure category, or a location. If a provider's numbers are getting better or worse, this section of the dashboard is a fruitful resource to search for explanations. Two key metrics, collections and productivity, are the focus of this section.

EXHIBIT 11.6 DASHBOARDS: PHYSICIAN TRENDS TRACKING SAMPLE

Physician Trends ($$ and wRvu)										
Physician	Curr Mo	Current 6	Last 6	Chg	Var	YTD	PYTD	Chg	Var
Receipts	$270,410	$1,535,548	$1,846,502	($310,954)	-16.8%	$2,211,735	$2,394,850	($183,115)	-7.6%
wRVUs	1,241	5,941	5,871	70	1.2%	7,842	8,756	(915)	-10.4%
Cases	86	334	355	(21)	-5.9%	450	493	(43)	-8.7%
Receipts	$54,127	$352,643	$353,335	($693)	-0.2%	$444,693	$472,651	($27,957)	-5.9%
wRVUs	79	2,103	2,268	(165)	-7.3%	2,985	3,659	(674)	-18.4%
Cases	3	108	130	(22)	-16.9%	152	164	(12)	-7.3%
Receipts	$6,503	$41,194	$35,310	$5,883	16.7%	$52,317	$46,884	$5,433	11.6%
wRVUs	50	311	236	75	31.6%	386	324	62	19.2%
Cases	0	0	0	0	0.0%	0	0	0	0.0%
Receipts	$123,038	$889,068	$864,561	$24,507	2.8%	$1,138,579	$1,622,930	($484,350)	-29.8%
wRVUs	878	6,746	5,952	794	13.3%	8,455	9,990	(1,536)	-15.4%
Cases	31	229	221	8	3.6%	293	351	(58)	-16.5%
Receipts	$52,984	$294,813	$300,014	($5,201)	-1.7%	$422,517	$366,396	$56,121	15.3%
wRVUs	676	3,534	3,734	(201)	-5.4%	4,838	4,759	79	1.7%
Cases	48	233	235	(2)	-0.9%	310	278	32	11.5%

This dashboard has been refined, tested, and improved over the years. As the management team has used the dashboard, they have requested additional filters and additional sections to identify areas for practice improvement. As stated in the introduction to this chapter, one size fits one. In other words, this dashboard is ideal for this practice because it was designed specifically for this practice. Your practice is different and your approach to a dashboard should be different, too.

After management was comfortable with the numbers and the way the data was presented, the practice automated a process to email a PDF version of the dashboard each month to the physicians. Simply automating the physician reporting saved the practice hours each month. Recall from Chapter 3 that SSRS allows users to schedule an email for delivery. Scheduling a report for delivery is called subscribing in SSRS. As part of subscribing to a report, users can enter any parameters needed as part of the subscription. For example, Dr. Smith's email is filtered to only show Dr. Smith's data. The dashboard is emailed to management several days before emailing the information to the physicians. Management uses that timeframe to understand variances and trends so they are prepared to answer questions when the physicians receive their copy.

ONE PAGE SAMPLE DASHBOARD WITH CHARGES, RECEIPTS, PAYER MIX AND REFERRING PHYSICIANS

This practice took a different approach to their senior management dashboard. They identified specific measures that were critically important to success and report accordingly. Rolling averages are a big part of this dashboard. Each measure is based on either an average of the previous three months or the previous six months. The prior year comparison is also based on a rolling average of the same number of months. Rolling averages are not very common in canned reports, but a rolling average is a fantastic way to understand trends while minimizing the effect of one good or bad month.

The payer mix section of this dashboard is also interesting. Rather than show all payer categories, this dashboard shows the five largest changes in payer mix for the rolling six-month average, compared to the prior year. The SQL Server logic feeding the dashboard takes the absolute value of the change (whether the change was positive or negative) to determine the five payers to display. The approach is like an exception report discussed throughout this book. The dashboard only shows the payer mix changes that the practice manager needs to see.

EXHIBIT 11.7 DASHBOARDS: ONE PAGE SAMPLE

Annualized Rolling 6 Month Average Charges

Company	Prior Year	Current Year	Change
	$192,693,954	$147,154,400	-23.6%
	$36,875,980	$33,926,854	-8.0%
Total	$229,569,934	$181,081,254	-21.1%

Annualized Rolling 6 Month Average Collections

Company	Prior Year	Current Year	Change
	$40,373,494	$40,884,974	1.3%
	$4,909,784	$4,802,877	-2.2%
Total	$45,283,278	$45,687,851	0.9%

Top 5 Payer Mix Changes (Rolling 6 Month Average)

Insurance Group	Prior Year	Current Year	Change
Major Insurance Groups Here	1.3%	3.0%	1.7%
	4.6%	6.0%	1.4%
	15.9%	14.5%	-1.4%
	3.1%	1.9%	-1.3%
	11.3%	12.4%	1.2%

Top 10 Referring Physicians by Collections (Rolling 3 Month Avg)

Referring Physician	Prior Year	Current Year	Change
Referring Physicians Listed Here	$196,322	$138,712	-29.3%
	$81,258	$101,616	25.1%
	$14,595	$72,689	398.0%
	$71,827	$47,680	-33.6%
	$21,368	$28,184	31.9%
	$26,182	$21,425	-18.2%
	$31,973	$21,097	-34.0%
	$24,962	$19,710	-21.0%
	$21,391	$19,562	-8.6%
	$17,218	$19,486	13.2%

Bottom 10 Referring Physicians by Collections (Rolling 3 Month Avg)

Referring Physician	Prior Year	Current Year	Change
Referring Physicians Listed Here	$18,195	$4,286	-76.4%
	$15,448	$4,920	-68.2%
	$10,555	$3,450	-67.3%
	$17,728	$6,060	-65.8%
	$12,166	$6,518	-46.4%
	$15,404	$8,519	-44.7%
	$14,895	$8,776	-41.1%
	$13,568	$8,233	-39.3%
	$14,123	$8,671	-38.6%
	$18,716	$12,011	-35.8%

The referring physician section on the right ranks the top ten referring physicians by collections and the bottom ten referring physicians to show what is happening on both ends of the referring physician spectrum.

THIS DASHBOARD IS DELIVERED BY EMAIL MONTHLY, BUT IS AVAILABLE THROUGHOUT THE MONTH IN THE REPORT MANAGER FOR SENIOR MANAGEMENT. REPORT MANAGER IS THE SSRS INTERFACE TO VIEW DASHBOARDS, AND IS DISCUSSED IN APPENDIX 1. REPORT MANAGER ORGANIZES REPORTS BY FOLDER AND OFFERS SECURITY OPTIONS BY FOLDER. IF THIS DASHBOARD IS ONLY DESIGNED FOR SENIOR MANAGEMENT TO SEE, THE ACTIVE DIRECTORY LOGIN TO WINDOWS CAN CONTROL WHICH SSRS FOLDERS IN THE REPORT MANAGER A USER CAN ACCESS.

SAMPLE DASHBOARD WITH FINANCIAL DATA

Exhibit 11.8 is another dashboard designed by a CPA. This dashboard replicated a manual process that required hours of running multiple PM reports and then saving the data in spreadsheets. The SSRS parameter filtering this dashboard is a drop-down list of all practice providers. The CPA's focus is on productivity (charges and work RVUs) and financial metrics, and includes some ratios this practice needs to the right of the dashboard.

This practice is very interested in departments, which are defined by procedure code. The underlying SQL Server code associates each procedure code to a specific department, and SSRS subtotals the data for each department. A similar approach could be made for locations, payers, groups of providers or other subtotals that matter to your practice. The bottom of the dashboard includes an overall summary either for all physicians or for the physicians selected in the dropdown list.

Like other dashboards in this chapter, this dashboard also features a version that summarizes data for each physician that is automatically emailed to the physician each month after the CFO has reviewed the data. Automatically sending information has saved this practice a significant amount of time preparing reports that is now spent acting on the information in the report.

EXHIBIT 11.8 DASHBOARDS: FINANCIAL DATA SAMPLE

SUMMARY Monthly Dashboard as of 10/31/2016

Month	Chg Count	Work RVUs	Charge	Adjustments	Payments	Refunds	Net Receipts	Chg/Enc	Pmt/Enc	Pay/Chg
Departments Entered Here										
January	7,844	14,181.14	$3,258,161.51	$1,907,584.20	$1,173,526.91	$10,872.18	$1,162,654.73	$415.37	$149.61	36%
February	7,194	12,192.92	$2,876,924.82	$2,039,359.33	$1,079,874.59	$14,860.46	$1,065,014.13	$399.91	$150.11	38%
March	6,139	15,869.20	$4,344,515.46	$2,607,619.01	$1,149,402.22	$13,163.47	$1,136,238.75	$707.69	$187.23	26%
April	5,338	14,845.87	$3,901,152.12	$2,790,128.82	$1,122,439.33	$4,221.56	$1,118,217.77	$704.43	$202.68	29%
May	5,526	14,998.31	$3,868,804.96	$3,061,652.27	$1,174,099.65	$18,492.51	$1,155,607.14	$700.11	$212.47	30%
June	5,941	15,592.34	$4,127,012.62	$2,751,526.98	$1,124,761.08	$4,312.12	$1,120,448.96	$694.67	$189.32	27%
July	5,161	13,463.22	$3,857,289.84	$2,651,585.08	$1,064,956.07	$3,380.03	$1,061,576.04	$747.39	$206.35	28%
August	5,497	13,976.91	$3,943,943.32	$3,271,046.33	$1,268,477.79	$18,510.28	$1,249,967.51	$717.47	$230.76	32%
September	5,260	14,025.38	$3,973,592.92	$2,433,364.13	$1,002,705.76	$14,829.10	$987,876.66	$714.67	$180.34	25%
October	4,937	12,482.47	$3,526,336.21	$2,811,226.07	$1,126,272.74	$13,501.59	$1,112,771.15	$714.26	$228.13	32%
Totals	**59,337**	**141,627.76**	**$37,677,723.78**	**$26,325,092.40**	**$11,286,516.14**	**$116,143.30**	**$11,170,372.84**			
Avg/Month	**5,934**	**14,162.78**	**$3,767,772.38**	**$2,632,509.24**	**$1,128,651.61**	**$11,614.33**	**$1,117,037.28**	**$634.98**	**$190.21**	**30%**
Departments Entered Here										
January	189	498.01	$173,842.00	$66,228.65	$148,186.02	$730.76	$147,455.26	$919.80	$784.05	85%
February	169	469.55	$159,335.00	$69,229.77	$82,406.07	$352.14	$82,053.93	$942.81	$487.61	52%
March	215	644.46	$192,410.00	$78,901.91	$131,318.44	$134.88	$131,183.56	$894.93	$610.78	68%
April	216	674.60	$202,526.65	$73,060.71	$125,071.99	$208.99	$124,863.00	$937.62	$579.04	62%
May	259	779.09	$233,094.80	$76,374.95	$121,997.44	$50.00	$121,947.44	$899.98	$471.03	52%
June	195	584.56	$172,511.35	$87,009.60	$134,584.05	$362.24	$134,221.81	$884.67	$690.17	78%
July	237	709.98	$223,479.91	$73,272.06	$107,171.89	$587.76	$106,584.13	$942.95	$452.20	48%
August	205	610.56	$190,830.00	$93,102.55	$119,956.73	$79.81	$119,876.92	$930.88	$585.15	63%
September	235	706.15	$223,937.78	$83,574.97	$137,763.62	$248.16	$137,515.46	$952.93	$586.23	62%
October	182	534.09	$165,826.00	$69,339.60	$118,791.42	$912.22	$117,879.20	$911.13	$652.70	72%
Totals	**2,102**	**6,211.03**	**$1,937,793.49**	**$750,084.77**	**$1,227,247.67**	**$3,666.96**	**$1,223,580.71**			
Avg/Month	**210**	**621.10**	**$193,779.35**	**$75,008.48**	**$122,724.77**	**$366.70**	**$122,358.07**	**$921.88**	**$583.85**	**63%**
Departments Entered Here										
January	5,098	45.08	$382,347.30	$100,818.71	$191,759.99	$2,698.48	$189,061.51	$75.08	$37.63	50%
February	5,148	38.00	$331,108.27	$115,916.97	$220,320.89	$0.00	$220,320.89	$64.33	$42.80	67%
March	4,205	44.95	$315,862.55	$96,174.22	$212,675.64	$0.00	$212,675.64	$75.12	$50.58	67%
April	5,920	45.38	$341,037.43	$118,325.16	$273,106.03	$1,624.40	$271,371.63	$57.61	$46.15	80%
May	6,881	43.21	$431,909.24	$113,336.35	$248,897.83	$4,234.22	$244,663.61	$62.77	$36.17	58%
June	4,985	45.73	$319,194.41	$118,697.03	$261,865.68	$18.00	$261,847.68	$64.03	$52.49	82%

ONE PAGE DASHBOARD FOCUSING ON RESOURCE UTILIZATION

A different physician group chose to start the dashboard process with a department-level dashboard instead of a senior management dashboard. A sample of the dashboard is included as Exhibit 11.9. The focus is on measures that departments have some control over, and are designed to be rolled up on a senior management dashboard. The top left section on Resource Utilization is discussed in more detail in Chapter 7.

The top middle section on referral sources examines ancillary services offered by the practice and the volume of internal and external referrals to those ancillary services. Some of the ancillary services are almost exclusively referred to by providers inside the practice, but other services have referrals from outside the practice. This chart measures that volume monthly. Earlier dashboards in this chapter included SSRS parameters that filtered by physician, location, or department code. A unique aspect of this dashboard is that it filters by month. The dashboard can be run with up to 13 months of prior data to help middle management identify and act on trends.

Even though most of this dashboard is focused on resource utilization, the top right section of the dashboard is a payer mix based on payments received that month. The primary objective of this data is to identify large shifts in the payer mix over time. Since the space available for the payer mix is relatively small, most payers are grouped in six major categories with the remaining payers are grouped in an "Other" category (10% on the chart) at the far right. The SQL Server code that feeds this dashboard is specially designed to force the other and patient categories to display at the right instead of in descending order like the rest of the chart is sorted.

Exhibit 11.9 Dashboards: By Departmental Levels

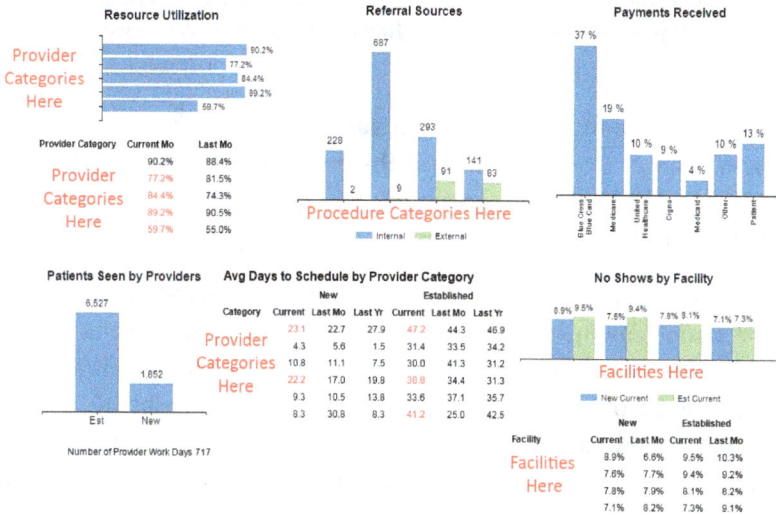

The bottom left section simply displays the number of established and new patients seen during the month. The practice executive who designed this dashboard explained it this way: "The percentage breakdown of new versus established patients for our practice should remain fairly constant over time. Noticeable changes in this data prompt a deeper dive into scheduling and resource templates to ensure the behavior is aligned with the expected service delivery and throughput." There is also a calculation of "Provider Work Days" below the chart. Management set rules to determine how many visits a provider must have for the day to be considered a "Provider Work Day." The number of provider work days gives context to the number of patients seen by providers. If the number of patient visits is down, fewer provider work days due to vacations or holidays may explain the variance. How many provider work days does it take to generate 8,000 total visits? What is the mix of established to new patients? Those are the types of questions answered in this section of the report.

Provider access is a major issue for this practice. The bottom middle section is a table calculating the average days to schedule an appointment for a new patient and an established patient, trended by current month, last month, and last year. For more information about this section of the dashboard, please see Exhibit 6.35 in Chapter 6.

The bottom right section of the dashboard is a chart with no-show information. Managing no shows is so important to this practice that the data is shown twice, once in a chart and once in a table. The practice uses PivotTables to help drill down and understand trends in no-show appointments.

The dashboard is designed to be consolidated into a higher-level dashboard for senior management, which only shows summary-level information. For example, the high-level dashboard may only show the overall no-show percentage instead of the percentages by location. The dashboard is also designed to be expanded further for front-line managers. For example, rather than show overall provider categories of resource utilization, a more-detailed dashboard would show specific providers in a department or location. Aligning dashboards so that senior management, middle management, and front-line managers all focus on the same metrics and objectives is a major initiative for this well-run medical practice.

ONE PAGE DASHBOARD FOCUSING ON VISITS AND CASH COLLECTIONS

Exhibit 11.10 is another custom dashboard designed for a specific practice situation. The management and ownership structure of this practice changed and this dashboard was created as part of the monitoring process after the change. The top left section focuses on patient visits (not necessarily procedure codes) for each revenue center in the practice. This dashboard focuses on weekly information and is delivered weekly.

Originally the dashboard was delivered on Monday morning. After a trial period, as management worked with the dashboard, the decision was made to track billed visits as opposed to counting appointments as visits. Appointments are spectacular for looking into the future, as described in Chapter 6. Appointments can be less reliable for historical data since historical appointments contain no shows and cancellations. Some practices are better than others at recording no shows and appointment cancellations, but there is the chance that historical appointment data contains visits that did not happen and will not be billed. Management decided to use visits but to schedule the weekly dashboard for Wednesday mornings to allow the billing department two days to record all visits in the PM system.

Working down the dashboard, the next section reports the same visit information by location instead of by revenue category. Note the YTD column. Originally the YTD number was the year-to-date count of visits. The management team suggested that the dashboard would be more useful if year-to-date was an average week year-to-date. An average week year-to-date calculation can get complicated, especially early in the year. If a year starts on Wednesday, is the average YTD for the first week the average of the short week (especially since the practice is closed on New Years' Day) or should the average be an average of the first five days in the year? What about holiday weeks? To keep things a little simpler, the dashboard calculates the total number of visits for the year and divides by the total number of weeks in the year so far. That math may make the January year-to-date numbers more volatile, but it is an easy to understand calculation throughout the year.

The next section of the dashboard trends accounts receivable. As discussed earlier in this chapter, accounts receivable can be difficult to trend. This dashboard takes all charges and subtracts all payments and adjustments based on the post date of last week and based on the post date of two weeks ago to generate the values. A year-to-date accounts receivable calculation would require recalculating accounts receivable for every week in the year. Rather than recalculate a year-to-date average every week, calculate accounts receivable weekly and store the data in the data warehouse to make the calculations more efficient and the dashboard run faster.

The bottom left section reports cash collections by revenue center, again based on last week, two weeks ago, a year-to-date average and a prior year-to-date average. This quick statistic helps senior management monitor cash collections with two weeks ago, year-to-date, and prior year-to-date as reference points. Any variances in this section are quickly researched.

A PIVOTTABLE WITH COLLECTIONS DATA BY PROVIDER, LOCATION, REVENUE CATEGORY, PAYER, AND OTHER METRICS SUPPORTS THIS SECTION OF THE DASHBOARD TO MAKE THE ANALYSIS EASIER. THE PIVOTTABLE IS A SEPARATE SPREADSHEET, NOT PART OF THE DASHBOARD. THE DASHBOARD DOESN'T READ DATA FROM THE PIVOTTABLE. BOTH THE DASHBOARD AND THE SPREADSHEET READ DATA FROM AN UNDERLYING DATASET STORED IN THE DATA WAREHOUSE. ONE DATASET FEEDING MULTIPLE REPORTS IS THE SECRET SAUCE OF BUSINESS INTELLIGENCE DESCRIBED IN CHAPTER 2.

EXHIBIT 11.10 DASHBOARDS: VISIT AND COLLECTION FOCUSED SAMPLE

Visits by Category	Last Week	2 Weeks Ago	YTD
	13	88	3,375
Procedure	62	124	6,385
Categories	164	662	29,246
Listed Here	55	254	12,451
	58	249	8,185
Total	352	1,377	59,642

Accounts Receivable	Last Week	2 Weeks Ago
	$1,591,695	$1,486,999

Upcoming Appointments	This Week	Next 30 Days
Appt Categories Here	1,194	3,293
	116	377
Total	1,310	3,670

Visits by Location	Last Week	2 Weeks Ago	YTD
Locations	140	363	16,348
	81	415	17,304
Listed Here	131	599	25,990
Total	352	1,377	59,642

Cash Collections	Last Week	2 Weeks Ago	YTD
Procedure	$62,207	$121,009	$4,599,507
Categories	$92,129	$196,684	$6,296,669
Listed Here	$35,472	$74,318	$2,968,496
	$3,354	$3,563	$261,357
Total	$193,161	$395,575	$14,126,029

Visits by Week

The top right section looks at future visits in the current week and the next 30 days. While historical visits were used on the left side of the dashboard, the right side of the dashboard uses appointment data to report the number of visits scheduled. It can be hard to compare visit data with appointment data since visits are often categorized differently than appointments. Visits may be categorized as new or established patients or by the procedure performed. Appointment categories may focus more on the resources, both staff and time, required to serve the patient. Though categories may differ, comparing past visits in aggregate to future appointments in aggregate does give managers a sense for how busy the practice will be compared to how busy the practice has been.

The bottom right section charts the number of patient visits in the past 11 weeks. This trend helps management get a sense for how the practice is growing over time. Management considers holidays that interrupt the visit schedule, but the overall trend is very important to them.

PARTNER MEETING DASHBOARD

The dashboard in Exhibit 11.11 is designed to be a topic of discussion at a monthly partner meeting. The dashboard shows that all providers are selected. Like other dashboards in this chapter, there is an SSRS parameter linked to a drop-down box that allows the practice administrator to filter the dashboard by provider. The approach of this dashboard is to list the current month first, followed by the prior 11 months.

The first line of the dashboard is the number of work days in the month. There are several ways to calculate the number of work days in a month. One is to instruct the data warehouse on which days the practice is open by essentially maintaining a calendar in the data warehouse. Another approach is to use logic to determine work days. This practice chose logic. Management's logic is to count days with more than five patient encounters as a work day. If there were more than five patient visits with any provider on that day, the clinic is considered open for purposes of calculating the number of work days. The next line is the average number of days each provider worked, using the same five visits per day standard applied at the provider level.

In addition to charges and payments, the dashboard calculates a quarterly net collection rate that matches the percentage of charges collected during the prior three months. Accounts receivable is so important to this practice that this dashboard includes aging buckets as part of the dashboard and some benchmark goals for the practice based on participating in MGMA surveys. This dashboard allows providers and administrators to monitor trends over time, as well as benchmark data within their practice. The practice administrator closely monitors accounts receivable to capture any potential cash flow issues quickly and efficiently.

The practice tracks the overall number of charges and counts charges for particularly important ancillary services. Relevant RVU information is also included.

Exhibit 11.11 Dashboards: By Providers

Providers: All

Indicators	Goal (MGMA)	Last 12 Months Here											
Days In Month		19	22	20	21	23	21	21	22	20	23	21	19
Days Worked		14.0	16.4	16.0	17.1	15.5	15.8	17.3	17.9	14.0	18.1	15.7	13.2
Total Charges		$2,358,856	$2,610,805	$2,443,366	$2,531,319	$2,772,760	$2,572,349	$2,439,755	$2,598,379	$1,844,454	$2,355,956	$2,071,973	$2,033,603
Total Collections		$985,808	$1,077,978	$963,135	$1,029,301	$1,181,911	$1,219,416	$1,135,960	$1,095,659	$1,005,137	$1,002,905	$984,450	$868,466
Net Collection Rate				90.9%				100.1%			107.0%		96.5%
% A/R > 121 Days	<19.5% (with LOP)	18.2%	18.8%	14.7%	11.3%	10.8%	12.7%	14.1%	13.8%	17.2%	16.2%	14.8%	14.4%
AR Aging Analysis		$2,164,338	$2,146,748	$2,303,492	$2,402,086	$2,509,488	$2,211,677	$2,114,231	$2,240,757	$1,878,857	$2,000,639	$1,839,350	$1,848,674
0-30	>49.6%	54.1%	56.3%	60.0%	56.9%	58.4%	52.1%	49.6%	60.3%	49.9%	57.6%	53.3%	55.4%
31-60	<17.14%	13.9%	15.0%	16.3%	19.9%	16.9%	20.2%	19.3%	11.8%	18.1%	11.3%	18.6%	14.5%
61-90	<8.36%	6.6%	5.3%	5.9%	8.9%	8.4%	9.4%	9.9%	8.2%	8.3%	9.7%	6.6%	10.6%
91-120	<5.43%	7.3%	4.6%	3.1%	3.2%	5.5%	5.6%	7.1%	5.9%	6.5%	5.2%	6.7%	5.0%
121-150	<19.49%	5.2%	5.3%	2.0%	2.4%	2.3%	4.3%	4.8%	3.5%	4.5%	4.3%	3.9%	4.7%
151-180		3.9%	4.1%	4.3%	1.3%	1.6%	1.7%	2.6%	3.2%	3.5%	3.2%	3.6%	3.6%
>181	excluding LOP	1.4%	1.4%	1.2%	1.1%	1.1%	1.2%	1.2%	1.1%	1.2%	1.0%	1.1%	1.1%
Days in A/R	38.56	27.6	27.3	29.2	30.5	32.0	28.1	26.3	28.1	23.8	25.2	23.5	23.7
Total Charge Count		11,326	13,935	12,750	13,115	16,699	15,975	13,819	14,621	10,631	14,615	12,806	11,417
		228	280	256	277	314	267	219	264	191	193	167	204
Procedures Here		1,360	1,498	1,670	1,838	1,874	1,953	1,557	1,639	1,182	1,722	1,485	1,297
		127	151	165	110	143	122	118	119	80	110	80	72
RVU		12,043	14,258	13,117	13,301	15,540	14,019	13,063	14,217	10,108	12,686	11,479	11,015

Aging percentages and accounts receivable data make this dashboard very calculation-intensive. This practice stores the monthly data over time in the data warehouse so SSRS only needs to calculate the current month each month. With all the historical data stored in the data warehouse, the dashboard runs very quickly.

PAYER CONTRACTING

Another version of this dashboard is included in Chapter 4 as Exhibit 4.10 on payer contracting. The dashboard is included in this chapter as an example of what one practice is doing to make sure claims are paid according to the negotiated contract terms. The dashboard is emailed daily to both staff and management to confirm that exceptions are resolved in a timely manner and payers pay appropriately.

EXHIBIT 11.12 PAYING CLAIMS NEGOTIATED IN CONTRACT TERMS TRACKING SAMPLE

From: Reports@yourpractice.com
Sent: Wednesday 6:45 AM

CPM Dashboard as of 4/12/2017

Yesterday's Exceptions

Insurance Group	$ Variance	Count
Medicare DMERC	$3013.27	8
Payer ABC	$232.25	2
Cigna	$2807.00	1
Work Comp	$67.19	1
Anthem	$60.79	1
Medicare Advantage	$40.83	1
Total	$6221.33	14

Top 10 Open Exceptions by Variance($)

CPT Code	Insurance Group	$ Variance	Count
29823	Medicare	$253.83	2
29824	Preferred PPO	$224.50	1
15275	Anthem	$209.94	2
29823	Preferred PPO	$208.25	1
95909	Cigna	$207.00	1
27676	Preferred PPO	$203.50	1
27650	Aetna	$177.90	1
64493	Medicare	$169.51	3
27659	Preferred PPO	$163.25	1
28270	Preferred PPO	$162.70	1
	Total	$1,980.38	14

Open Exceptions

Insurance Group	$ Variance	Count
Preferred PPO	$1,293.44	10
Medicare	$669.94	13
Medicare Advantage	$630.87	110
United Healthcare	$536.82	21
Work Comp	$517.64	6
BCBS	$335.38	3
Cigna	$331.38	4

Top 10 Open Exceptions by Count

CPT Code	Insurance Group	$ Variance	Count
27447	Blue Cross	$3535.90	14
27447	Medicaid	$3001.59	9
27130	Cigna	$2000.08	8
20610	Medicare	$500.45	8
72100	Medicare Advantage	$750.14	7

TRACKING LINES OF BUSINESS

This practice wanted a spreadsheet-based dashboard tool to supplement an SSRS dashboard. The spreadsheet includes more detail than the SSRS dashboard and is designed with a tab for each provider and each location. Each tab is designed to print on one page so that the practice can combine summary pages and detail for each location into one PDF to email monthly. Because the dashboard is a spreadsheet instead of an SSRS report, management can interact with the Excel formulas and copy/paste data to another spreadsheet for additional analysis.

The focus of this dashboard is based on lines of business. Management carefully divided the procedures offered by the providers into categories and then subcategories so those lines of business can be compared to other providers, locations, and even other practices over time. The dashboard in Exhibit 11.13 compares visits and revenues by lines of business over a two-year period.

EXHIBIT 11.13 DASHBOARDS: BUSINESS LINE TRACKING SAMPLE: PART 1

		YTD 2016	YTD 2017	VARIANCE	%
	NEW	11,462	11,608	146	1.3%
	ESTABLISHED	27,495	27,230	(265)	-1.0%
Visits	PROCEDURES A	5,800	7,434	1,634	28.2%
	PROCEDURES B	6,167	5,936	(231)	-3.7%
	PROCEDURES C	2,915	3,148	233	8.0%
	TOTALS	53,839	55,356	1,517	2.8%

		YTD 2016	YTD 2017	VARIANCE	%
	NEW PATIENT VISITS	$ 1,598,183	$ 1,547,447	(50,736)	-3.2%
E&M	EST PATIENT VISITS	$ 2,644,044	$ 2,714,749	70,705	2.7%
	TOTALS	$ 4,242,227	$ 4,262,197	19,969	0.5%
	SUBCATEGORY 1	$ 138,467	$ 261,963	123,496	89.2%
	SUBCATEGORY 2	$ 1,242,163	$ 1,450,085	207,922	16.7%
	SUBCATEGORY 3	$ 259,740	$ 237,568	(22,171)	-8.5%
	SUBCATEGORY 4	$ 367,960	$ 350,893	(17,067)	-4.6%
PROCEDURES A	SUBCATEGORY 5	$ 673,397	$ 690,004	16,607	2.5%
	SUBCATEGORY 6	$ 443,781	$ 506,088	62,308	14.0%
	SUBCATEGORY 7	$ 967,825	$ 1,147,120	179,295	18.5%
	SUBCATEGORY 8	$ 1,029,067	$ 1,089,284	60,217	5.9%
	TOTALS	$ 5,122,399	$ 5,733,006	610,607	11.9%
	SUBCATEGORY 1	$ 1,183,131	$ 1,206,921	23,791	2.0%
	SUBCATEGORY 2	$ 654,659	$ 676,413	21,754	3.3%
	SUBCATEGORY 3	$ 593,655	$ 432,441	(161,214)	-27.2%
PROCEDURES B	SUBCATEGORY 4	$ 112,746	$ 97,268	(15,478)	-13.7%
	SUBCATEGORY 5	$ 75,250	$ 66,431	(8,819)	-11.7%
	SUBCATEGORY 6	$ 244,634	$ 245,910	1,275	0.5%
	TOTALS	$ 2,864,074	$ 2,725,383	(138,692)	-4.8%
	SUBCATEGORY 1	$ 10,636	$ 14,373	3,736	35.1%
	SUBCATEGORY 2	$ 32,592	$ 37,251	4,658	14.3%
	SUBCATEGORY 3	$ 121,057	$ 105,983	(15,074)	-12.5%
PROCEDURES C	SUBCATEGORY 4	$ 11,001	$ 8,790	(2,212)	-20.1%
	SUBCATEGORY 5	$ 1,677	$ 15,075	13,398	799.1%
	SUBCATEGORY 6	$ 58,478	$ 65,650	7,173	12.3%
	TOTALS	$ 235,441	$ 247,120	11,680	5.0%
	GRAND TOTAL	$ 12,464,141	$ 12,967,706	503,565	4.0%

Page two of the dashboard is shown in Exhibit11.14. The same lines of business in the same order (visits, then revenues) are shown to make it easy for management to quickly scan the dashboard. The dashboard also uses color to make the lines of business easier to identify. Exhibit 11.14 displays charges and collections as opposed to just showing collections like the first page of the dashboard showed. The additional detail helps management understand whether variances in collections are based on changes in productivity or changes in the amount of charges that are collected.

EXHIBIT 11.14 DASHBOARDS: BUSINESS LINE TRACKING SAMPLE: PART 2

		YTD 2016		YTD 2017	
		CHARGES	COLLECTIONS	CHARGES	COLLECTIONS
E&M	NEW PATIENT VISITS	$ 1,208,433	$ 1,185,398	$ 1,450,878	$ 1,211,122
	EST PATIENT VISITS	$ 2,233,826	$ 2,104,983	$ 3,311,961	$ 2,197,941
	TOTALS	$ 3,442,259	$ 3,290,381	$ 4,762,839	$ 3,409,063
Procedures A	SUBCATEGORY 1	$ 396,204	$ 202,689	$ 502,777	$ 219,285
	SUBCATEGORY 2	$ 2,445,155	$ 1,133,767	$ 2,831,987	$ 1,095,689
	SUBCATEGORY 3	$ 207,459	$ 164,786	$ 232,784	$ 148,953
	SUBCATEGORY 4	$ 627,173	$ 243,388	$ 829,832	$ 364,308
	SUBCATEGORY 5	$ 1,188,716	$ 523,122	$ 1,272,409	$ 559,414
	SUBCATEGORY 6	$ 828,652	$ 487,604	$ 1,309,550	$ 635,633
	SUBCATEGORY 7	$ 2,437,890	$ 846,827	$ 2,664,975	$ 906,188
	SUBCATEGORY 8	$ 2,856,393	$ 842,654	$ 2,814,129	$ 818,845
	TOTALS	$ 10,987,642	$ 4,444,835	$ 12,458,443	$ 4,748,315
Procedures B	SUBCATEGORY 1	$ 919,520	$ 978,840	$ 1,002,097	$ 1,105,266
	SUBCATEGORY 2	$ 511,185	$ 397,213	$ 382,526	$ 275,253
	SUBCATEGORY 3	$ 443,391	$ 443,391	$ 375,462	$ 375,462
	SUBCATEGORY 4	$ 77,235	$ 77,235	$ 78,074	$ 78,074
	SUBCATEGORY 5	$ 53,770	$ 53,770	$ 60,744	$ 60,744
	SUBCATEGORY 6	$ 280,224	$ 265,401	$ 445,905	$ 431,767
	TOTALS	$ 2,285,325	$ 2,215,850	$ 2,344,809	$ 2,326,567
Procedures C	SUBCATEGORY 1	$ 11,140	$ 11,140	$ 8,855	$ 8,855
	SUBCATEGORY 2	$ 31,712	$ 31,712	$ 31,437	$ 31,437
	SUBCATEGORY 3	$ 86,375	$ 86,375	$ 42,557	$ 42,557
	SUBCATEGORY 4	$ 6,991	$ 6,991	$ 6,732	$ 6,732
	SUBCATEGORY 5	$ 11,796	$ 11,796	$ 9,970	$ 9,970
	SUBCATEGORY 6	$ 54,178	$ 54,178	$ 35,911	$ 35,911
	TOTALS	$ 202,192	$ 202,192	$ 135,463	$ 135,463
	GRAND TOTAL	$ 16,917,418	$ 10,153,258	$ 19,701,553	$ 10,619,408

The third page of the dashboard compares payer mix based on charges and payments. An example is shown in Exhibit 11.15.

EXHIBIT 11.15 DASHBOARDS: BUSINESS LINE TRACKING SAMPLE: PART 3

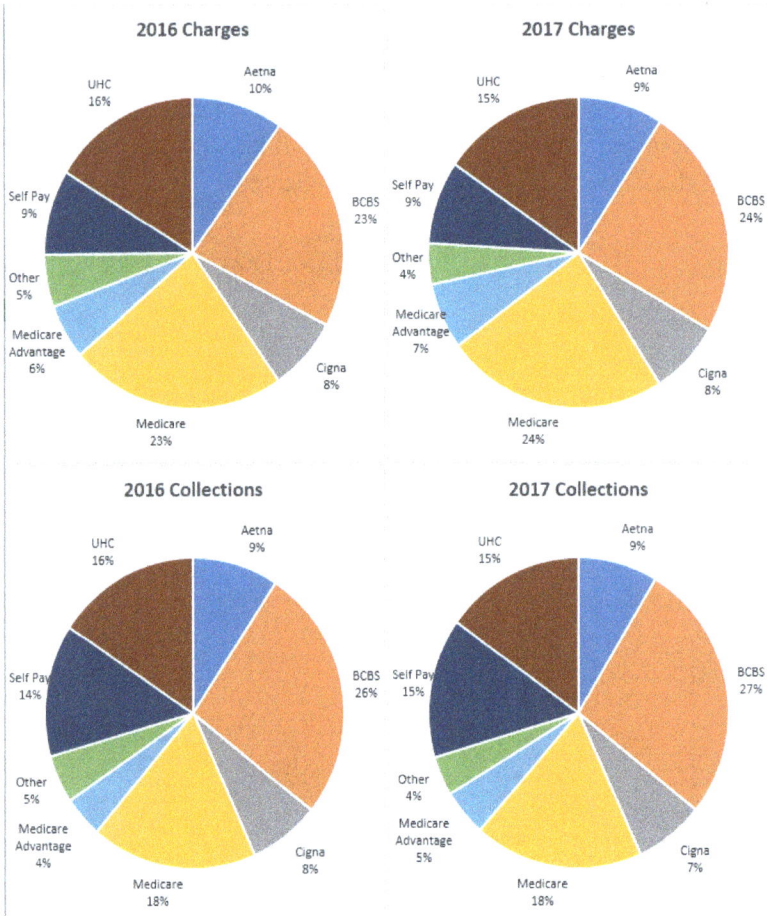

There is a balance to grouping the payers into enough categories to see differences without having so many little categories that it is hard to analyze the practice. This practice grouped the payers into eight categories. An easy way to start grouping is to group similar products from the same payer. Some big national payers have multiple plan types and claims addresses so practices have multiple insurance carriers set up in the PM system even though the payer is the same. You might also group similar contracts, even though the payers are different. Medicare Advantage plans or workers' compensation may fall in this category. Another grouping could include local payers.

The "Other" category in this example is a catch-all category that includes all payers that cannot be easily categorized elsewhere. Sometimes practices may choose to exclude the other category from an analysis like this. An advantage of excluding small payers is that the payer mix only represents payers you are likely to spend time to manage. A disadvantage of excluding small payers is that the sum of the parts will not add up to the whole. For example, assume small payers constitute 15% of the payer mix and Payer A is 34% of the payer mix. Removing small payers from the denominator would decrease the denominator from 100% to 85%, making Payer A 34/85 = 40% of the adjusted payer mix. Payer A is 34% of the overall payer mix and 40% of the payer mix the practice is focusing on. If everyone involved understands that distinction, removing small payers may be helpful when analyzing payer mix.

ACCOUNTS RECEIVABLE AND PAYMENTS POSTED

The practice that designed the next three exhibits had been frustrated with issues in the billing office and was behind in collecting accounts receivable. In the words of the practice administrator, "The request for these dashboards stemmed from wanting to get a feel for how each representative was working their accounts receivable and how many claims were in the older buckets. The accounts receivable is assigned at the beginning and the rep is given certain areas to concentrate on first. This dashboard allows for trending as well as measuring staff production. The aging grid allows us to see if we are having success with the old accounts as well as keep track of the aging buckets. The grid by site allows me to see how well each location is collecting demographics as well as over the counter collections (surgery deposits, co-insurance and copayments). If the demographics are entered correctly it improves the pass-through rate so the claim gets paid right the first time. The goal is to increase collections within 60 days and decrease the balances in older aging buckets."

The dashboard captures each day of the month in rows and the major insurance carriers in columns. The administrative team can quickly track trends in payment posting to ensure that payments are being posted promptly. The dashboard makes it easy to see if the practice is behind on posting specific payers' payments. Columns to the far right are the daily deposit total, the cumulative total for the month, a comparison to last year's month-to-date total, and a variance column. The comparisons to last year are especially helpful to track improvement over where the practice was when the problems were acute.

EXHIBIT 11.16 DASHBOARDS: MONTHLY PAYMENTS BY INSURANCE GROUPS

EXHIBIT 11.16 ALSO DISPLAYS AN ACCOUNTS RECEIVABLE AGING SUMMARY THAT PRINTS ON THE SAME PAGE AS THIS DASHBOARD. SOME DASHBOARDS ARE DESIGNED TO FIT ON A PRINTED PAGE, BUT THEY DON'T HAVE TO BE. USERS WHO COMMONLY SEE THE DASHBOARD ON A COMPUTER MONITOR MAY CHOOSE TO SCROLL AND ULTIMATELY HAVE MORE INFORMATION DISPLAYED THAN WOULD FIT ON A PRINTED PAGE. USERS WHO COMMONLY READ THE DASHBOARD ON A MOBILE DEVICE OR WHO USE A PRINTED VERSION OF THE DASHBOARD MAY PREFER A MORE COMPACT DASHBOARD.

EXHIBIT 11.17 DASHBOARDS: MONTHLY PAYMENTS BY INSURANCE GROUPS APPLIED TO OLD ACCOUNTS RECEIVABLES

AR Payments posted as of

Charge Plan Type	Current	31-60 Days	61-90 Days	91-120 Days	121-150 Days	151-180 Days	Over 180 Days	UnApplied	Total
	$90,098	$50,467	($108)	($287)	$1,162	($902)	($1,093)		$139,338
	$18,826	$5	$15		$145		$2,400		$21,391
	$28,106	$16,430	$592	$117		$0	$496		$45,742
	$372,679	$73,389	$8,960	$4,324	$3,011	$949	$6,214		$469,527
	$6,800								$6,800
	$131	$140			$284		$38		$593
	$293,594	$32,990	$4,837	$980	$860	$274	$3,121		$336,656
	$8,540	$29,558	$7,317	$1,505	$765	$272	$912		$48,869
	$147,652	$213,656	$46,361	$33,557	$10,307	$12,238	$41,509		$505,281
Insurance	$228	$3,255	$4,879	$6,507	$2,315	$2,591	$3,353		$23,128
	$40,240	$30,989	$1,917	$0	$0	$1,381	($1,390)		$73,137
Groups					$0				$0
Displayed	$10,269	$3,555	$1,380	$495	$110	$178	$91		$16,078
	$915	$130					$260		$1,305
Here	$3,170								$3,170
	$1,983	$3,078	$276	$0	$1,684	$0	$114		$7,135
	$338,223	$85,629	$12,555	$3,476	$1,088	$3,356	$3,116		$447,442
	$231	$4,155	$207	$46	$224	$14	$14		$4,891
								$9,443	$9,443
	$320,538	$41,438	$64,279	$26,540	$14,224	$10,832	$36,654	$69,001	$583,505
	$25,324	$14,749	$3,774	$312	$230	$93	$1,577		$46,058
	$800		$942	$177	$20	$20	$1,821		$3,779
	$84,844	$19,427	$2,668	$355	$1,067	$1,442	$451		$110,255
	$292,459	$74,056	$36,273	$9,040	$1,774	$1,467	$5,775		$420,844
Total	$2,078,721	$703,887	$197,263	$87,142	$39,271	$34,205	$105,432	$78,444	$3,324,365

As the practice gets caught up on old accounts receivable, the dashboards can change to focus on other metrics. Exhibit 11.18 is an example. This practice expanded their dashboard to include a page tracking payment posting by service location.

EXHIBIT 11.18 DASHBOARDS: PAYMENT TRACKING BY SERVICE LOCATION

AR Payments posted by Location for Charges in the Past 60 Days as of

Location	Total
	$121,183
	$144,394
	$138,806
	$49,817
	$34,911
	$10,499
	$12,247
	$41,549
	$60,135
	$43,168
Each Location Where Services	$86,336
	$180,380
are Rendered is Listed Here	$150,891
	$186
	$52,636
	$389,499
	$90,330
	$7,036
	$38,291
	$126,867
	$205,864
	$230,887
	$566,697
Total	$2,782,609

Like examples throughout this book, these accounts receivable exhibits are customized to the specific needs of this practice. Your practice will likely focus on different metrics, time periods, and approaches to measuring accounts receivable. These dashboards are each emailed daily. You may want your dashboard delivered weekly or monthly, or there may be a daily dashboard that goes to the billing department followed by a weekly or monthly summary to management. Once you have the data and some metrics you want to measure, it's not hard to build dashboards to get the information you need when you need to see it.

Canned accounts receivable reports from PM systems can easily be hundreds or thousands of printed pages. Of course, a printout is outdated almost before the ink dries. It doesn't take long for billing offices who need and use this information to appreciate how Business Intelligence can make their department more efficient. These summary-level dashboards provide a much better presentation of how a practice is doing. When these dashboards are combined with actionable tools for the staff to work accounts receivable, practices will have much better results that improve the bottom line.

DASHBOARD SUMMARY

This chapter includes a wide variety of dashboards, but none of these examples are a simple cut-and-paste solution to your practice, for several reasons. First, a number of these dashboards will change in the future as practices focus on different strengths, weaknesses, opportunities, and threats. The "set-it-and-forget-it" approach works well in many areas, but not Business Intelligence. The practice environment is far too fluid to succeed by measuring the same things we have always measured. Both external and internal industry changes will mean that every practice must constantly update their Business Intelligence tools to stay competitive and at the top of their game.

Second, your unique practice environment is different than the practices that have shared their examples in this book. These practices' ownership structure, physician compensation, and competitive environment are different than any other practice. No two practices have the same payer contracts, staffing model, overhead structure, and management style. The practices that shared the dashboard in this chapter vary in specialty, location, size, and business environment. One of these practices competes aggressively with another similarly sized practice in the same community. Those two practices are the only choices for that specialty. Another practice competes with a major integrated health system. Several practices compete with large teaching universities. One practice is trying to grow dramatically and manage that growth. Another practice is trying to digest a period of growth. It may take a numbers-focused CPA to benefit from some of these dashboards. Your practice may need a transformation in leadership style or different staffing to leverage this information. The dashboard you need might require more resource allocation in the billing office or a change in practice workflow to be successful.

Third, the business factors that these practices can manage and influence are different than your practice. A dashboard reporting things you cannot control may as well be a dashboard reporting the weather. These practices report and focus on areas they want to manage. Design metrics that measure your practice's progress toward these goals.

Ideally, as you finish reading this chapter you already have several dashboard ideas for your practice. It all started with this question. "If you could have one page of information automatically emailed to you every day, what would be on that page?" Now you can better visualize what that email looks like and how that email would immediately change priorities and results in your practice. The examples in this chapter and throughout the book capture a practice's numbers at a point in time, but they also capture a practice's priorities at a point in time. What is critical now may be automatic a year from now, or it may not be important at all. Dashboards evolve over time in response to changes in the business environment.

Most of these dashboards have gone through several iterations to get to the point they are today, but the initial versions were still very useful. Start with something. Test the data on the dashboard for accuracy and relevance. If the information on the dashboard isn't actionable, or if it's disregarded for weeks at a time, it is time for a change. Even if the dashboard tells you everything is normal and operations are within expected parameters, it has told you something valuable. You now know you can start putting out the day's fires and managing the rest of the practice. What is on your one-page email?

CHAPTER 12

BUSINESS INTELLIGENCE IN YOUR PRACTICE

B y now you have plenty of ideas on how other practices are currently using Business Intelligence to change the way they manage their business of medicine. It can be overwhelming to see so many examples that would make an incredible difference in your practice. It isn't surprising to suddenly have several ideas and want several similar tools immediately. As you begin, here are some thoughts on how to get started.

Start small. As hard as it is, choose one area to focus on. Focus on receivables, productivity, patient collections, or any other pain point in your practice. Pulling the data from your PM or EMR system to answer that first question may well give you data for several more questions. For example, if the issue is productivity, you might pull billed charges data from the PM system. Pull charges and work RVUs by provider, location, patient, procedure code, diagnosis code, referring physician, date of service, posted date, primary insurance, secondary insurance, modifiers, and more. Pull all the data around your first issue and use that dataset for future projects.

Let the boss win. Sometimes the best way to secure approval and funding for a Business Intelligence project is to focus on what is most important to the physicians, owners, or administrators in your group. Even if you are certain that reducing no-show appointments, collecting more at the front desk, or improving patient scheduling would bring more value to your practice, start with what motivates the boss. How are they compensated? Where are their frustrations? What data have they always asked for but never received? Start there. Prove the value of Business Intelligence for a project that matters to the boss. Let them see return on investment and they will be much more willing to continue to invest.

Don't bite off more than you can chew. You and your team can only consume so much information. New reports will require downstream work and workflow changes. Rather than creating dozens of emails or spreadsheets that staff don't have time to read, let alone act on, start with one email or spreadsheet that has a clear path to action. Once that email has demonstrated its effectiveness, the workflows have changed, and the habits are in place, take a moment to celebrate your success and then start a second project. A physician group in the Northeast wanted quality data. They came up with hundreds of fields to track. The problem was that as most of the data did not exist in the EHR, the physicians had to report all the new data points. Even with scribes, the task was so daunting the project stalled until they simplified the list of data to a manageable amount.

Manage expectations. Most Business Intelligence expectations tend to err on the side of too much time and too much cost. Business Intelligence projects should produce actionable data within a few weeks, not months or years. Starting small often means that the cost is reasonable; it shouldn't take a lot of time or money to get started. If this isn't the case, your project is likely too large. Can you make a smaller, trial-size version of your project to test whether it will deliver what you need? If successful, add to your trial-sized success. Use tools like Excel and SSRS that you already own. It is much easier to talk the practice's decision-makers into a Business Intelligence project if you can leverage what the practice already owns. The right Business Intelligence project should pay for itself several times over, and quickly.

As discussed throughout this book, a Business Intelligence project is never the last tool your practice will need. Every Business Intelligence project eventually needs to be freshened up to meet new needs. Payers will constantly be changing reimbursement models. Compliance will change. Your competition will change. Business Intelligence is a magnificent tool to manage those changes.

Track your successes. Practices have been very successful showing a before and after view of their Business Intelligence projects. Just seeing the before and after view of their Business Intelligence projects is all the proof they need to see how far they have come. Celebrate these side-by-side comparisons to build staff morale. Share the successes and savings with management to reinforce the return on investment that will get the next Business Intelligence project approved.

Exhibit 12.1 shows the number of open pre-authorization cases for a busy practice. The vertical axis shows the number of cases needing pre-authorization. The horizontal axis shows the number of days until the patient appointment. Gold cases have not been started. Blue cases in are progress, meaning the pre-authorization has been requested but the payer has not responded. There are 36 cases two days out where the pre-authorization has not been started. The pre-authorization department was often full of drama and crises.

EXHIBIT 12.1 OPEN PRE-AUTHORIZATIONS CHART: BEFORE

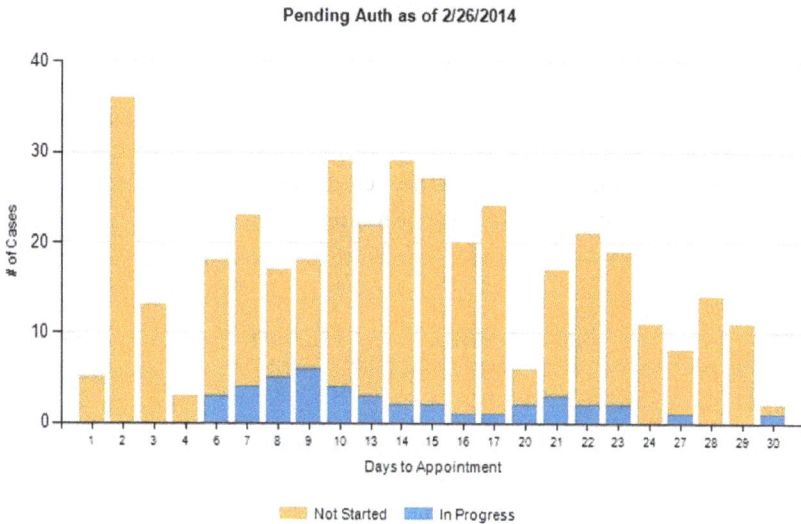

Exhibit 12.2 is the same chart, 30 days later. The practice built a tool to help the pre-authorization department better see and manage the workload. Some of the cases do take longer to pre-authorize. The tool balances time-consuming pre-authorizations with time-sensitive pre-authorizations. Exhibit 12.2 is a daily email for the department to track improvement. The progress the department made in 30 days with hard work and the right tools is remarkable.

EXHIBIT 12.2 OPEN PRE-AUTHORIZATIONS CHART: AFTER

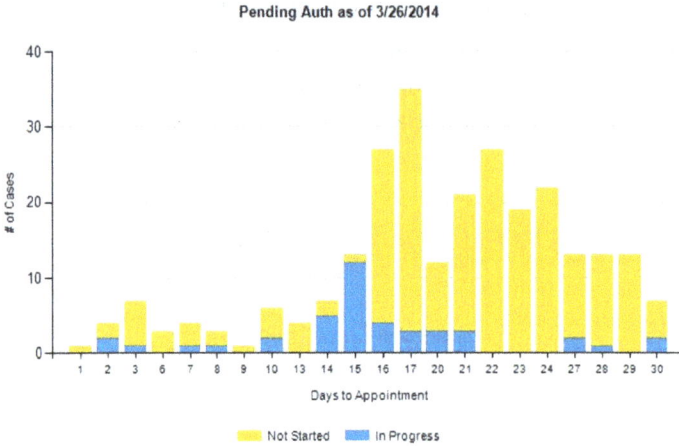

Pending Auth as of 3/26/2014

The pre-authorization department has continued to refine and improve their processes. Exhibit 12.3 is a version almost three years after the chart was created.

EXHIBIT 12.3 OPEN PRE-AUTHORIZATIONS CHART: 3 YEARS LATER

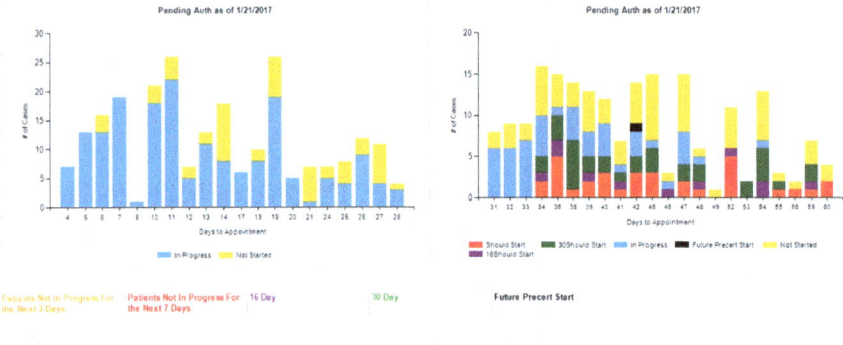

Pending Auth as of 1/21/2017

The chart on the left is the next 30 days, similar to the charts we just reviewed. Notice all the blue, in-progress cases. The chart starts at Day 4 since earlier cases are authorized and ready to go. The chart on the right tracks pre-authorizations for cases 31 to 60 days in the future. That chart has several more colors tracking cases that have been scheduled but the pre-authorization process has not started yet, even though the case is at least a month away. The section at the bottom of the dashboard lists all the patients who fall into each colored category above. The section also lists the patient number and appointment time to make it easy for the pre-authorization team to work the report.

Charts like this make it easy to show physicians and management value and return on their Business Intelligence investment. The charts also make it easy to show the pre-authorization team how much better they are doing. Examples throughout this book have made similar differences for their practices. What will make a difference in your practice?

If you are doing way too much manual analysis, dumping data to Excel, cleaning the data, and then recreating the same analysis from last month, find a way to automate that process. Think again about what could be on a one-page email to you, your staff, your administrators, and your physicians. What information is most actionable and most influential for each group? How often will the emails be delivered, and who needs to be copied on the email to make sure the information is acted on?

I close almost all my Excel videos by thanking people for watching. I will close this book the same way. Thanks for purchasing and reading this book. I hope you have discovered the direction and the motivation you need to move forward with Business Intelligence in your practice. Medical practice management has never been more complex, more time-consuming, or more intellectually challenging than it is right now. The good news is that there are tools available to manage that complexity and thrive in the business of delivering medicine. You likely own most of those tools. Please use this book to put new tools to use and improve profits and patient care in your practice.

Appendix 1

SQL Server Reporting Services

These appendices are technical discussions about how to use tools beyond spreadsheets to see your data. If you have an IT department or an outside consultant who will create these reports, feel free to turn these sections over to them. Even if someone else implements the report development, it may still be helpful to review these appendices for a sense of what is possible.

Practices that store their own data in SQL Server also own SSRS, a product that comes with almost every version of SQL Server. SSRS is a fantastic way to create dashboards and to email those dashboards throughout your organization. Physicians, administrators, and staff need to remember to run reports or open spreadsheets. The beauty of SSRS is that you can push critical information via email to staff instead of relying on them to pull that information. Now they can access your reports on any device they use to receive email.

The ability to push data without buying any additional software is very powerful, but SSRS is more complicated than a traditional spreadsheet. This appendix is designed as an introduction to SSRS, starting from a blank canvas and building an interactive report that analyzes CMS data on providers' charges by procedure code by state. The demonstration will not include every SSRS feature or be a step-by-step SSRS instruction manual. There are entire books on SSRS and the end of this chapter will recommend an author of helpful SSRS books.

You will probably need some IT help to get started, but there's plenty than an average practice manager can do, especially if that practice manager is Excel-savvy. The more you can do, the faster you can get reports in a format you like and the faster you will have emails you can send. The more you understand about SSRS, the better you can communicate your needs with your IT department. And the more you learn about what can be done, the closer you'll be to getting started. By being graphics heavy and technical detail light, this section means to motivate more medical practice managers and the IT teams that support those practices to become more familiar with SSRS.

GETTING STARTED

To get started, you need a dataset. Chapter 2 calls datasets the secret sauce for Business Intelligence in medical practices, and that is as true in SSRS as anywhere. Report Builder will let you join multiple tables to create your own dataset, datasets that you can even share with other SSRS reports. But building that dataset is generally beyond the scope of a practice manager's experience. Building a dataset requires a thorough understanding of the structure of the underlying PM or EHR data and SQL skills that are usually best outsourced to IT. The dataset in our example is publicly available CMS data that shows all billed charges to Medicare by procedure code, provider specialty, and state. At the time of this writing (early 2017), the latest CMS data available is for the year 2014.

You need a tool to build SSRS reports, and SSRS is unique in that it provides two separate tools that can build the same report. This section will cover Report Builder. Report Builder is a free download, though you need SSRS to make Report Builder work. IT will need to install and configure SSRS and help you connect Report Builder to SSRS, but once you have a dataset and the configuration, you can get started.

For reference, you can also use a version of Microsoft's Visual Studio® to build SSRS reports. Depending on the version of SQL Server, the Visual Studio version might be called Business Intelligence Development Studio (BIDS) or SQL Server Data Tools (SSDT). The Visual Studio version of SSDT for SQL Server 2012 is shown in Exhibit 13.1.

Exhibit 13.1 Report Builder

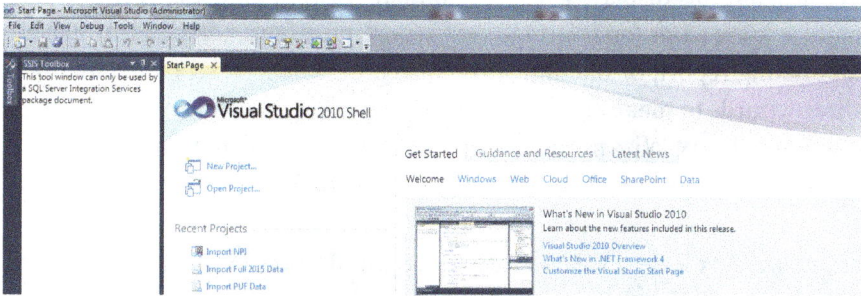

While Visual Studio is an option, Report Builder is a friendlier environment for developing reports. Report Builder is designed to look and feel like a Microsoft Office® application to make it less intimidating and more approachable than Visual Studio, but don't get your hopes up. Report Builder isn't quite as easy to use as Excel or Microsoft Word®, but there is a wizard that can help you get started.

SSRS WIZARD

Once IT has SSRS configured, Report Builder installed, and a dataset for you to work with, you are ready to launch Report Builder. The screen captures in this appendix are from the SQL Server 2012 version of Report Builder. The first screen looks like Exhibit 13.2.

Exhibit 13.2 Report Builder: First Screen

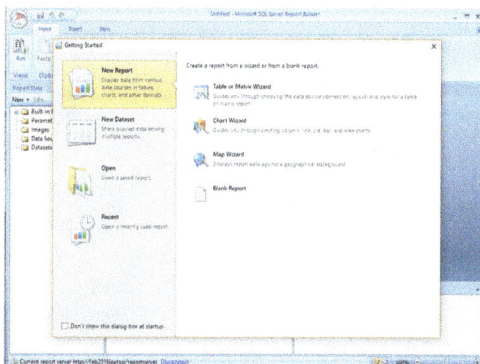

You can hide this startup window as you get more familiar with the Report Wizard, but this displays a helpful summary of your choices. Down the left-hand side are icons for creating a new report, creating a new dataset, opening an existing report, or opening a recent report. The new report menu offers three wizards to make creating your first SSRS report easier. We will use the Table or Matrix Wizard to create a new report. Choosing Table or Matrix Wizard brings us the screen shown in Exhibit 13.3.

EXHIBIT 13.3 REPORT BUILDER: TABLE OR MATRIX WIZARD

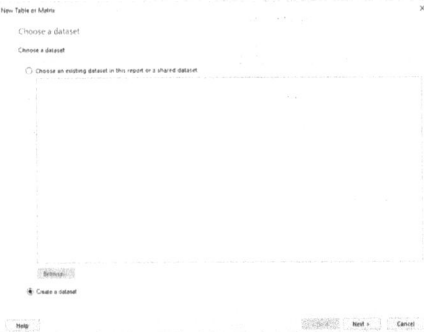

Datasets are the foundation of every SSRS report, so the first screen wants to know what data you will use to build your report. The Report Wizard will list existing datasets. We will build a new dataset. Clicking Next brings up the screen in Exhibit 13.4.

EXHIBIT 13.4 REPORT BUILDER: REPORT WIZARD

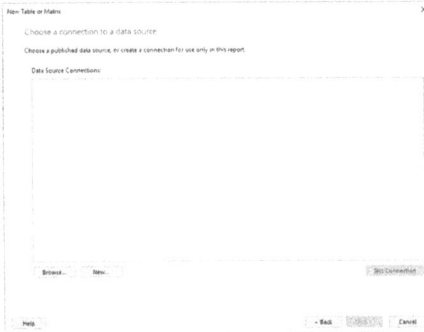

A Data Source is the location where the dataset is stored. The CMS data contains over nine million rows and is stored in SQL Server. We need to connect to SQL Server to use the dataset stored there. Exhibit 13.5 shows the screen to connect to the Data Source.

EXHIBIT 13.5 REPORT BUILDER: CONNECTING TO THE DATA SOURCE

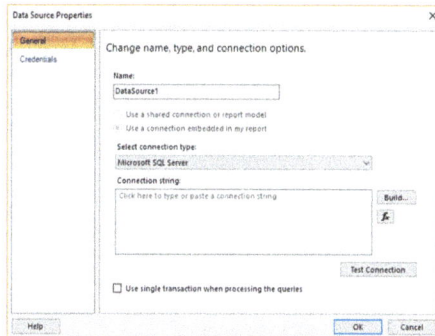

There are two ways to connect to SQL Server to access data stored there. Windows Authentication allows you to connect with the same login you use to access Windows. SQL Server Authentication is a login specific to SQL Server. For SSRS to run a report based on SQL Server data, Report Builder needs to tell SQL Server how to connect to the data. The screen in Exhibit 13.6 has the details SSRS needs.

EXHIBIT 13.6 REPORT BUILDER: CONNECTING TO SQL SERVER: PART 1

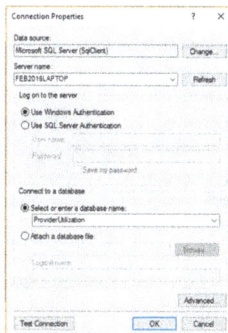

We will connect to a SQL Server installation called FEB2016LAPTOP using Windows Authentication. On that server is a database called ProviderUtilization that has been downloaded from the CMS website. You can test the connection from this screen to ensure that SSRS will be able to access the provider utilization data as shown in Exhibit 13.7.

EXHIBIT 13.7 REPORT BUILDER: CONNECTING TO SQL SERVER: PART 2

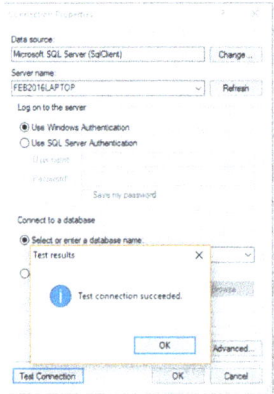

Now that we can connect to the data, the next step takes us back to the Data Source Properties window. The completed Data Source Properties is shown in Exhibit 13.8.

EXHIBIT 13.8 REPORT BUILDER: DATA SOURCE PROPERTIES

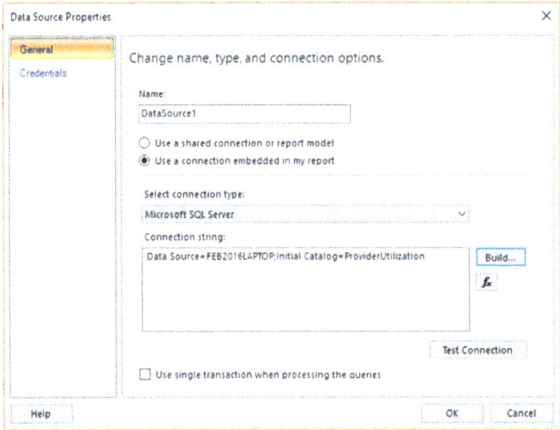

Exhibit 13.9 shows the Credentials tab (the menus are on the left of the window) from the Data Source Properties window. Microsoft requires credentials to connect to data stored in SQL Server. When you build an SSRS report you need to ensure that any user who needs to run the report has the credentials to connect to SQL Server to refresh the data. The internal SSRS dashboard is called Report Server. The question on the credentials screen is how you want other users to connect to SQL Server when they use the report. Your IT department can take the lead in answering this question. Consider creating a SQL Server Authentication login with just enough rights to run SSRS reports and use that login to connect to SQL Server to refresh the data. If you do not save a password and instead prompt users for login credentials every time they access the SSRS dashboard, users may get frustrated.

EXHIBIT 13.9 REPORT BUILDER: DATA SOURCE PROPERTIES: CREDENTIALS

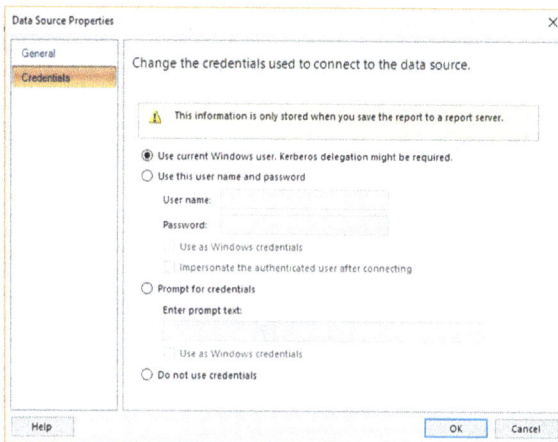

Once you have a connection to SQL Server, you can refresh your report with data stored on SQL Server. The next screen of the wizard (shown in Exhibit 13.10) allows us to select the Data Source we just created as the source for this report.

EXHIBIT 13.10 DATA SOURCE CONNECTIONS

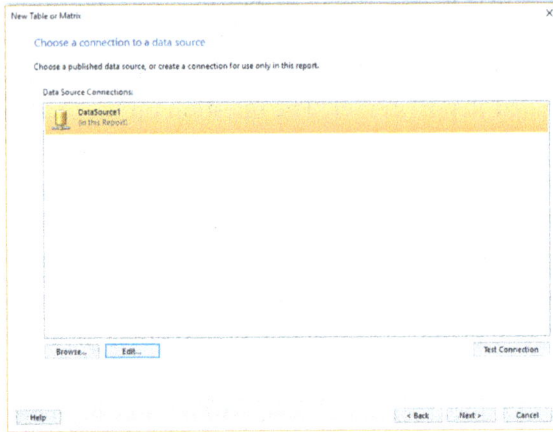

In our example, all our data is on the same SQL Server, so one connection is plenty. Now that we have access to data, the next step is to query that data. The wizard in Exhibit 13.11 will help us do that.

EXHIBIT 13.11 REPORT BUILDER: DATA QUERY

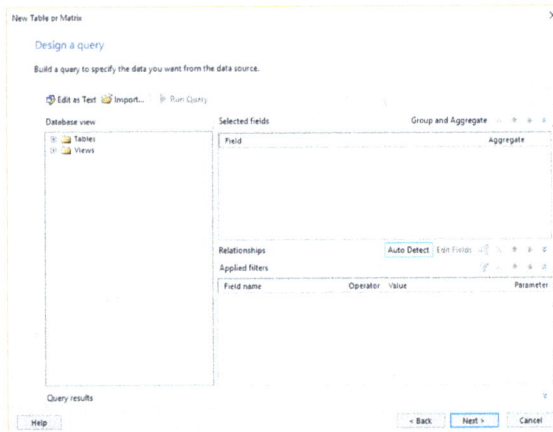

Note on the left of the window that the query can be composed of Tables or Views. For our purposes, a view is simply a group of tables joined together into one table we can query. In Exhibit 13.12 the Tables node is expanded to show a table called PUF2014. That table's node is expanded to show the fields in the table. Each of the 9.3 million rows in the table represent CMS billing history for a procedure code for a provider in a state. Each column in the table represents information about that row. For example, the NPI column has the National Provider Identifier of the provider in the row. Further down, the hcpcs_code field shows the procedure code billed.

It might seem overly complex to have so many columns or fields in a dataset, but this is part of what makes datasets so powerful while reducing IT's workload. Rather than create a separate dataset to support each report, IT creates one dataset with many fields that might support a wide variety of reports. Once you understand what data is in each field, you can choose which data you need for your specific application and that dataset can support many reports.

EXHIBIT 13.12 REPORT BUILDER: TABLES

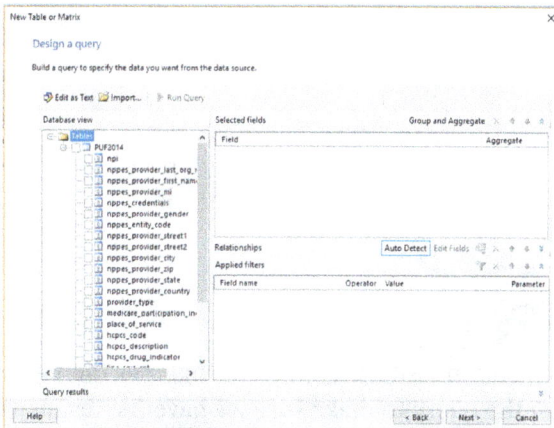

In Exhibit 13.13, four fields have been chosen to use in our dataset, hcpcs_code (procedure code), provider_type (providers' specialty), bene_unique_cnt (the number of unique beneficiaries billed), and average_submitted_chrg_amt (the average charge submitted to Medicare). You might ask your IT team to give the fields more user-friendly names than this CMS dataset has.

The Query Designer allows us to group and aggregate the data. The report groups the data by procedure code and provider specialty. The report also sums the number of unique beneficiaries and takes the average submitted charge. The Report Builder modifies the field names to reflect the way we aggregate the data. For example, bene_unique_cnt became Sum_bene_unique_cnt.

On the bottom half of the window, the filter only shows new patient procedure codes (99201-99205) and to only show providers in the state of California. We do not have to include the nppes_provider_state field in the data to filter by state. The only fields that will appear in our data are the four selected fields at the top of the window.

Exhibit 13.13 Report Builder: Query Designer

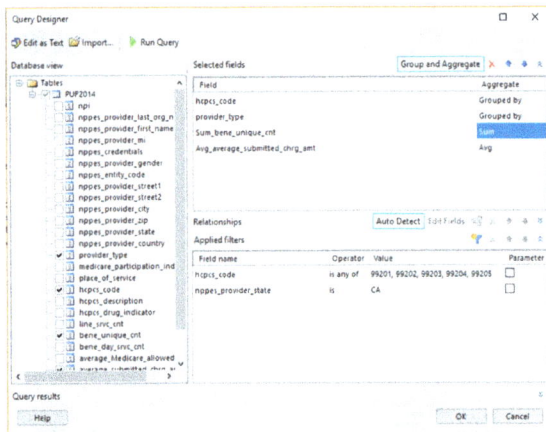

The Run Query button (with the green triangle) at the top of the window allows us to run the query to make sure we have the results we need in our dataset. An example of the query is shown in Exhibit 13.14.

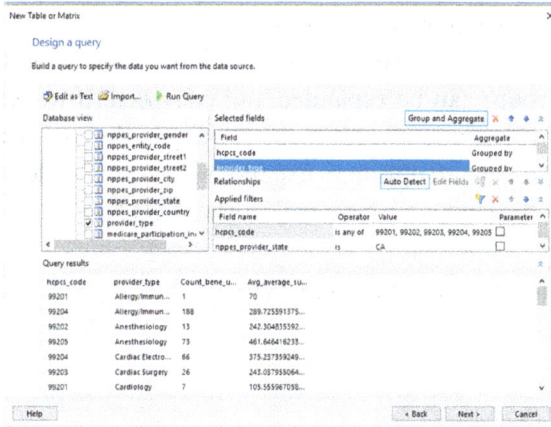

Now that we have data, the next step (shown in Exhibit 13.5) helps us arrange the fields in our report. Two of the main ways to display text in SSRS are a Tablix or a Matrix. (You can also build a list, for things like mailing labels.) A Tablix is like an Excel Table, while a Matrix is like an Excel Pivot Table. A Tablix can display details, while a Matrix allows you to aggregate the data displayed. Since we are summing the unique beneficiary count and averaging the billed charges, the Matrix format will work well. The two aggregate fields are in the Values section of the Matrix. The provider_type field will show provider specialties in rows. The new patients' procedure codes will be shown in columns.

EXHIBIT 13.15 ARRANGE FIELDS

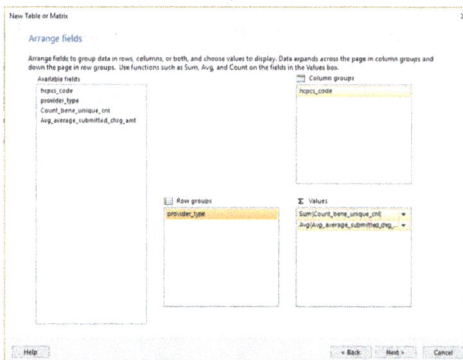

Now that we have a connection to SQL Server, a dataset, a query, and a structure for our report, we are almost done with the wizard. The wizard will help us with two more steps: choosing a layout and a style. The layout is shown in Exhibit 13.16. Layout options include where subtotals are shown and whether groups can be expanded and collapsed. If we wanted to show individuals providers underneath each specialty in the row groups in the last exhibit, we could have an option to expand or collapse that level of detail. For the time being, the layout we have will work. Select Next.

Exhibit 13.16 Report Builder: Layout

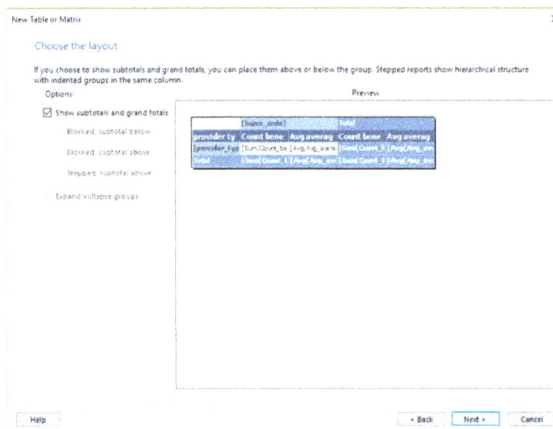

The section of the wizard helps you with a choice of six default styles. Styles control the colors and fonts used in the report. Styles are a solid way to make all the reports you create for your practice look consistent. You might also start with a common style and then change the default colors so that the practice can quickly distinguish which email they are looking at.

EXHIBIT 13.17 REPORT BUILDER: LAYOUT STYLES

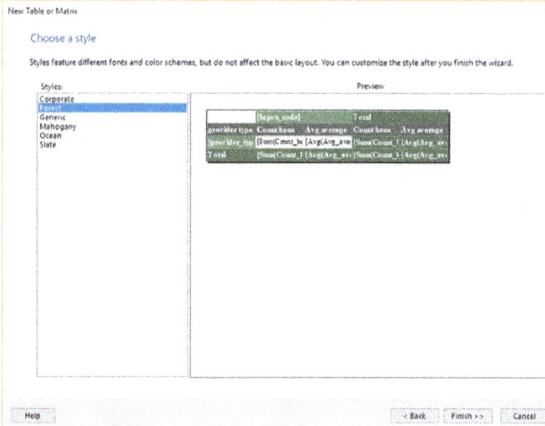

After selecting a style, the wizard closes leaving us with a draft of our report. We aren't finished yet, but the wizard has done a lot of the work for us. The Run button, circled in red in Exhibit 13.18, will preview the report.

EXHIBIT 13.18 REPORT BUILDER: RUN REPORT

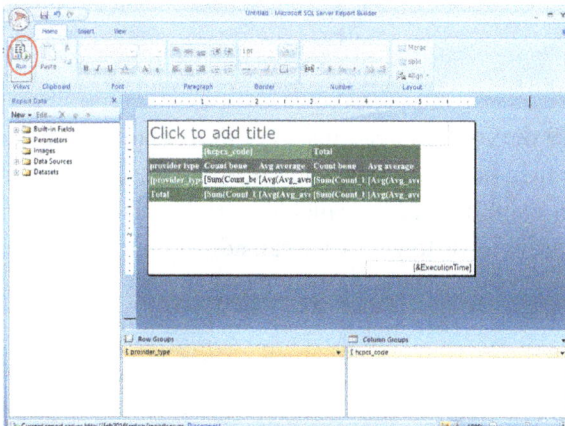

FORMATTING REPORTS IN SSRS

Exhibit 13.19 shows a preliminary result. The wizard did much of the groundwork, but a lot of formatting remains. The averages are displayed with way more decimals than our users need, for example. Some of the column widths need adjustment as well. Report Builder has replaced the Run button highlighted in the last exhibit with the Design button. Click the Design button to return to designing the report.

EXHIBIT 13.19 REPORT BUILDER: FORMATTING

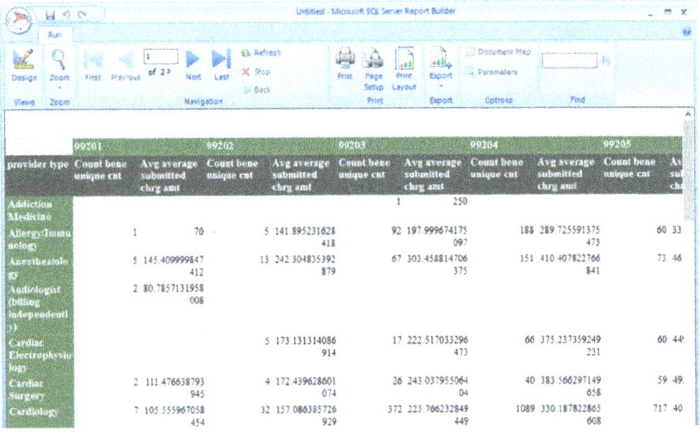

In Exhibit 13.19 the column headings have been made much shorter and the average charge field has been selected in order to fix the number format. The menu shown in Exhibit 13.20 is available by right-clicking the field. Selecting Text Box Properties leads to where we can adjust the numeric format.

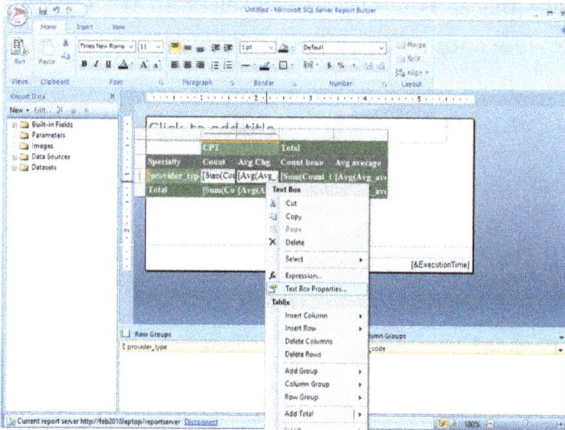

Exhibit 13.21 shows text box formatting options box in Report Builder. You can change the numeric format, font, border, fill, and more from here. The [fx] button will also appear frequently in these menus. That button allows you to write formulas to customize the field, like conditional formatting in Excel, only much more powerful.

EXHIBIT 13.21 REPORT BUILDER: TEXT BOX PROPERTIES: MENU

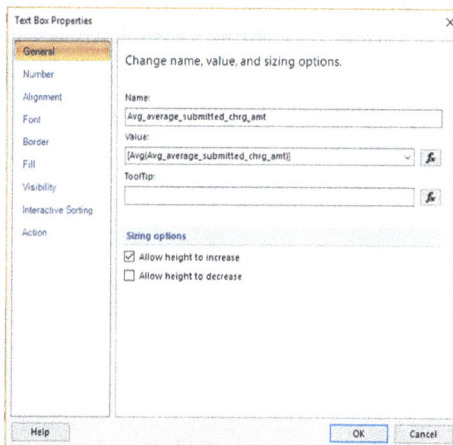

323

Selecting Number brings up the window shown in Exhibit 13.22. This menu is very similar to formatting a number in Excel. Simply choose the format you need, the number of decimal places, and whether to show a comma in the thousands place. You will see the selection is currency, two decimal places, and showing commas.

EXHIBIT 13.22 REPORT BUILDER: TEXT BOX PROPERTIES: NUMBER

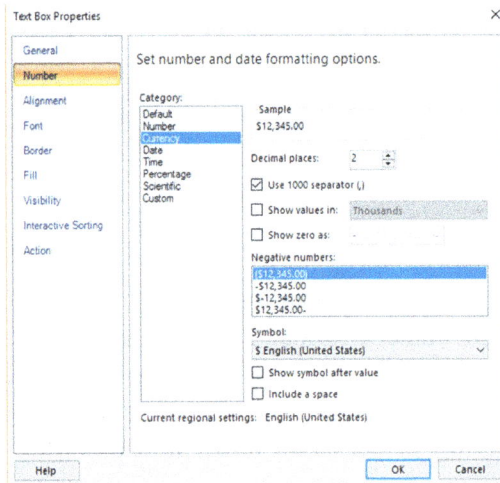

Another way to access properties of Report Builder components is the properties window. To display the properties window, check the properties box on the View tab, as shown in Exhibit 13.23. This window displays the properties of whatever SSRS element you select. The property window in Exhibit 13.23 shows the properties of the report body.

EXHIBIT 13.23 REPORT BUILDER: VIEW TAB AND REPORT BODY PROPERTIES

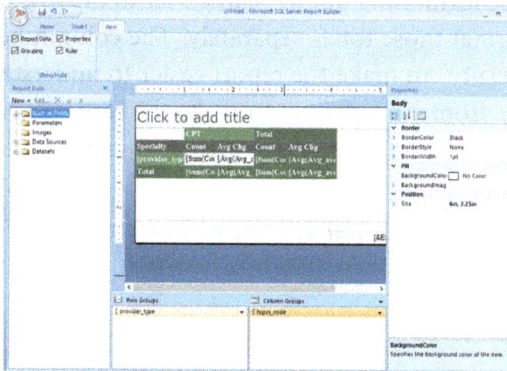

Exhibit 13.24 shows the beneficiary unique count selected and the size of the field is highlighted in the properties window. Though you can drag columns to resize them, it helps to use the size window to get the exact dimensions of the columns and match columns sizes across the report. Properties are grouped in the properties window. Some report elements have a lot of options. You can also show the options in alphabetical order if that makes it easier to find what you are looking for.

EXHIBIT 13.24 REPORT BUILDER: RESIZING WINDOWS AND COLUMNS

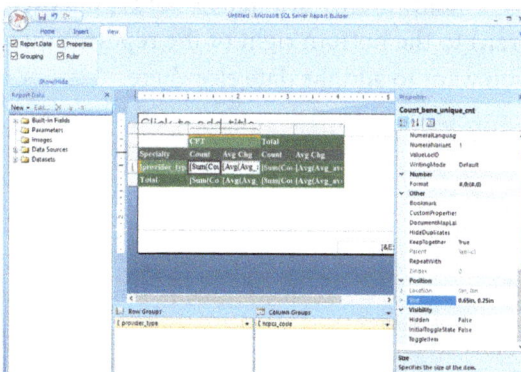

Our report is formatted and a lot closer to what we need in the preview shown in Exhibit 13.25. When we format a number like the average billed charge, that format carries over to each time the average billed charge is used in the Matrix. The formatting doesn't carry over to the row or column totals of the report. Format those totals separately. The column heading has been changed to "Specialty" to make the report easier to understand. It is easy to rename the fields from your dataset to make the report easier for your end users to understand. The next step is to give the report a title.

Exhibit 13.25 Report Builder: Report Preview

	99201		99202		99203		99204		99205		Total	
Specialty	Count	Avg Chg	Count	Avg Chg	Count	Avg Chg	Count	Avg Chg	Count	Avg Chg	Count	Avg Chg
Addiction Medicine					1	$250.00					1	$250.00
Allergy/Immunology	1	$70.00	5	$141.90	92	$198.00	188	$289.73	60	$337.71	346	$207.47
Anesthesiology	5	$145.41	13	$242.30	67	$303.46	151	$410.41	73	$461.65	309	$312.65
Audiologist (billing independently)	2	$80.79									2	$80.79
Cardiac Electrophysiology			5	$173.13	17	$222.52	66	$375.24	60	$449.14	148	$305.01
Cardiac Surgery	2	$111.48	4	$172.44	26	$243.04	40	$383.57	59	$492.78	131	$200.66
Cardiology	7	$105.56	32	$157.09	372	$225.77	1,089	$330.19	717	$405.55	2,217	$244.83
Clinical Laboratory					1	$112.05					1	$112.05
Colorectal Surgery (formerly proctology)	3	$93.55	20	$154.40	66	$228.91	52	$348.47	24	$456.90	165	$256.44
Critical Care (Intensivists)	1	$64.09	1	$156.14	12	$228.42	39	$326.42	25	$402.20	78	$235.46
Dermatology	108	$85.10	750	$138.11	1,030	$184.31	158	$255.89	11	$329.83	2,057	$198.65
Diagnostic Radiology	7	$133.39	11	$197.65	34	$281.91	27	$404.95	14	$530.33	93	$309.65
Emergency Medicine	13	$91.74	112	$171.92	263	$218.43	163	$294.86	53	$353.38	604	$226.06
Endocrinology	2	$124.01	5	$173.89	60	$233.99	239	$345.98	198	$427.54	504	$261.08

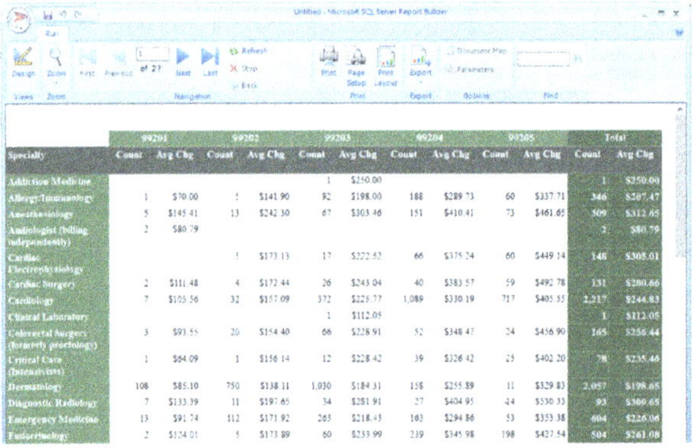

In Exhibit 13.26 we have switched back to design view to add a title. Simply type a title into the box that says, "Click to add title" (we will customize the title later on). By default, the wizard added the report execution time (the time the report ran) to the bottom right of the report. You can easily delete that text box if you want to add the date elsewhere.

EXHIBIT 13.26 REPORT BUILDER: ADDING A TITLE

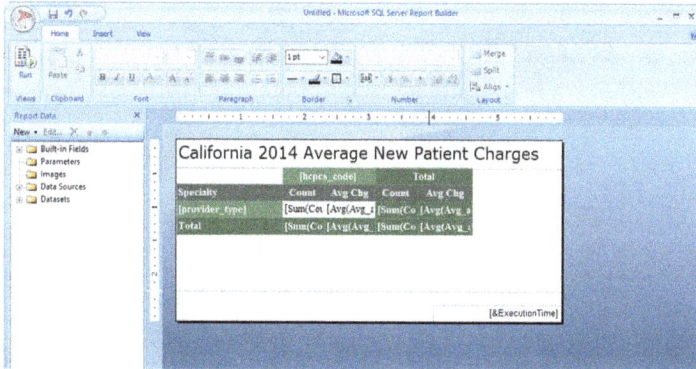

As Exhibit 13.27 shows, our report is looking good. Now it's time to save it. The interesting thing about saving SSRS reports in Report Builder is that rather than saving it to folder on your network, Report Builder saves to a specific folder for Report Manager to use in the dashboard.

EXHIBIT 13.27 REPORT BUILDER: TITLE RESULTS

Exhibit 13.28 shows the save location. There will be more information about Report Manager later in the appendix, but Report Manager is the home for all the dashboards you create. The folders shown are those that allow users to navigate through your dashboard. Report Manager also lets you email any dashboard report you create. For reference, Report Builder saves reports in an .rdl file format, which Excel cannot open.

EXHIBIT 13.28 REPORT BUILDER: SAVING THE REPORT

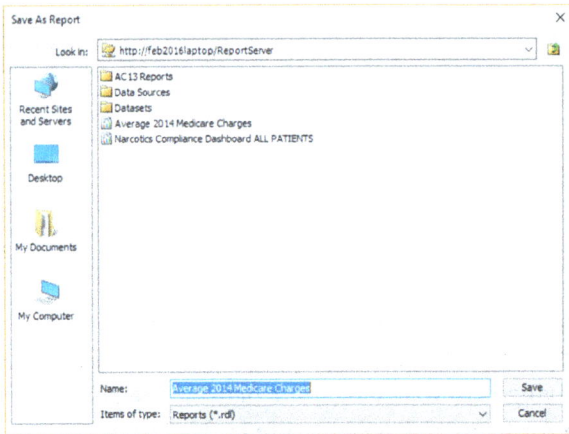

Exhibit 13.29 is our saved report. The formula has been changed to sum unique beneficiaries instead of counting the beneficiaries, but the title header is still Count. This report reflects our data and if we only wanted California data, we would be finished.

EXHIBIT 13.29 REPORT BUILDER: SAVED REPORT

California 2014 Average New Patient Charges

Specialty	99201		99202		99203		99204		99205		Total	
	Count	Avg Chg	Count	Avg Chg	Count	Avg Chg	Count	Avg Chg	Count	Avg Chg	Count	Avg Chg
Addiction Medicine					26	$250.00					26	$250.00
Allergy/Immunology	16	$70.00	79	$141.90	3,388	$198.00	7,623	$289.73	1,812	$337.71	12,918	$207.47
Anesthesiology	127	$145.41	387	$242.30	4,294	$303.46	10,833	$410.41	3,286	$461.65	18,927	$512.65
Audiologist (billing independently)	86	$80.79									86	$80.79
Cardiac Electrophysiology			95	$173.13	462	$222.52	3,745	$375.24	3,520	$449.14	7,822	$305.01
Cardiac Surgery	142	$111.48	118	$172.44	1,175	$243.04	1,462	$383.57	2,371	$492.78	5,268	$280.66
Cardiology	132	$105.56	949	$157.09	17,690	$225.77	66,503	$330.19	37,149	$405.55	122,423	$244.83
Clinical Laboratory					18	$112.05					18	$112.05
Colorectal Surgery (formerly proctology)	41	$93.55	1,084	$154.40	4,228	$228.91	2,830	$348.47	963	$456.90	9,146	$256.44
Critical Care (Intensivists)	11	$64.09	21	$156.14	360	$228.42	1,886	$326.42	1,136	$402.20	3,414	$235.46
Dermatology	3,682	$85.10	54,359	$138.11	91,331	$184.31	6,994	$255.89	260	$329.83	156,626	$198.65
Diagnostic Radiology	192	$133.39	203	$197.65	1,309	$281.91	646	$404.95	463	$530.33	2,813	$300.65
Emergency Medicine	404	$91.74	3,330	$171.92	16,804	$218.43	9,017	$294.86	2,006	$353.38	31,561	$226.06
Endocrinology	37	$124.01	129	$173.89	1,843	$233.99	11,432	$345.98	10,305	$427.54	23,746	$261.08

MAKE SSRS DASHBOARDS INTERACTIVE WITH PARAMETERS

The report we just created works. Because of the connection we created, if the underlying data in SQL Server changed (as PM and EHR data does constantly), the report would refresh with those changes. The next step is to make our report interactive so users can choose which state they wish to analyze instead of being limited to California. In Exhibit 13.30 the dataset that feeds our report has been right-clicked. Select "Query" to edit the query underlying the report.

EXHIBIT 13.30 REPORT BUILDER: INTERACTIVE QUERY

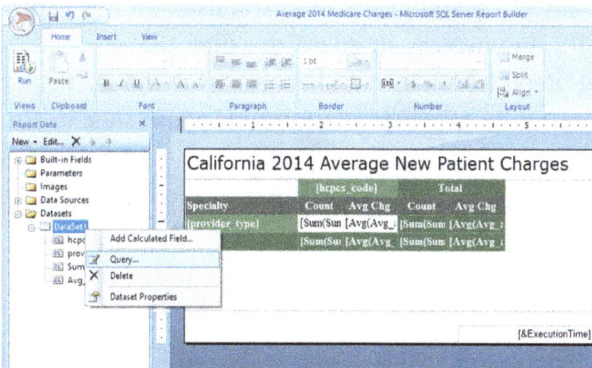

Exhibit 13.31 shows the query designer we used when we created the query. The state filter that limits the data to CA has been selected.

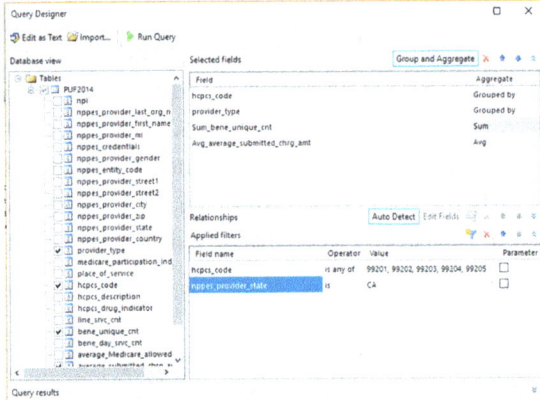

Remove the CA value and check the parameter box, as shown in Exhibit
13.32. An SSRS parameter is an interactive filter that allows users to change
filters via the Report Manager dashboard. Now the query that drives the
report will look to the state field to determine which state to display.

EXHIBIT 13.32 REPORT BUILDER: QUERY DESIGNER: INTERACTIVE
FILTER

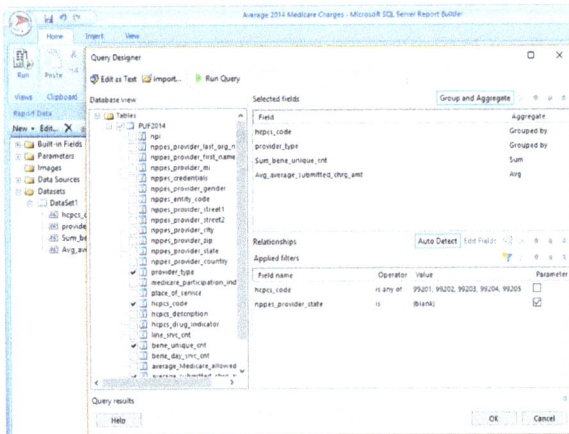

The next step is to provide a list of options for users to choose a state from
in a dropdown box as part of the report. One way to create this parameter

would be to list all 50 states, but it's generally better to use the underlying data to develop the list of parameters. In this example, if CMS did not have data for a state, we would not want that state in our list of options. If our report instead allowed users to select procedure codes, we would not want to list every possible procedure code, but only those procedure codes included in the CMS data. We will provide that list of states as a new dataset. In Exhibit 13.33 Datasets has been right-clicked. Choose Add Dataset from the following menu.

EXHIBIT 13.33 REPORT BUILDER: ADDING A DATASET

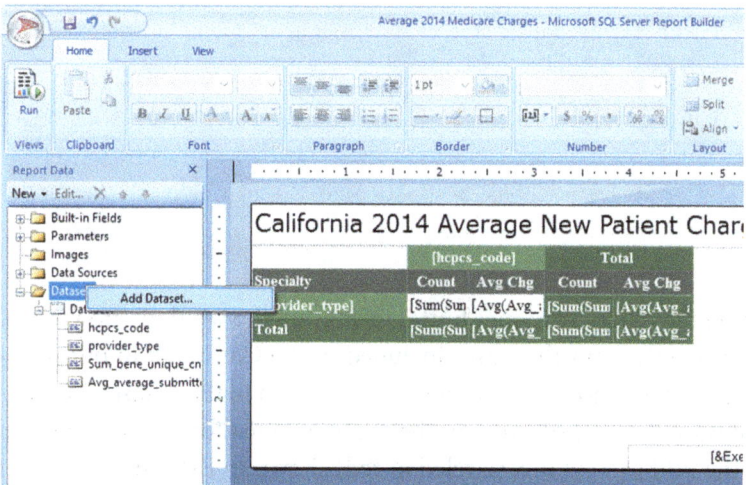

Thankfully, we have already built a connection to SQL Server when we used the wizard to initially develop our report. We select the "Use a dataset embedded in my report" button, and then select DataSource1 as the data source, as shown in Exhibit 13.34.

EXHIBIT 13.34 REPORT BUILDER: SELECTING DATA SOURCE

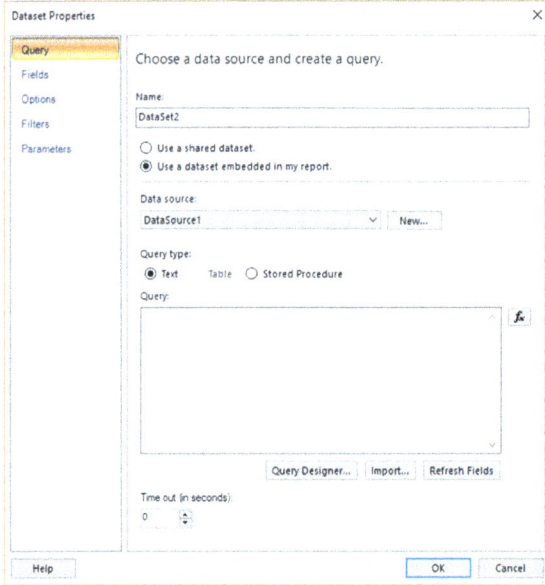

Selecting the Query Designer button brings up the window shown in Exhibit 13.35. We only want the states included in the CMS data in our query. The problem is that there are 9.3 million rows of data in the dataset. We definitely do not want 9.3 million rows in the dropdown list for users to choose from. Click the Edit as Text box (circled in red) shown in Exhibit 13.35.

EXHIBIT 13.35 REPORT BUILDER: BUTTON TO EDIT QUERY DESIGNER
RESULTS

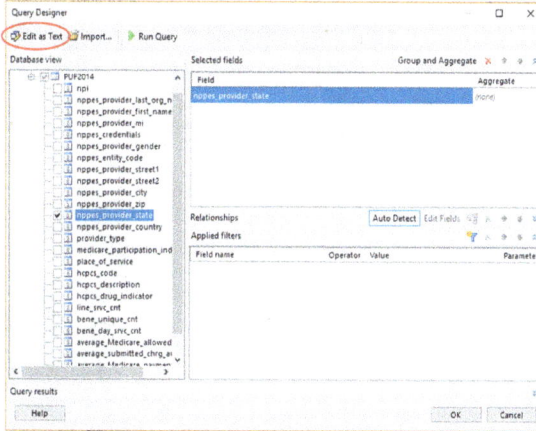

The next window, shown in Exhibit 13.36, allows us to edit the SQL text
created by the Query Designer. Two pieces of code have been added to the
SQL statement. First, the keyword DISTINCT has been added so the query
will only select unique states. Second, the ORDER BY clause has been added
in order to sort the states in alphabetical order. The query results are displayed
at the bottom of the window. The CMS data includes locations besides the
50 states. If we wanted to, we could filter these territories and other locations
out of our dropdown box.

Exhibit 13.36 Report Builder: Editing Query Designer Results

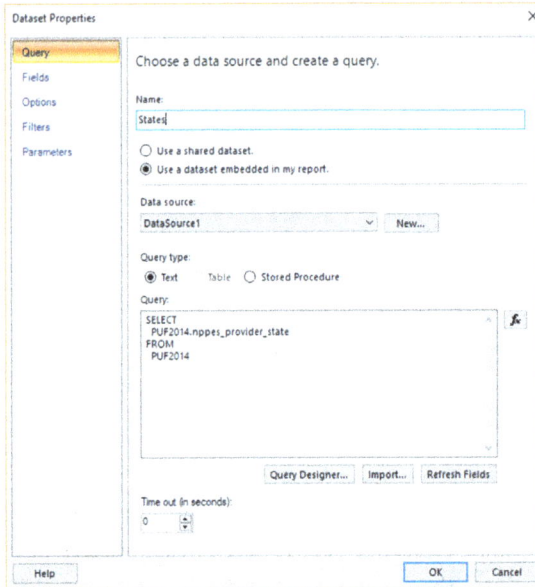

Finish editing the query, and the window will return you to the Dataset Properties screen, as shown in Exhibit 13.37. To make the parameter easier to work with, the dataset has been renamed "States" instead of Dataset2. Now we have our underlying query, Dataset1, set to look at the parameter to see which state to use. We also have a dataset called States available to populate the dropdown box.

EXHIBIT 13.37 REPORT BUILDER: RENAMING DATASETS

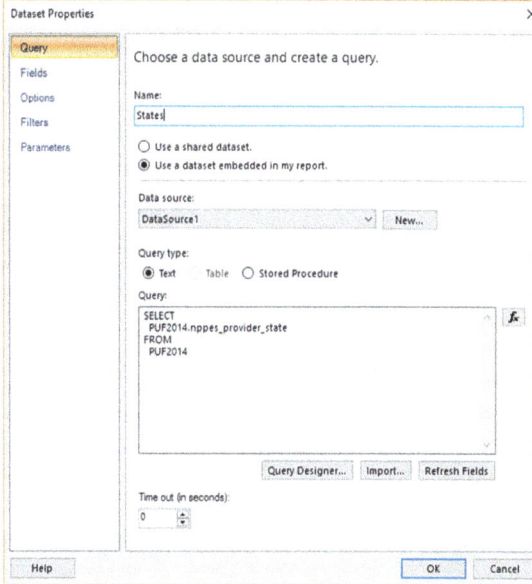

The next step is to build a parameter to allow users to interact with the report. Exhibit 13.38 shows the parameter in the parameters section of the Report Data window. The parameter is named nppes_provider_state from when we checked the box in the original query to set that field as a parameter.

EXHIBIT 13.38 REPORT BUILDER: BUILDING PARAMETERS

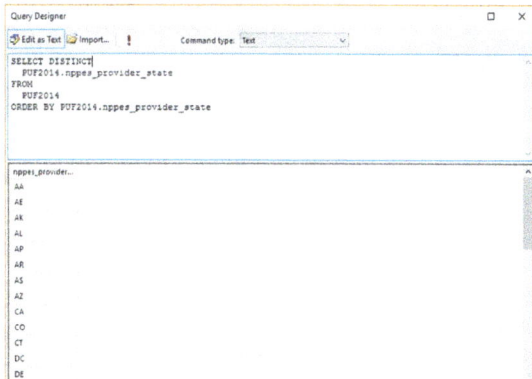

Right-click the parameter, as shown in Exhibit 13.40, to access the Parameter Properties window.

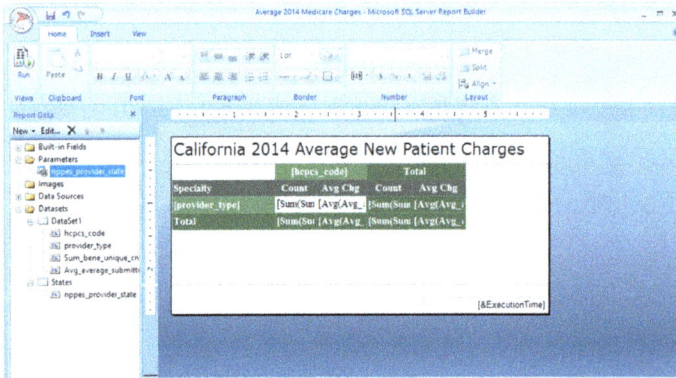

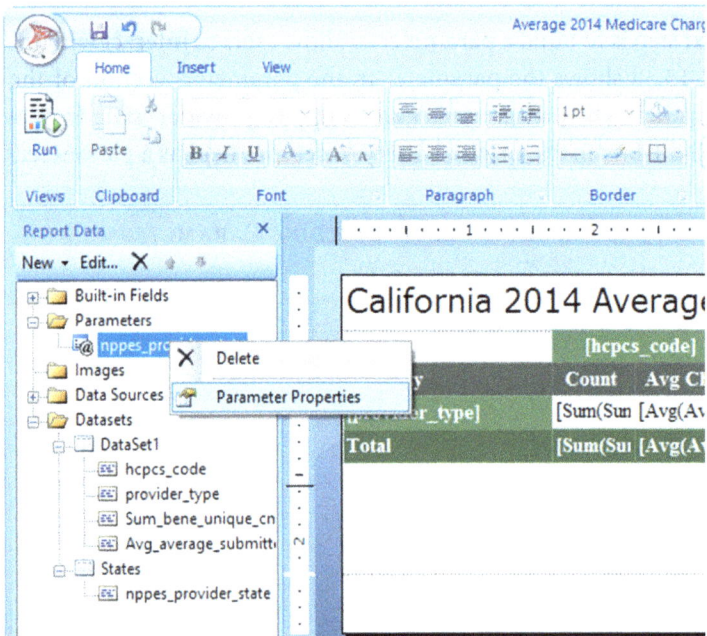

EXHIBIT 13.41 REPORT BUILDER: PARAMETERS PROPERTIES WINDOW

We need to change two things on the menu for our states parameter, as shown in Exhibit 13.41. First, the Prompt is what the end user will see when the parameter is displayed in the Report Manager. "State" is much easier to understand than "nppes provider state." Second, we do not want to allow blank values in this report. Often it makes sense to allow a summary report to run with all providers, all locations, all procedure codes, etc. For this report, we want to make sure users always choose a state, so uncheck "Allow blank value." We could allow users to select multiple states by checking "Allow multiple values," but to keep things simple, we will require only one state in the parameter. Parameters can be much more involved. You can choose date/time as a data type and Report Manager will display an interactive calendar icon. You can also choose boolean (true/false) and numeric parameters. The revised Report Parameter Properties window is shown in Exhibit 13.42.

EXHIBIT 13.42 REPORT BUILDER: REVISED REPORT PARAMETERS

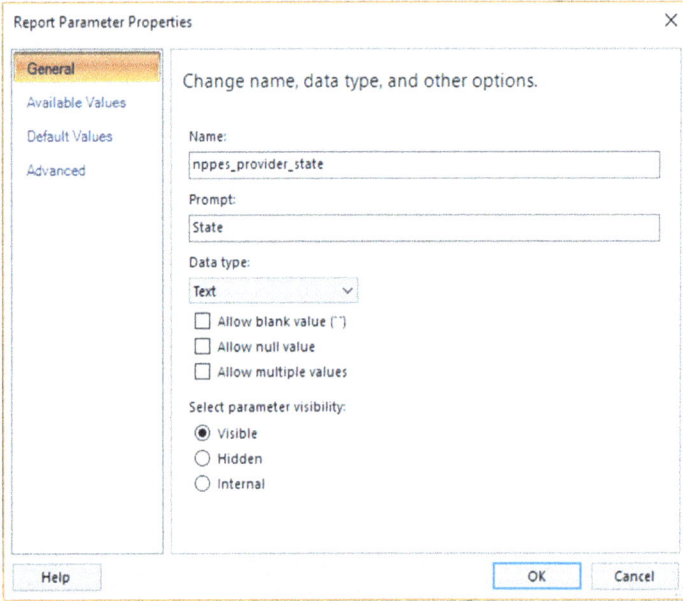

Now that the parameter is set up, the next step is to use the States dataset to populate the dropdown box of choices the user will see. On the Available Values tab, "Get values from a query" has been selected and the dataset States is chosen. The value field is the value of the parameter that feeds back into the filter we created for Dataset1. The label field is what the user will see in the parameter. In our example, the value field and the label field are the same. If our dataset had "CA" in one column and "California" in another column, we could make CA the value field, since CA is what the CMS data needs to filter on. We would make California the label field, which is what the user would see in the dropdown list. The Available Values tab is shown in Exhibit 13.43.

EXHIBIT 13.43 REPORT BUILDER: AVAILABLE VALUES TAB

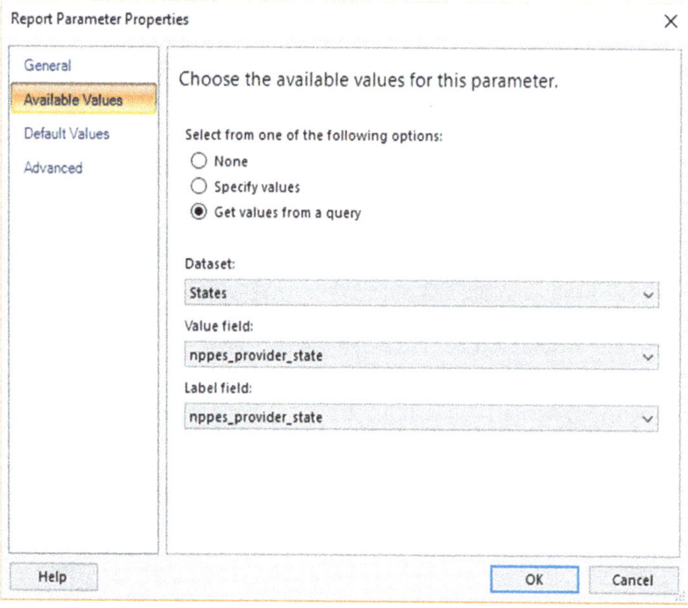

Report Parameter Properties   ✕

General

Available Values

Default Values

Advanced

Choose the available values for this parameter.

Select from one of the following options:

○ None
○ Specify values
◉ Get values from a query

Dataset:

States   ⌄

Value field:

nppes_provider_state   ⌄

Label field:

nppes_provider_state   ⌄

Help   OK   Cancel

The last window to visit is the Default Values window, which sets the default value for our States parameter. "Specify Values" is chosen and CA is the default value. Every time the report opens, SSRS will choose CA as the parameter until the user chooses differently. If we wanted to email this report, the SSRS term is to subscribe to the report. When you subscribe to a report with parameters, you can set up the subscription with a parameter. For example, we could subscribe to the report and select FL as the default parameter for that subscription, even though the report default is California. We could then email that version of the report to providers in Florida. The Default Values tab is shown in Exhibit 13.44.

EXHIBIT 13.44 REPORT BUILDER: DEFAULT VALUES TAB

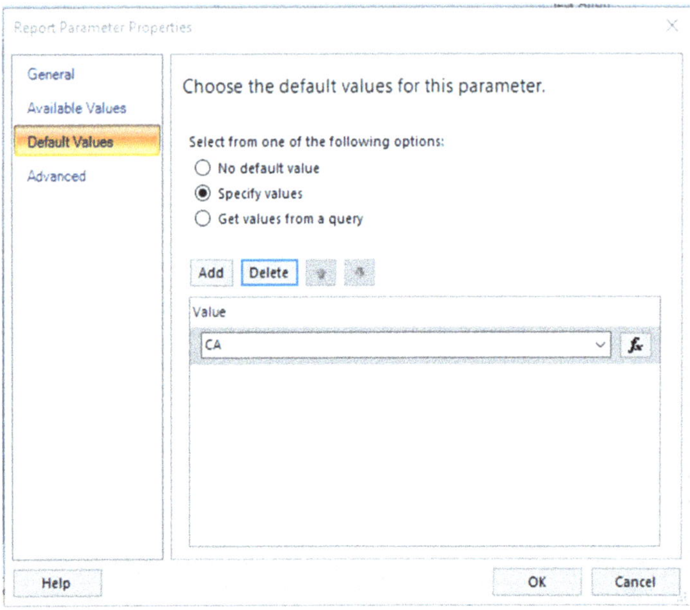

Now that the parameter is set up, we need to change the title of the report. Our report used to be "California 2014 Average New Patient Charges." Now we want the user's choice of parameter that is feeding the report's filter to feed the report's title as well. Right-click the title, as shown in Exhibit 13.45, and choose Expression. Expressions control what is displayed in the text box.

EXHIBIT 13.45 REPORT BUILDER: EXPRESSION DROP DOWN

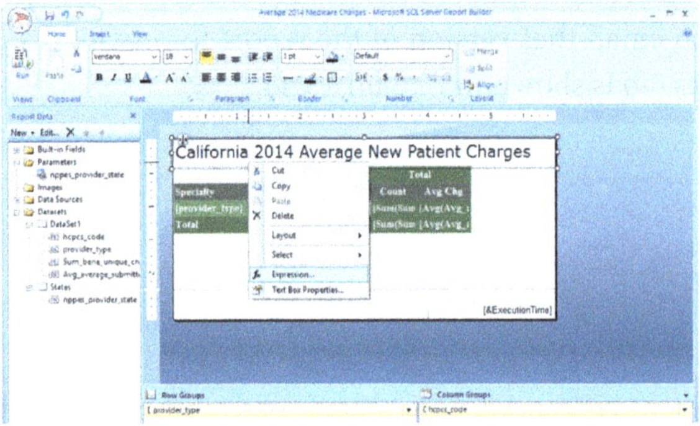

The formula in the top of the Expression window captures the parameter value and then adds the words "2014 Average New Patient Charges." Expression formulas are very powerful and flexible and are beyond the scope of this appendix. To give you a sense of what can be done with expressions, the category section in the lower left of the Expression window lists the categories available for expressions. There are plenty of math related functions, ways to interact with the report and the datasets on the report, dates and times, and much more. For example, we could put the date the report is run in the report title, which is a very common request. Your title might be something like "Billed Charges as of February 18, 2018."

EXHIBIT 13.46 REPORT BUILDER: EXPRESSION MENU

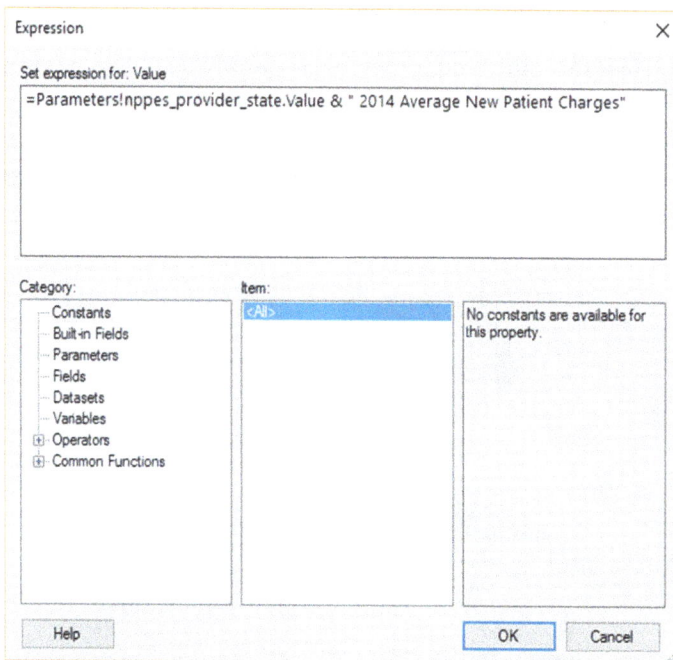

Click OK to close the Expression window. The report title now shows "Expr" instead of the actual title in Exhibit 13.47. SSRS uses Expr to indicate that there is an expression in that text box.

EXHIBIT 13.47 REPORT BUILDER: TITLE REPLACED WITH EXPRESSION

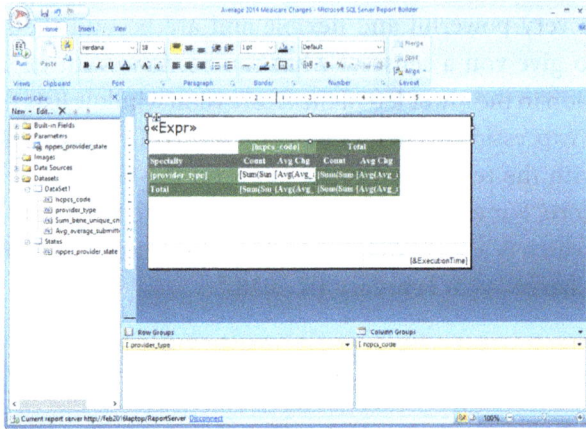

Exhibit 13.48 shows the final report with parameters. The parameters are circled in red in the top left. The default state is CA and that CA is included in the title. To change to different a different state, simply select the new state from the dropdown menu and then click View Report (circled in red on the right of the report).

EXHIBIT 13.48 REPORT BUILDER: FINAL REPORT WITH PARAMETERS

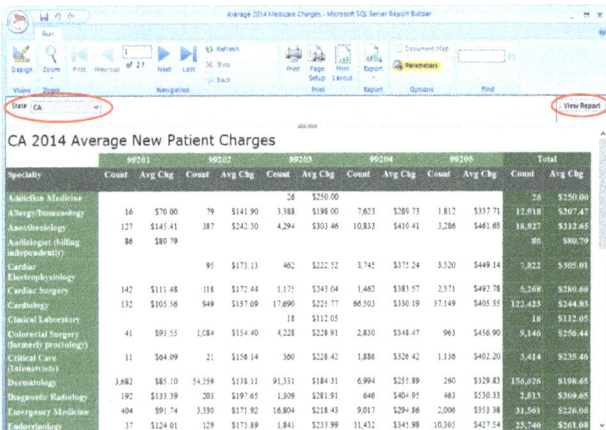

Finally, Exhibit 13.49 shows the same report with Florida selected instead of California.

That high-level overview is the process to create a report. As you save the changes, the changes automatically feed the Report Manager dashboard and are available to any end users with access to the dashboard. Any email subscriptions to the report will also reflect the latest version.

OTHER SSRS FEATURES

One example cannot do justice to all the reporting options available in SSRS through Report Builder. Exhibit 13.50 is the Home tab of the Report Builder toolbar. There are simple ways to change the font, paragraph, border, and number settings. The Align options in the Layout section make it easy to line everything up. Some of the alignment settings take a little practice. Because the same report must be rendered in a browser and in email, the settings can be less forgiving than a typical Office product. Emailed reports can be delivered in the body of the email or as an attached PDF or spreadsheet. The flexibility in delivering reports is very helpful and is worth the efforts to format the report properly.

Exhibit 13.50 Report Builder: Home Tab for Report Builder Toolbar

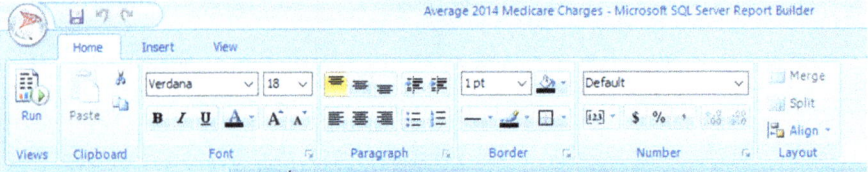

Exhibit 13.51 is the Insert tab. Report Parts is a visual list of the components of a report. We have discussed the Data Regions section. The Table (sometimes called a Tablix in SSRS) and Matrix options are very commonly used. The dropdown arrow underneath the Table, Matrix, Chart, and Map options opens a wizard like the wizard we used earlier. We have not spent any time on the available Data Visualizations. The Chart options are very similar to what is available in Excel.

Exhibit 13.51 Report Builder: Insert Tab for Report Builder Toolbar

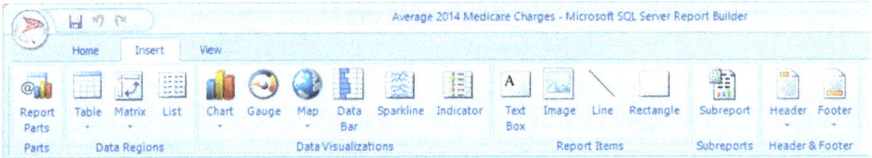

Gauges are dials and thermometer-like indicators. Examples of gauges are shown in Exhibit 13.52. There are options unlike anything available in Excel, but the gauges consume a lot of space relative to the information they provide.

EXHIBIT 13.52 REPORT BUILDER TOOLBAR: GAUGES

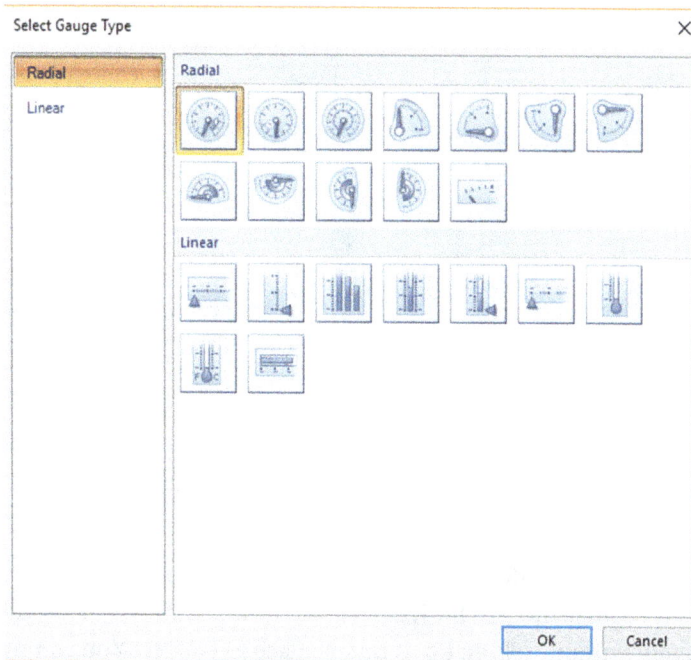

Available Sparklines are shown in Exhibit 13.53. You may be familiar with Sparklines from Excel, where a Sparkline is a miniature chart designed to fit in a cell. As of early 2017, Excel offers three different Sparklines. There are several more options available in SSRS. Sparklines generally convey information much more efficiently than gauges do.

Exhibit 13.53 Report Builder Toolbar: Sparklines

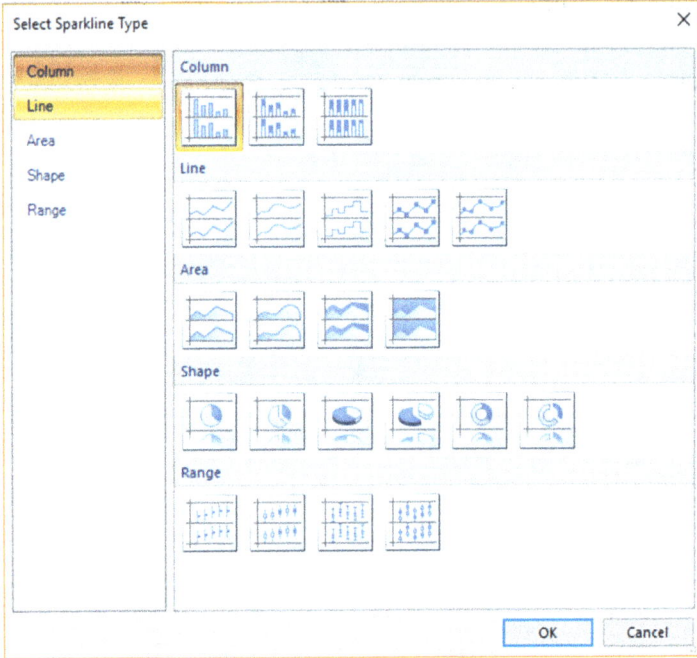

Exhibit 13.54 shows SSRS Indicators. Savvy conditional formatting users in Excel will recognize this list. Indicators are icon-like ways to quickly designate trends, again without taking up as much space as gauges. You can use some of these indicators, but often the report is cleaner if you simply change the color of the font (using an fx formula) to indicate increases or decreases.

EXHIBIT 13.54 REPORT BUILDER TOOLBAR: INDICATOR TYPES

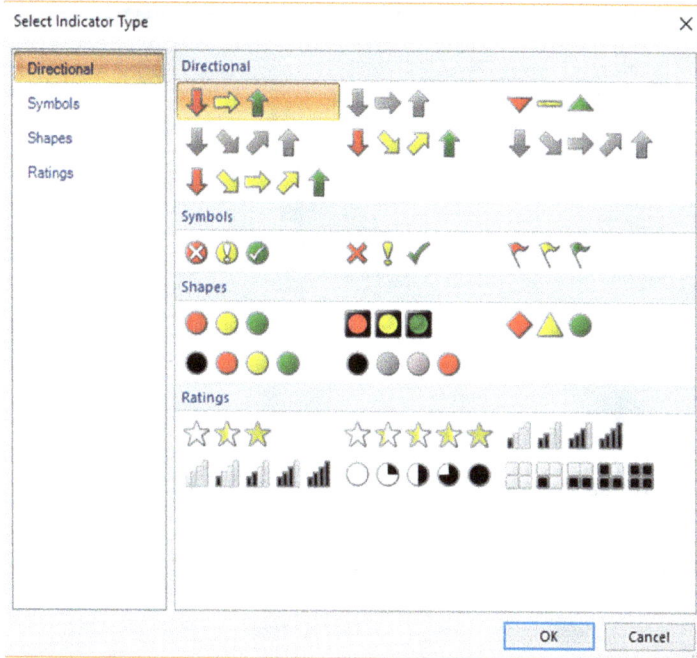

The other thing to mention on the Insert tab is Subreports. A Subreport is an SSRS report designed to fit inside another SSRS report. Subreports can be used to show drilldown detail behind a main report. You might also create a top-level dashboard report to display related Subreports. PivotTables in a supporting spreadsheet are another way to drill down on information rather than creating Subreports.

REPORT MANAGER

Report Manager is the dashboard SSRS uses to access and display reports. Exhibit 13.55 is an example of what Report Manager might look like.

Exhibit 13.55 Report Manager

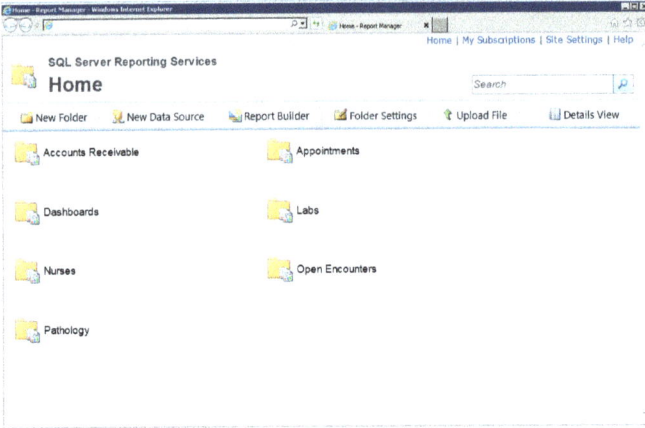

Each folder holds several dashboards, as shown in Exhibit 13.56.

Exhibit 13.56 Report Manager Folders

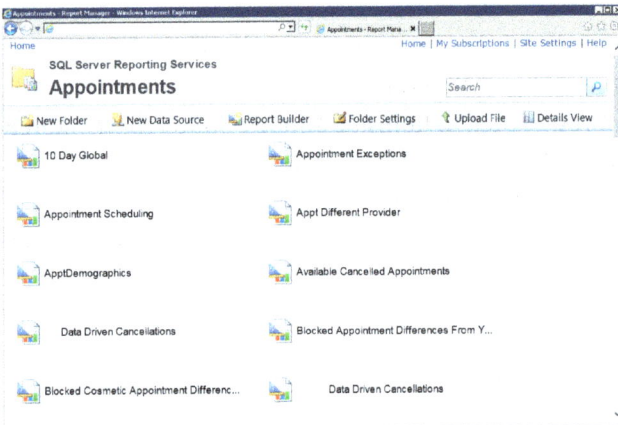

Even though Report Manager is accessed through a web browser, use Internet Explorer (IE). Practices have had trouble trying to use browsers other than IE with SSRS.

To subscribe to a report means to receive the report via email. Exhibit 13.57 is an example of a subscription screen. There are a variety of ways the report can be delivered. Choose the MHTML option to embed the report in an email. For complex, involved reports, choose PDF to better control how the final report will appear.

EXHIBIT 13.57 REPORT MANAGER: SUBSCRIBING TO A REPORT

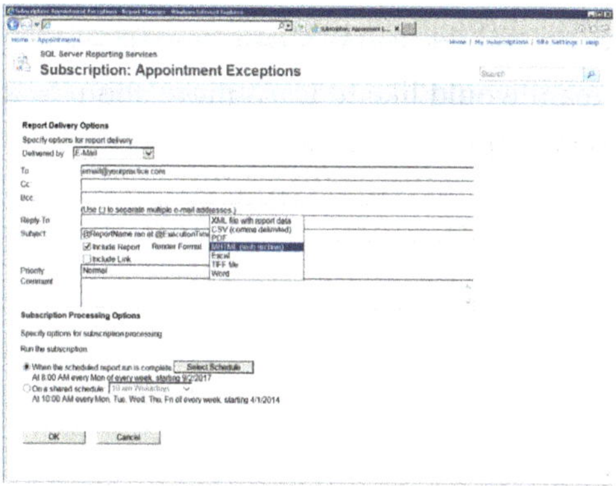

Subscriptions can be delivered on a very flexible schedule. The scheduling options are shown in Exhibit 13.58.

EXHIBIT 13.58 REPORT MANAGER: SUBSCRIPTION SCHEDULING OPTIONS

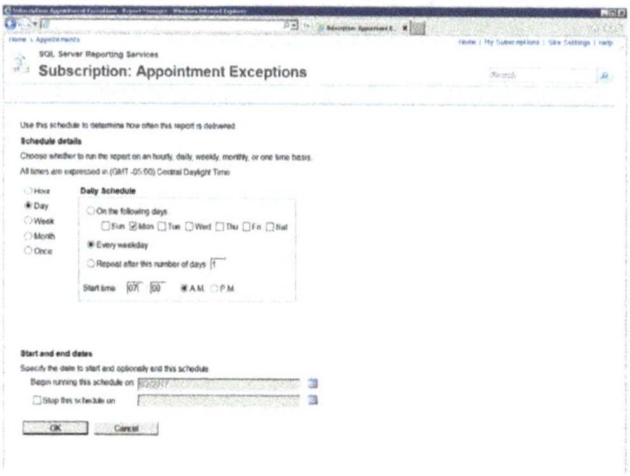

Hopefully this general overview has encouraged you to get started with SSRS. Imagine a daily email showing exactly what your providers, administrators, or front desk staff need to see to be most productive. It might take several datasets before they get all the data they need, and it will take time to get the reports exactly the way you want them, but keep at it. Good reporting is an iterative process. Keep trying until you get something that will change the way your practice runs for the better. The ability to push that data to whoever needs to see it, whenever they need to see it, on any device that can receive email, is a major breakthrough for practices.

If you or your IT team would like to learn more about SSRS, Brian Larson's books have been very helpful to get started.

APPENDIX 2

MORE BUSINESS INTELLIGENCE TOOLS TO CONSIDER

The first book in this series, *Better Data Better Decisions,* introduced PivotTables and the previous appendix in this book introduced SSRS. Those two tools go a long way toward giving medical practices powerful tools to analyze and report on their data. This section will review six other Business Intelligence tools that practices can use to either report on or interact with their data.

The first three tools, Power BI, PowerPivot, and the Excel Data Model are all interrelated. Power BI is Microsoft's new approach to self-service Business Intelligence. Power BI allows users to access reports and dashboards via the internet on mobile devices and browsers. Microsoft is making a concerted effort to upgrade Power BI often and add a variety of new features not available in tools like Excel. One especially interesting feature is a tool called natural language Q&A.

Power Pivot is like PivotTables on steroids. PivotTables run in the traditional Excel environment with a one million row limit. Approaching that million-row limit can slow PivotTables down. Power Pivot can analyze millions of rows of data, but some of the features of PivotTables are different in a Power Pivot environment.

The Excel Data Model was introduced in Excel 2013. Traditional PivotTables run off one table of data. The Excel Data Model is a way to manage multiple tables of data in one PivotTable by establishing relationships between the tables. PM and EHR systems are structured as relational databases, meaning data is stored across many different tables. Relational databases and how to work with the Excel Data Model will be discussed later in this appendix.

Maps are a new feature in Excel, beginning with Excel 2013. Called Power Map, this feature is only found in the Excel 2013 Professional version. When Excel 2016 and Office 365 debuted, the feature was renamed 3D Map and made available in both Professional and Standard Editions. The ability to show patient data geographically can be very powerful. Chapter 5 has examples of how practices have mapped data to better understand where patients are coming from.

The last two tools are included with most versions of SQL Server (much like SSRS). Practices that own their data in SQL Server also have access to these tools. SQL Server Integration Services (SSIS) is a tool that can import data into or export data out of SQL Server. If you have data in a non-SQL Server format that you want to integrate with SQL Server data, SSIS can make that happen. SSIS can also export data out of SQL Server to meet formatting requirements of outside vendors. This appendix includes examples of both importing and exporting data using SSIS.

SQL Server Analysis Services (SSAS) also comes with SQL Server. SSAS can do two things to help medical practices. First, SSAS can build cubes. A cube is a very compact way to store a lot of summarized data. SSAS can also be used for data mining to look for patterns in your data. This appendix demonstrates using predictive analytics and data mining to analyze patterns in no shows.

Practices can make tremendous strides with PivotTables and SSRS. Those two tools and a few datasets are an excellent place to start changing the way your practice uses data. Once your practice has those tools in place, utilizing one or more of these other tools can help make more data available to analyze or make it easier to consume that data.

POWER BI

Power BI is a tool to analyze data and share that analysis with users who can interact with the it via their phones, tablets, and browsers. Microsoft released Power BI in 2015 and has been frequently updating Power BI since. Because Power BI is a different platform than a traditional Excel spreadsheet, it's possible to perform actions in Power BI that you could never do in Excel. Conversely, some actions that Excel has been performing for 25 years simply can't be done in Power BI.

Exhibit 14.1 is a list of the visualizations available in Power BI in early 2017. Since Microsoft is adding functionality Power BI on a monthly basis, the list will likely grow over time.

EXHIBIT 14.1 POWER BI: VISUALIZATIONS

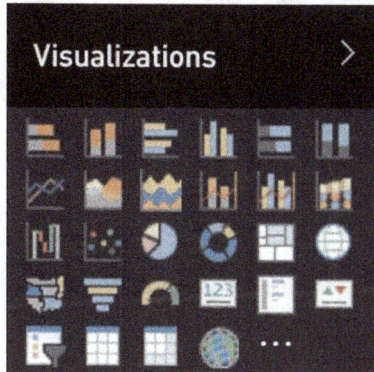

The first row of visualizations contains charts you will be familiar with from using Excel. In order, the graphics represent stacked bar and column charts, clustered bar and column charts, and 100% stacked bar and column charts. The second row will also be familiar to Excel users, including a line chart, an area chart, a stacked area chart, a combination line and stacked column chart, a combination line and clustered column chart, and a waterfall chart. A waterfall chart is a way to display a running total as values are added or subtracted over time.

The third row has a scatter chart and a pie chart, followed by a treemap. Microsoft uses treemaps to display hierarchical data. You might examine new patient referrals as hierarchical data by grouping major referring physicians by group (physician group, hospital, university, etc.) and then making each physician within the group a branch. The tree starts with a branch, represented by a rectangle in the chart that is proportional to the size of the data being displayed. Branches can be subdivided into rectangles or leaves, also proportionally sized, representing the data inside components of the branch. Users can visualize hierarchical data using the colored rectangles. An example of a treemap is shown in Exhibit 14.2.

EXHIBIT 14.2 TREEMAP SAMPLE

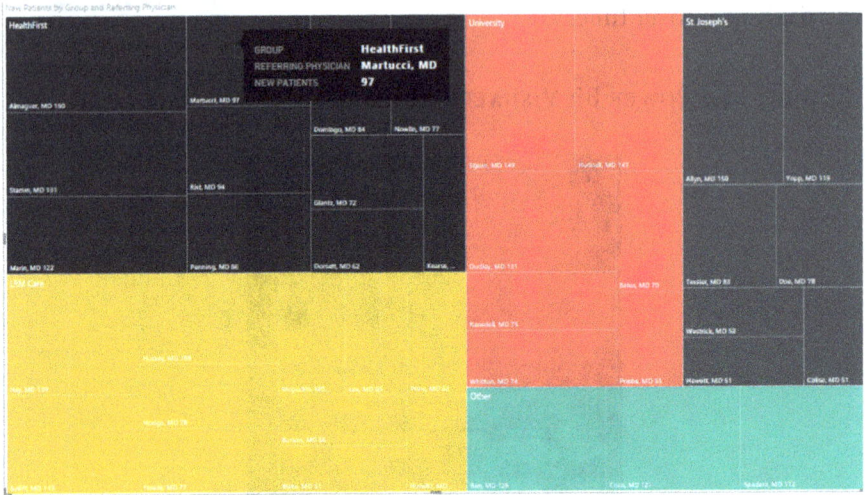

Each of the major groups is shown as a branch in a different color. Physicians in the HealthFirst group are the largest group of referring physicians, so they are shown in the top left of the treemap. Referring groups sending fewer patients are shown to the right and down in the treemap. The exhibit hovers over Dr. Martucci to see she sent 97 new patients to the practice last year.

It is generally not a good idea to use chart types that are unfamiliar to users. Users can be intimidated by new chart types and fail to ask questions and understand how to interpret the data. That said, if we tried to show all 39 providers in this treemap on one bar or column chart, the data would be too small to be of much value. We could not display both the referring physician group and the referring physician on the same chart. A pie chart would be even worse. If there is a need for an application like a treemap in your organization, it may be worth teaching providers how to use it.

Power BI is a work in progress. As clever and helpful as you might find a treemap, you have limited options for the data labels (the physician name and number displayed at the bottom left of each rectangle):

- You can change the color of the data labels.
- You can display the number in thousands, millions, billions or trillions.

- You can decide how many decimal places to show in the number of new patient referrals.

Those are your choices. You cannot:

- Change the font size of the data labels
- Move the data labels to a different corner of the rectangle, or
- Show the number of referrals before the physician name.

Most visualizations have similar limitations. The good news is that Microsoft is continually adding new features and options to make Power BI more user friendly and flexible.

Returning to the third row of the visualizations, the last three options are a map, a table, and a matrix. The map is another area where more functionality and features will be added over time. A table is like an Excel table. A matrix is like an Excel PivotTable, where data can be aggregated to show sums, counts, averages, and more.

The fourth row of visualizations starts with a filled map, sometimes known as a choropleth. A filled map shades regions to indicate higher or lower values. For example, if more patients are coming from New Jersey than New York, New Jersey would be shown in a darker color. The next visualization is a funnel chart. Microsoft designed a funnel chart to show sequential flows. The example Microsoft uses is sales. The sales process starts with a lead, then a prospect, a qualified prospect, a commitment, and then a sale. A funnel chart shows how many potential customers are in each stage of the process. A funnel chart takes up a lot of precious space on a dashboard relative to the information the chart conveys.

The fourth row of visualizations continues with a gauge. A gauge is like a speedometer that can track progress toward a goal. A gauge also takes up a lot of precious space. The next two visualizations are a multi-row card and a card. Cards show a single number. A multi-row card shows more than one piece of information on a card. You may find cards helpful to track a critical piece of data on a dashboard, realizing the tradeoff between the importance of the information and the space on your dashboard. Exhibit 14.3 shows a card, and Exhibit 14.4 shows a multi-row card.

Exhibit 14.3 Card Sample

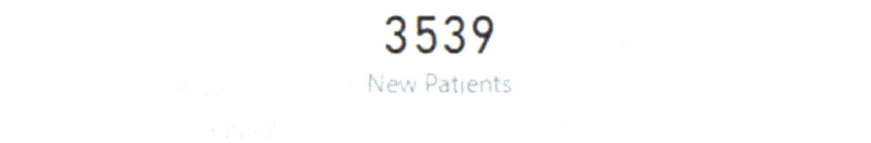

3539
New Patients

Exhibit 14.4 Multi-row Card Sample

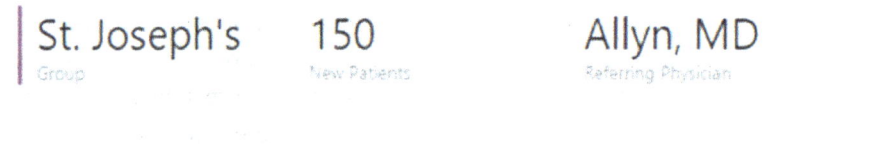

St. Joseph's	150	Allyn, MD
Group	New Patients	Referring Physician

The last visualization on the fourth row is a KPI indicator. The KPI is another gauge to show progress toward a goal. The goals must be loaded in addition to your data. Some practices may like the white space on a dashboard and want funnels, gauges, cards, and KPI indicators on a dashboard. Many commercially available dashboards are filled with these types of indicators.

The bottom row of Power BI visualizations starts with a slicer. Excel users may be familiar with slicers. A slicer is a dashboard filter that allows users to interact with the data. In our treemap example, a slicer could allow users to only show the HealthFirst doctors. The next visualization is a donut chart, which is like a pie chart. The R launches an R script editor. R is a statistical program that is way beyond the scope of this book. The three dots as the last visualization allow access to custom visualizations. Microsoft allows interested IT developers to build their own visualizations for Power BI. Custom visualizations are also way beyond the scope of this book.

Many of these visualizations can drill down to detailed levels. The drill down works on mobile devices, so users can focus on specific areas of concern. The data is fed by a model like the Excel Data Model, discussed later in this appendix. Power BI reports can be built using a tool called Power BI Desktop. You can also interact with the reports online at powerbi.microsoft.com.

Saving the report as a dashboard online gives more options to interact with the data. Exhibit 14.5 is our treemap online. Pay particular attention to the gray section at the top titled, "Ask a question about your data."

EXHIBIT 14.5 TREEMAP ONLINE SAMPLE

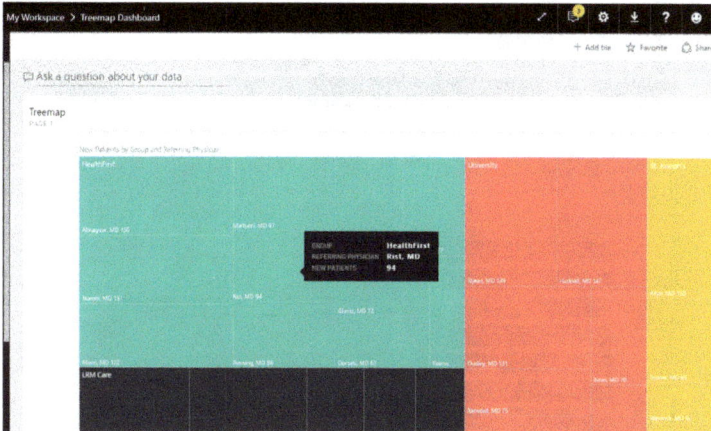

The ability to ask a question about your data using Power BI's natural language question and answer tool is something unique to the Business Intelligence tools described in this book. Using our treemap as an example, look at the ask a question section in Exhibit 14.6. Users can ask a question using fields from the underlying data and Power BI will answer the question.

- Assume that you want data from the University physicians, so include the "University" keyword.
- Assume you want to see the total number of new patients. Since the dataset has a column called New Patients, Power BI knows what data we want.
- The keyword "bar" tells Power BI you want the data displayed as a bar chart.
- The words "referring physician" also reference a column in the dataset that has the name of each referring physician.

Power BI built a bar chart showing the new patients by referring physician from University physicians. The Q&A section is a very powerful way for end users to understand your data without having to understand how to build visualizations in Power BI. The syntax takes a little getting used to and the users must know the names of the fields (University, Referring Physician, New Patients, etc.) in the data. Once users get used to Q&A, they can build their own reports, and they can pin reports they like to a dashboard.

EXHIBIT 14.6 TREEMAP Q&A SAMPLE

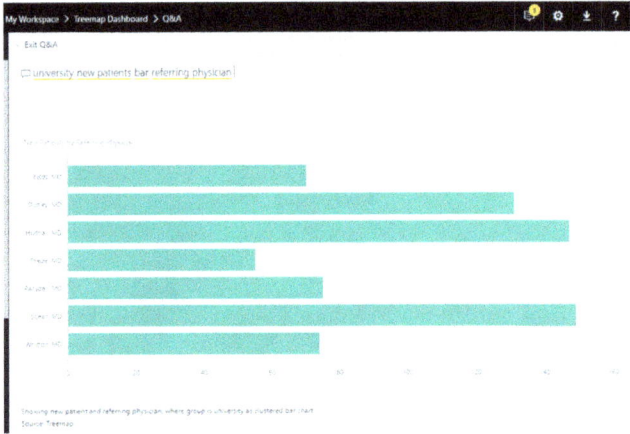

The data is also available on tablets. Exhibit 14.7 is the same dashboard on an iPad.

EXHIBIT 14.7 TREEMAP ON IPAD SAMPLE

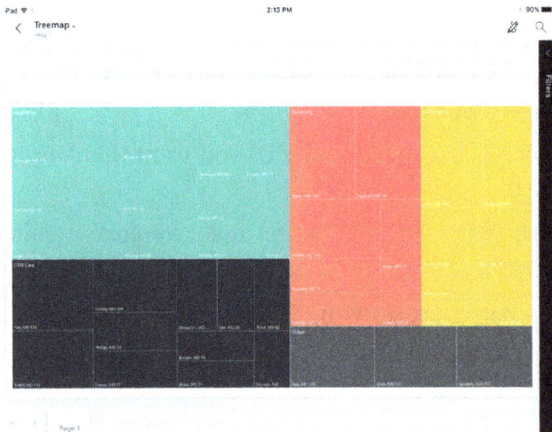

362

The iPad app also offers Q&A functionality, as shown in Exhibit 14.8.

EXHIBIT 14.8 TREEMAP Q&A ON IPAD SAMPLE

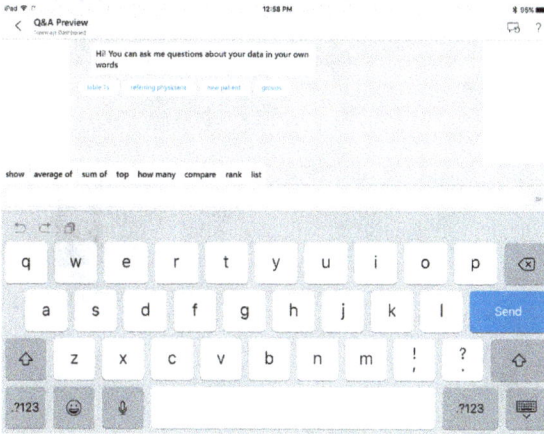

The Q&A results are shown in Exhibit 14.9.

EXHIBIT 14.9 TREEMAP Q&A ON IPAD RESULTS SAMPLE

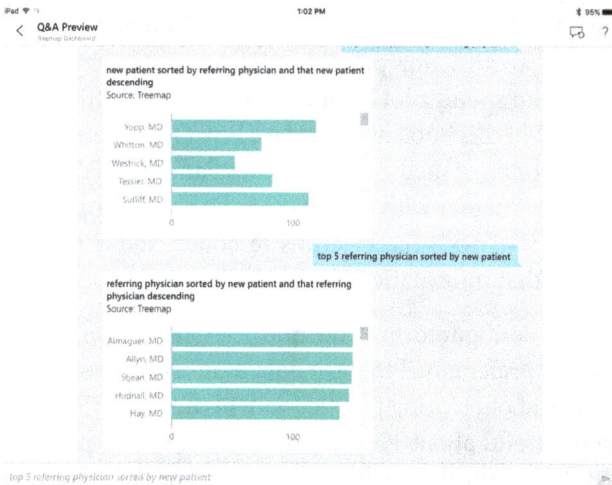

These examples used our treemap data. Medical practice data can be displayed in a near infinite number of ways on a Power BI dashboard. Exhibit 14.10 is a sample dashboard with duration of appointments data.

EXHIBIT 14.10 POWER BI APPOINTMENT DURATION DASHBOARD SAMPLE

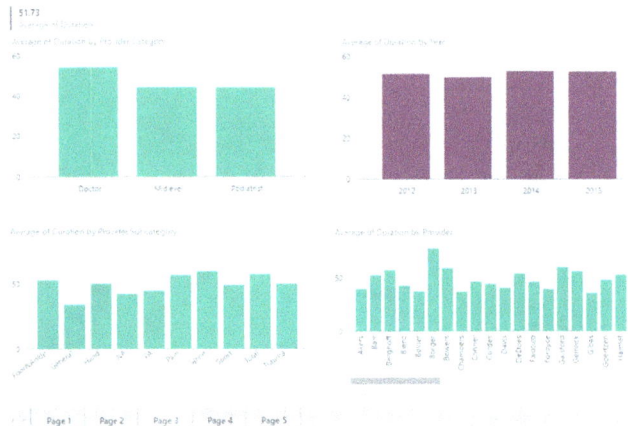

Power BI is free to start with. In early 2017, the professional version cost $9.99 per user per month, but it refreshes data from your practice's data source. SSRS is likely already available at no additional cost. The additional cost may be well worth it for practice administrators and key physicians, especially those who spend a lot of time away from the office. Almost all the examples in Part 2 of this book are based on PivotTables and SSRS. Consider using those tools for most medical practice staff and save Power BI for people who really need to interact with high level data. For example, send an email to the front desk staff with the balances to collect today rather than using Power BI to send that information.

Power BI can be configured to send notifications to a mobile device, but practices may still prefer email to push data to most end users. Practices may be uncomfortable about storing practice data in the Power BI cloud, and need to be especially careful about PHI. Even if the Power BI platform is secure, practices have less control over how and where mobile devices access that data. Email on personal devices carries similar risks though Power BI has the potential to expose more data. Power BI is a rapidly evolving technology that can be expected to become more powerful over time.

POWER PIVOT AND THE EXCEL DATA MODEL

Power Pivot is an add-in for Excel Professional (2010 or higher) that allows Pivot Tables to go far beyond Excel's million-row limit. Power Pivot is only available in Excel Professional versions (which means practices using standard versions will need to upgrade). Power Pivot comes included in Office 2016, but Microsoft's pricing strategy with the ad-in otherwise has been fluid (the Excel 2010 add-in was free), so confirm that the version you plan to purchase has access to Power Pivot.

Power Pivot uses the Excel Data Model. After enabling the Power Pivot add-in, Power Pivot is added to the Excel ribbon and the Manage button opens the Excel Data Model. The ribbon looks like Exhibit 14.11.

EXHIBIT 14.11 EXCEL DATA MODEL TOOLBAR

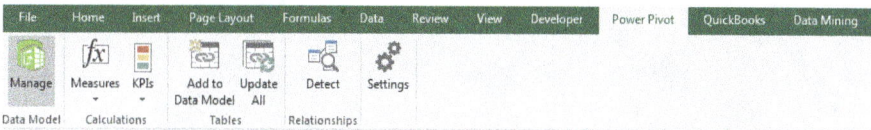

The Manage button brings up the Power Pivot for Excel window. From the Get External Data button, we will connect to SQL Server, as shown in Exhibit 14.12.

EXHIBIT 14.12 EXCEL DATA MODEL TOOLBAR: GET EXTERNAL DATA BUTTON

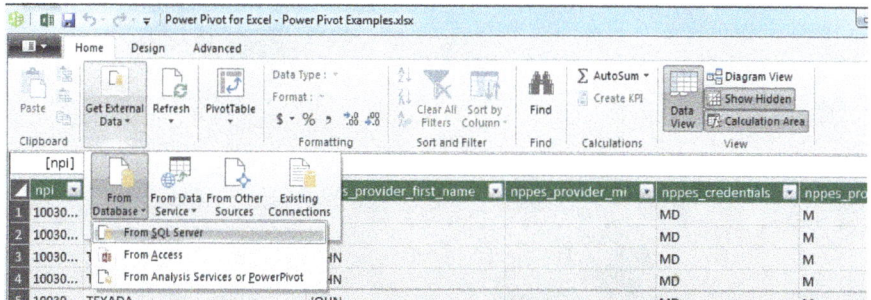

The From SQL Server button opens the Table Import Wizard window, as shown in Exhibit 14.13. The connection is like connecting SSRS to a SQL Server database in Appendix 1.

EXHIBIT 14.13 TABLE IMPORT WIZARD

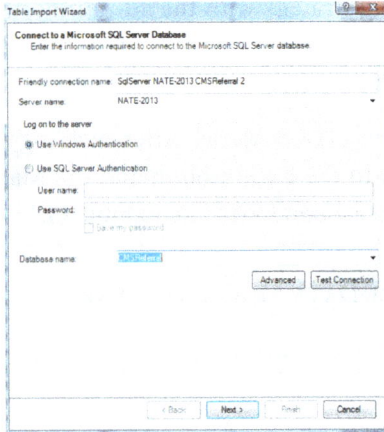

In Exhibit 14.14 we will select from a list of tables and views to choose the data to import. One of the big advantages of the Excel Data Model compared to traditional Excel is the ability to import and pivot multiple tables.

EXHIBIT 14.14 TABLE IMPORT WIZARD: SELECT LIST OF TABLES

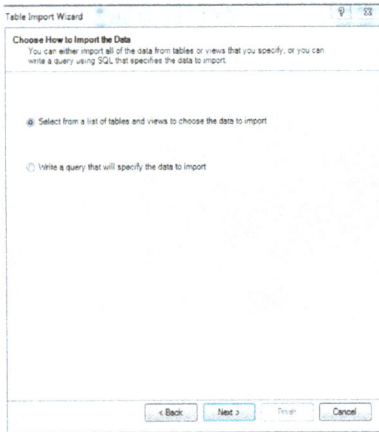

There are several tables of data selected to import in Exhibit 14.15. Clicking Finish will complete the wizard and return to the Excel Data Model. For reference, the bottom table checked contains over 55 million rows of data.

EXHIBIT 14.15 TABLE IMPORT WIZARD: FINISH

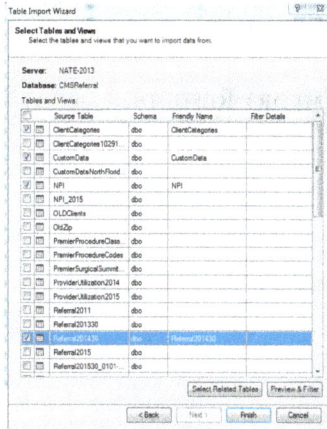

The successful import is shown in Exhibit 14.16. We have imported six tables totaling over 60 million rows. Traditional Excel has no chance at importing that much data, but Power Pivot can. The tables represent data used to analyze referring physician trends as described in the CMS Data section of Chapter 5.

EXHIBIT 14.16 SUCCESSFUL TABLE IMPORT

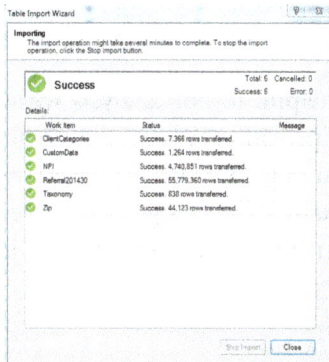

Now that we have data, Excel opens the main Power Pivot for Excel window. Our six tables are shown along the bottom of Exhibit 14.17. The main table, Referral201430 is selected. The table has over 55 million rows, but only five columns. Each row represents a shared relationship that CMS has identified where two providers render services to the same Medicare beneficiary. The From NPI number and the To NPI number are the NPI numbers of the first and second providers, respectively.

EXHIBIT 14.17 TABLE IMPORT RESULTS

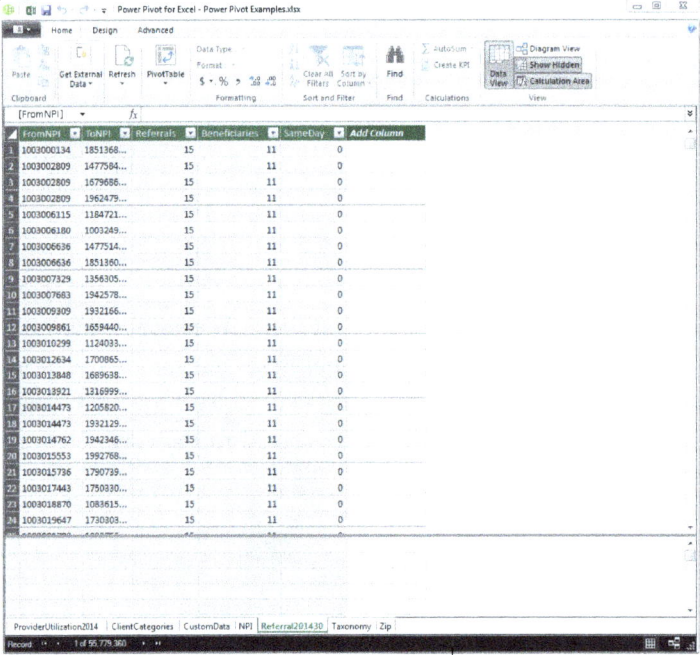

The NPI number isn't helpful to our analysis without converting the NPI numbers to the names of providers. We need to create a relationship between the From NPI number in our CMS data (the Referral 201430 table) and the NPI number in the NPI table. The Design tab on the Power Pivot ribbon has a Create Relationship button that brings up the window shown in Exhibit 14.18.

EXHIBIT 14.18 CREATE A RELATIONSHIP

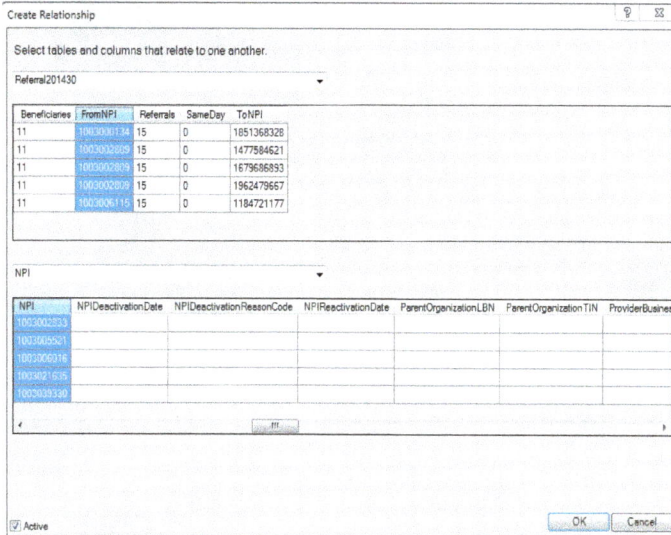

Creating relationships is Excel's way of integrating multiple data sources into one Power Pivot analysis. Similarly, a relational database stores information in tables. For example, providers are stored in one table, patients are stored in another table, and charges are stored in a third table. If a patient moves and changes her address, a relational database will only have to change her address one place, in the patients table. Since every claim, statement, letter, and other information in the PM or EHR obtains her address from the patients table, users only need to change her address in one place for the address to be updated throughout the database. A practice management database maintains relationships between tables like providers, patients and charges to make the system work. Power Pivot can create relationships to maintain similar relationships between the tables imported into the Excel Data Model.

Exhibit 14.19 shows the PivotTable Fields area in Power Pivot from the combined data. We have several different tables available to pivot compared a traditional PivotTable that only pivots fields from one table.

EXHIBIT 14.19 POWER PIVOTTABLE FIELDS

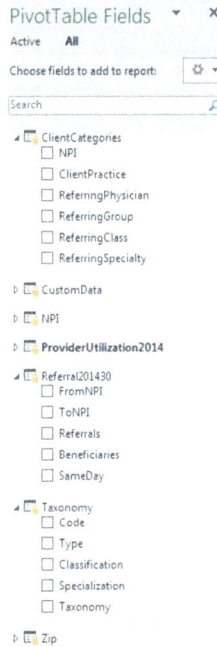

Another advantage to the Excel Data Model is the ability to create relationships between information from different systems. If you cannot import the other data into SQL Server using SSIS (discussed later this appendix), the Excel Data Model might be a solution.

There are some calculations, especially date-related calculations, that work well in the Excel Data Model, offering functionality beyond traditional Excel. The Excel Data Model is also very helpful if you do not have access to SQL Server data or if you cannot import data into SQL Server. If you do have access to SQL Server, use SQL Server to combine data and to write formulas to interact with that data. Utilize Power Pivot to analyze the data.

Exhibit 14.20 is an example of Power Pivot analyzing over 9 million rows of data to get the average charge by state and zip code for a colonoscopy procedure. Analyzing that much data is way too much with a PivotTable, but Power Pivot handles that much data just fine.

EXHIBIT 14.20 POWER PIVOT TABLE SAMPLE

Row Labels	Average of average_submitted_chrg_amt
AK	$1,768.74
AL	$830.73
AR	$836.86
AZ	$918.23
CA	$1,296.08
CO	$1,038.69
CT	$1,091.39
DC	$946.40
DE	$1,015.44
FL	$974.16
GA	
30005	$2,163.00
30012	$818.67
50024	$816.50
30030	$1,303.00
30032	$1,466.67
30033	$688.26
30041	$799.20
30045	$884.18
30046	$941.10
30052	$531.26
30058	$1,200.00
30060	$877.50
30067	$1,073.50
30076	$747.00
30078	$747.00
30084	$763.37

While it may sound appealing to analyze millions of rows of data in a PivotTable, most small to mid-size practices don't need that much data. Start by pulling the current year and the prior one or two years. That is usually plenty of data for analysis. For practices that want more than 600,000 or 700,000 rows of data, there are a couple of choices. Power Pivot is an option, but that requires a more expensive version of Excel. Another choice is to summarize the data by month, procedure code, provider, referring physician, location, or any other required fields. Summarizing the data results in a much smaller dataset for analysis. If a group wants patient-level detail for every charge or payment, another choice is to have a new dataset every year or two. For example, there may be a dataset with 2017-2018 billed charges, a separate dataset with 2015-2016 billed charges, and so forth. As with any Business Intelligence project, there are advantages and disadvantages to each approach. The key point is that are several ways to get enough data for a practice to analyze and the amount of data you need to analyze can drive whether you use PivotTables or Power Pivot. If you want even more data to analyze, the SSAS section on cubes offers another solution.

MAPS

The ability to see geographic data on a map can yield deep insights for practice managers. With Office 365 or Excel 2016, the 3D Map feature is now included in the standard edition of Excel and is easy to use. For this example, we will use the Power Pivot data we just created, though 3D Map data doesn't have to be in Power Pivot. A simple Excel table works just fine. To start, click any cell inside the data and choose 3D Map from the Insert menu on the Excel ribbon, as shown in Exhibit 14.21.

EXHIBIT 14.21 3D MAPS

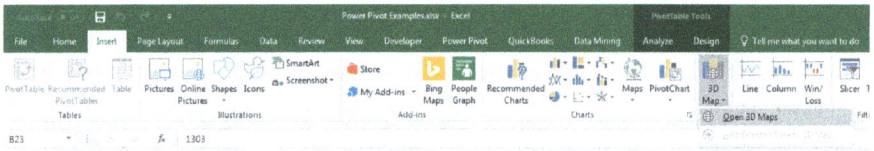

The window that appears on the right looks like a PivotTable field list. The fields are listed separately in 3D Maps, but it's easy to drag the state field to the location Area and the average charge amount to the Height area, as shown in Exhibit 14.22. The nppes_provider_state field is a state and we are averaging the average submitted charge field.

EXHIBIT 14.22 3D MAP FIELDS

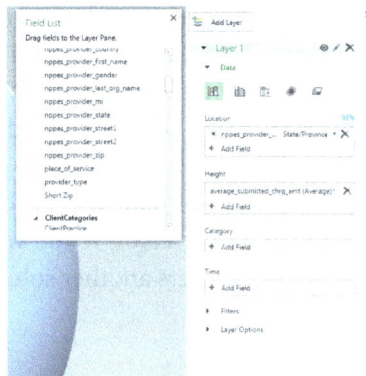

With those data fields in place, our map looks like Exhibit 14.23.

EXHIBIT 14.23 3D MAP RESULTS

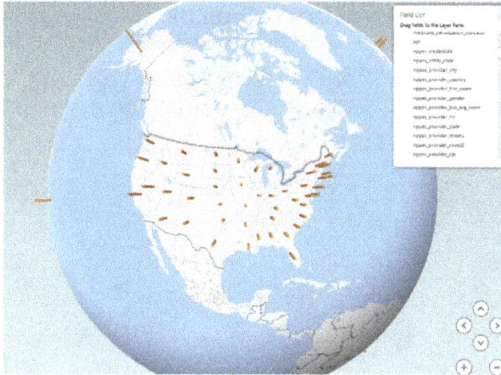

Several of the markers are outside the United States since some of the CMS data is outside the United States. We can filter those locations out by adding a filter for the nppes_provider_state field, as shown in Exhibit 14.24.

EXHIBIT 14.24 3D MAP: FILTERING FIELDS

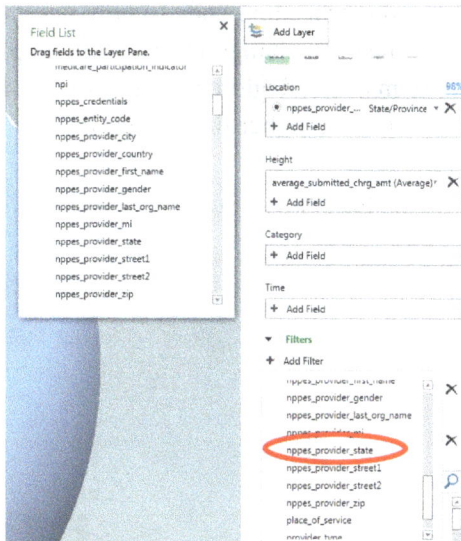

After clicking the plus and adding the nppes_provider_state field, we can uncheck any territories we want to exclude from our analysis, as shown in Exhibit 14.25.

EXHIBIT 14.25 3D MAP: EXCLUDING FIELDS

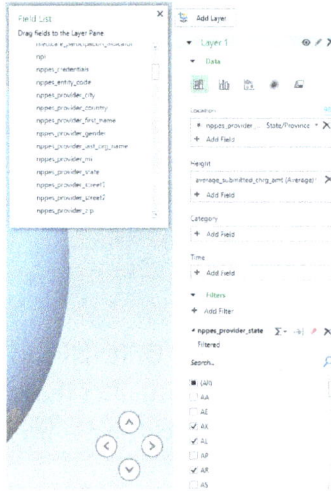

Now that we have narrowed the map to the list of states we want to include, the next step is to filter the procedure code to only select code 45378. After applying that filter, we need to change the way the map displays the data from a Stacked Column map to a Region map, as shown in Exhibit 14.26. The darker the shade of orange, the higher the average charge.

EXHIBIT 14.26 3D MAP: FILTERING FIELD RESULTS

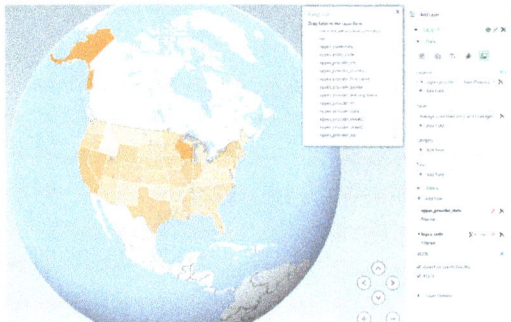

If we zoom in and hide the Tour Editor, Layer Pane, and Field List, we can more easily see charge variations for a single procedure across the United States. The results are illustrated in the map in Exhibit 14.27. Based on the colors on the map, it's easy to see a large disparity (a Power Pivot analysis of the data shows the disparity is over $900) between the average charge in Wisconsin and the average charge in Michigan. Having the geographic information makes it easier to compare a state to neighboring states. Having the raw data in Power Pivot shows that there are over three times as many Medicare beneficiaries with that service in Michigan compared to Wisconsin. What would mapping your major procedure codes in your geographic area tell you? What would a map of your new patients or major procedures by zip code reveal?

EXHIBIT 14.27 3D MAP RESULTS: ZOOMED IN

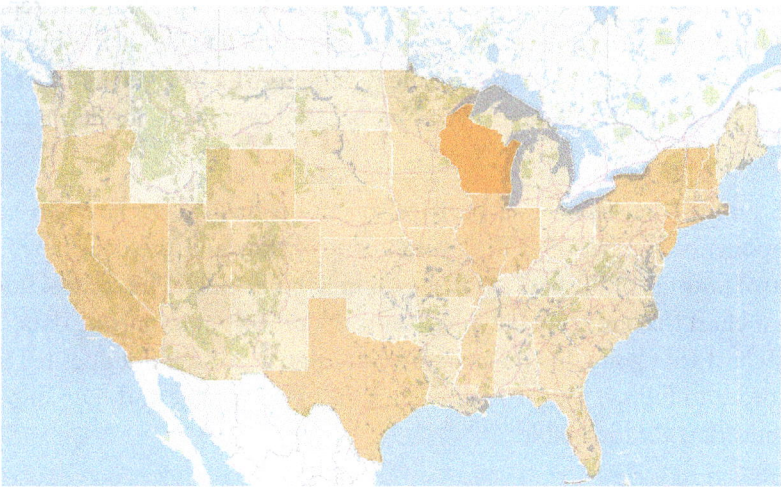

For more information about 3D Maps, watch the playlist of Excel Videos at https://mooresolutionsinc.com/3dmaps/.

SQL SERVER INTEGRATION SERVICES

If you want to take advantage of SSRS, you need your data stored in SQL Server. Practices may have some software in SQL Server but need to merge that data with other software that isn't based in SQL Server. For example, a dermatology practice had a PM system based in SQL Server for the medical side of the business but a specialty software that was not SQL Server based for the cosmetic side of the business. The reports in the cosmetic software did not have all the reporting information they needed. Management also wanted to combine the dermatology and cosmetic data to search for trends and opportunities between the two sides of the business. The practice used SQL Server Integration Services (SSIS) to import the cosmetic data into SQL Server. The staff entered the patients' identification numbers from the PM system in the cosmetic software so that the two systems could be linked. With combined data, the practice has one dashboard in SSRS that reports trends from both the dermatology and the cosmetic side of the business. Management can search for dermatology patients who have not had cosmetic services and cosmetic patients who may be good candidates for dermatology services.

SSIS builds what is called a package to import data. There are two main components of a package, the overall control flow and the data flow. The control flow tab of the package is shown in Exhibit 14.28. The control flow is a flow chart that controls and documents the process of importing data. The flow chart isn't going to win any graphic design awards, but it does tell SSIS the order to follow. The process deletes the existing table and then imports the new data for each table.

EXHIBIT 14.28 PACKAGE IMPORT DATA: CONTROL FLOW

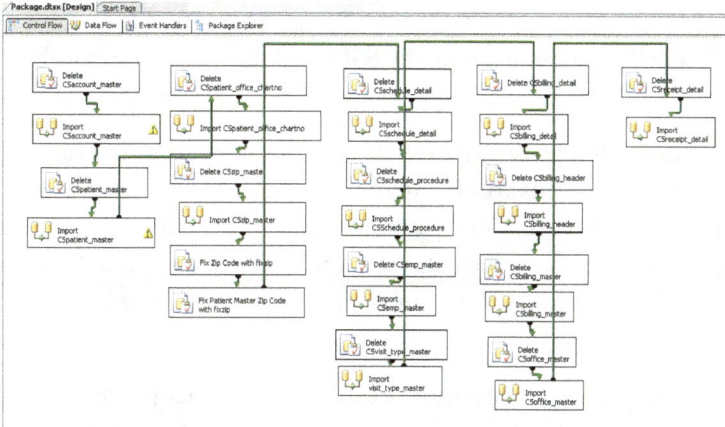

Each import process has a related data flow that controls how the data is imported. Exhibit 14.29 is an example that takes the raw data, derives columns (this derivation deals with a date formatting issue in the raw data), converts columns from the raw data to a format SQL Server will accept, and then imports the data to a destination.

EXHIBIT 14.29 PACKAGE IMPORT DATA: DATE FLOW

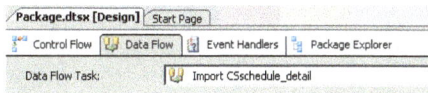

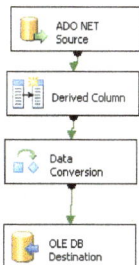

Once created, SSIS packages can be saved and run on a schedule. The key is to have the raw data saved to the same folder with the same name every night before the import package runs. Because the data file is always in the same place with the same name, the SSIS package can automatically import the data.

The same dermatology practice tracks pathology data in a different software package that also needs to be entered into SQL Server. Like the cosmetic software, the staff enters the patients' medical account number into the pathology software. Once the data from the cosmetic and pathology software is uploaded, SQL Server code can combine and integrate data into SSRS reports.

Practices using cloud-based software can create a similar process in SSIS. The practices receive a scheduled file each night with data from the cloud. An SSIS process can delete the old data and import the new data from the cloud into a SQL Server database on the practice's local network. SSIS may be your best chance to get better reports from cloud-based data.

SSIS can also export data from SQL Server into a different format. This package exports data in a bank-approved csv format to help a practice allow their patients to pay their bills online. The data flow task simply deletes the old csv file and then launches the data flow to create a new csv file for the bank. Exhibit 14.30 has the control flow page.

EXHIBIT 14.30 EXPORTING PACKAGE DATA

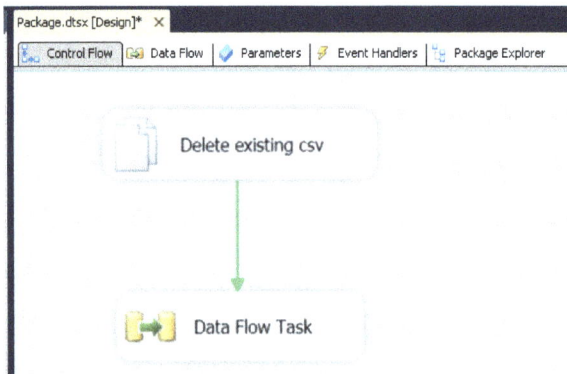

Instead of starting with raw data, the data flow section of the package in Exhibit 14.31 takes SQL Server data (the OLE DB Source) and runs a script that formats the csv file in the format the bank needs to import the data into their system. The package runs on a set schedule so that the csv file is always ready when the bank expects it.

EXHIBIT 14.31 PACKAGE DATA FROM SQL SERVER

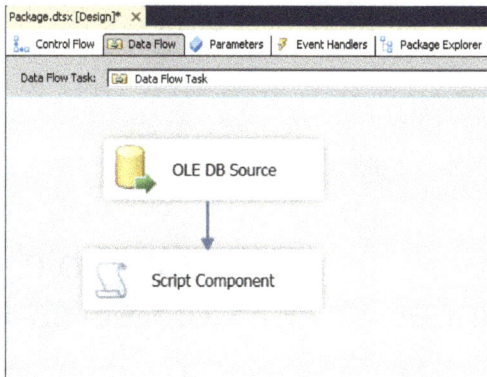

Anesthesia groups have used similar processes to export quality data to a QCDR and meet reporting requirements. A multispecialty practice uses SSIS to export appointment data nightly to a patient survey organization. If your practice is constantly downloading, re-formatting, and sending data, SSIS may be a big timesaver.

SQL SERVER ANALYSIS SERVICES

SSAS is probably the most complicated of the three SQL Server tools we have discussed. A multispecialty group really wanted all transaction level data going back 10 years. Every single billed charge. Every single payment. They wanted lots of detail for each charge and payment, including quantity, dates of service, dates of entry, work RVUs, patient information, rendering physician information, referring physician information, procedure codes, diagnosis codes, primary insurance, and more. There are over 40 providers in this group. There is no way to analyze that much data in Excel. The Excel

Data Model could manage the data, but the spreadsheet file was large and unwieldy. The practice built a cube and created a very small, manageable spreadsheet. Cubes are designed to hold data very compactly and Excel is good at efficiently pulling only the data requested from the cube. Exhibit 14.32 shows a comparison of a typical spreadsheet with a cube in terms of the size of the spreadsheet. The cube holds four times the data in less than one two-hundredth of the space on your server.

Exhibit 14.32 Connecting to Cube Data

Name	Date modified	Type	Size
2014 Billed Charges Connected to Table	7/5/2013 10:35 PM	Microsoft Excel Worksheet	3,804 KB
Billed Charges Connected to Cube	7/5/2013 10:35 PM	Microsoft Excel Worksheet	14 KB

Pivot Table	Pivot Table
Spreadsheet Table	Connected to Cube
500K records	2.1 M records

A cube stores a table for all the charges, payments, adjustments, and refund transactions that links to tables for patients, providers, referring physicians, procedure codes, diagnosis codes, insurance carriers, and more. The cube tracks relationships between the transactions and the other tables so tools like PivotTables can quickly navigate through the cube structure to get exactly the data this practice needed.

SSAS can also work on a wide variety of data mining projects. An orthopedic practice captured 300,000 historical appointments and then used SSAS to look for common factors that led to no shows. The process works by separating out a portion of the appointments and scanning the rest of the appointments for factors leading to a no show. The historical data knows whether a patient showed up for their appointment. SSAS looks for factors in that history that may predict a no show. Once factors are determined and a model is built, the model is tested on the held back portion of the data to see if the model accurately predicts no shows.

For example, the model looked at factors like:

- patients' primary insurance
- copay amount
- appointment time
- appointment location
- age
- appointment type (new vs. established patient)
- the number of days between the date the appointment was scheduled and the date of the appointment
- home zip code
- day of the week (do Monday morning appointments not show more than Tuesday afternoon appointments)
- provider
- history of no shows (number of no shows, percentage of no shows compared to kept appointments)
- gender
- referral source

One of the ways SSAS can analyze the data is to build a decision tree. For example, first determine if the patient is between 18 and 30. If they are between 18 and 30, check if they have missed more than 3 appointments in the past year. If both of those factors are true, then check the primary insurance. Each path down the decision tree leads to an estimated probability of missing the appointment.

The actual decision tree for the practice in this example showed patients between the ages of 24 to 36 were most likely to not show for their appointment, more than three times the rate of elderly patients. If the patient was between the ages of 24 to 36 and had missed more than half of their previous appointments, the no-show probability jumped to 27 percent.

Some larger practices do use cubes, and some vendors like GE's Centricity® product sell analytics products based on cubes. Data mining is probably not the first Business Intelligence priority for most practices. That said, SSAS is a product you already own that may be a good option to start with data mining if you have successfully implemented Business Intelligence projects described in Part 2.

The reports in Part 2 of this book will probably be a higher priority for most practices. The issues addressed and opportunities available in Part 2 are generally lower hanging fruit with a quick return on investment. Once Part 2 is well underway in your practice, the advanced Business Intelligence tools in this appendix can take your practice to an even higher level.

Index

www.ingramcontent.com/pod-product-compliance
Lightning Source LLC
Chambersburg PA
CBHW060748220326
41598CB00022B/2364